AF746016

Macrophages - Molecular Pathways and Immunometabolic Processes

Edited by Soraya Mezouar and Jean-Louis Mege

Published in London, United Kingdom

Macrophages - Molecular Pathways and Immunometabolic Processes
http://dx.doi.org/10.5772/intechopen.1000415
Edited by Soraya Mezouar and Jean-Louis Mege

Contributors
Abid Hamid Dar, Chia-Sheng Chu, Elena Shmakova, Irina Larionova, Jaishree Sharma, Julia Kzhyshkowska, Li-Ling Wu, Liyang Pan, Léa Paolini, Mai Mohamed Bedeir, Mohammad Muzamil Shah, Najia Jeroundi, Nissar Ahmad Wani, Nitish Arun Kulkarni, Owais M. Bhat, Pascale Jeannin, Rakeeb Ahmad Mir, Richard Stratton, Sandra Lopez Garces, Som Gowda Nanjappa, Tatiana Sudarskikh, Yuzuru Ninoyu

© The Editor(s) and the Author(s) 2024

The rights of the editor(s) and the author(s) have been asserted in accordance with the Copyright, Designs and Patents Act 1988. All rights to the book as a whole are reserved by INTECHOPEN LIMITED. The book as a whole (compilation) cannot be reproduced, distributed or used for commercial or non-commercial purposes without INTECHOPEN LIMITED's written permission. Enquiries concerning the use of the book should be directed to INTECHOPEN LIMITED rights and permissions department (permissions@intechopen.com).

Violations are liable to prosecution under the governing Copyright Law.

CC BY

Individual chapters of this publication are distributed under the terms of the Creative Commons Attribution 3.0 Unported License which permits commercial use, distribution and reproduction of the individual chapters, provided the original author(s) and source publication are appropriately acknowledged. If so indicated, certain images may not be included under the Creative Commons license. In such cases users will need to obtain permission from the license holder to reproduce the material. More details and guidelines concerning content reuse and adaptation can be found at http://www.intechopen.com/copyright-policy.html.

Notice

Statements and opinions expressed in the chapters are these of the individual contributors and not necessarily those of the editors or publisher. No responsibility is accepted for the accuracy of information contained in the published chapters. The publisher assumes no responsibility for any damage or injury to persons or property arising out of the use of any materials, instructions, methods or ideas contained in the book.

First published in London, United Kingdom, 2024 by IntechOpen
IntechOpen is the global imprint of INTECHOPEN LIMITED, registered in England and Wales, registration number: 11086078, 167-169 Great Portland Street, London, W1W 5PF, United Kingdom

British Library Cataloguing-in-Publication Data
A catalogue record for this book is available from the British Library

Additional hard and PDF copies can be obtained from orders@intechopen.com

Macrophages - Molecular Pathways and Immunometabolic Processes
Edited by Soraya Mezouar and Jean-Louis Mege
p. cm.
Print ISBN 978-0-85466-932-5
Online ISBN 978-0-85466-931-8
eBook (PDF) ISBN 978-0-85466-933-2

We are IntechOpen,
the world's leading publisher of
Open Access books
Built by scientists, for scientists

7,300+
Open access books available

192,000+
International authors and editors

210M+
Downloads

156
Countries delivered to

Our authors are among the
Top 1%
most cited scientists

12.2%
Contributors from top 500 universities

CLARIVATE ANALYTICS
BOOK CITATION INDEX
INDEXED

WEB OF SCIENCE™

Selection of our books indexed in the Book Citation Index
in Web of Science™ Core Collection (BKCI)

Interested in publishing with us?
Contact book.department@intechopen.com

Numbers displayed above are based on latest data collected.
For more information visit www.intechopen.com

Meet the editors

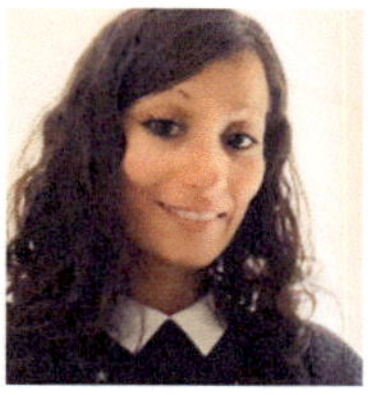

Soraya Mezouar started her research on the macrophage with Prof. Jean-Louis Mege's team. She participated in the investigation of the role of the macrophage in Q fever, an infectious disease caused by the bacterium *Coxiella burnetii*. She has addressed this theme in simple cellular models and with a translational approach with patient samples. She quickly switched to the study of the macrophage and its polarization profile within the placenta in connection with the vertical transmissions of this infection, including infection by *C. burnetii*. In this theme, she evaluated the role of this macrophage in the placental environment of a normal pregnancy but also patients suffering from obstetric complications related or not to infections. During the COVID-19 pandemic, she and her team will be able to highlight the key role of the macrophage located within the feto-maternal interface in the obstetric complications of pregnant women infected with SARS-CoV-2. Her research activities focus on the role of the macrophage and its polarization profile within the placental environment.

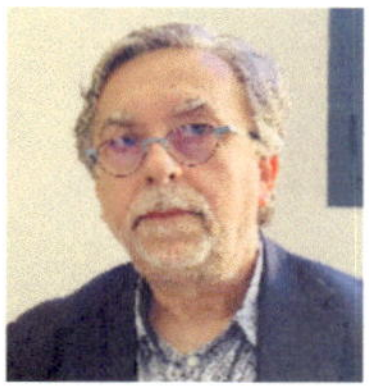

Jean-Louis Mege started his research with the investigation of the adhesive properties of macrophages and oriented this approach to the physiology of human macrophages. Around 1990, he joined a research unit involved in the study of intracellular pathogens including emerging. Hence, he was a leader in the role of macrophages in Q fever, an infectious disease due to *Coxiella burnetii*. This basic research of the intracellular traffic of *Coxiella* was completed by investigation of infected patients. Such an approach permitted to identify IL-10 as a biomarker of the chronic evolution of Q fever. The approach was extended to Whipple's disease, an infectious due to *Tropheryma whipplei*. More recently, his research project was oriented to the anti-infectious activity of macrophages in the context of tissue. Hence, he developed different methods to study placenta macrophages and their response to the infection. The pandemic pushed him to investigate macrophage response to SARS-COV2 infection. The major topic with the highest citations was macrophage polarization with a deep reflection on the meaning of polarization including in pathological samples and the development of tools to investigate this polarization in patients.

Contents

Preface

Macrophages are key cells of the immune system. They have varied roles at the homeostasis level. Due to their plasticity, they can modulate their activation profile, or polarization profile, which gives them the possibility of adapting to different stimuli within a tissue. They are thus involved in the pathophysiology of many inflammatory diseases, infections, and cancer. This book offers chapters that give an overview of the function of macrophages from their physiological role to their involvement in pathologies. Each chapter offers a future perspective and also opens this theme of macrophages to new investigations. The book will be of great use to students and researchers in immuno-biology, immuno-oncology, and translational immuno-infectiology. I would like to thank all those who have contributed to the success of this book.

Soraya Mezouar and Jean-Louis Mege
Anthropologie bio-culturelle, droit, éthique et santé (ADES),
Marseille, France

Section 1

The Mechanisms Associated to Macrophages Functions

Chapter 1

Macrophages: Molecular Pathways and Immunometabolic Processes

Rakeeb Ahmad Mir, Owais M. Bhat, Abid Hamid Dar, Mohammad Muzamil Shah and Nissar Ahmad Wani

Abstract

Macrophages, key players in the myeloid series, are vital for innate immunity, inflammation, pathogen elimination, host defense, and tissue repair. Their polarization can produce M1 and M2 phenotypes. At locations of tissue damage, M1 macrophages are triggered by TLR agonists or IFN-γ, leading to the production of pro-inflammatory cytokines such as IL-1β, TNF-α, IFN-γ, and IL-12, as well as reactive oxygen species (ROS). In contrast, M2 macrophages that IL-4 and IL-13 have stimulated produce TGF-β, IL-6, and IL-10, which are anti-inflammatory cytokines. Additionally, these cells transform arginine into ornithine, which stimulates the production of collagen and cell division, which are essential for wound healing, neoangiogenesis, and tissue remodeling. The regulation of damage, inflammation, and tissue repair depends on macrophages' capacity to dynamically alter their phenotype in response to external stimuli, including signals from pathogens, dying cells, and activated lymphocytes. M2 macrophages sustain tumor microenvironments, encourage endothelium development, and progress malignancy in neoplastic tissues. This chapter delves into the complex interplay of macrophage polarization, metabolism, and the advancement of illness. It emphasizes the molecular pathways, activation states, and potential therapeutic applications in conditions such as inflammation, cancer, cardiovascular diseases, and other afflictions.

Keywords: macrophage polarization, M-1 macrophages, inflammation, immunometabolism, disease pathogenesis

1. Introduction

Macrophages are part of the Myeloid series that play an essential role in innate immunity, apart from other responsibilities like acute and chronic inflammation, pathogen killing, host defense, and tissue repair. Macrophages can polarize into two main phenotypes, M1 and M2, which are also non-sensical. M1 macrophages release cytokines such as IL-1β, IFN-γ, TNF- α, and IL-12 [1]. In contrast, M2 macrophages secrete cytokines that play the function of anti-inflammation, which include IL-6, IL-10, and TGF-β [1].

Macrophages are highly versatile cells with multifunctional characteristics, and they also readily change their phenotypes depending on the signals readily available or existing within a particular milieu, for instance, signals from dying cells, microorganisms, or activated lymphocytes [2]. The above signaling makes macrophages polarize and become activated. M1 macrophages are induced through TLR agonists or IFN-γ in response to pathogens and produce inflammatory cytokines and ROS at the site of tissue injury [3]. This M1 process is flagged in the occurrence of injuries and inflammation at the response site, while M2 macrophages are activated by the cytokines IL4 and IL13. M2 macrophages can alter the metabolism of arginine, which results in the production of ornithine [4]. As for ornithine, when its levels rise, the productivity of collagen synthesis and cell division also rises [5]. During the process of converting M1 to M2 during wound repairing, a change in phenotype from M1 to M2 causes tissue remodeling, neoangiogenesis, and wound healing [6]. In neoplastic tissue, self-renewal of M2 macrophages involves being part of endothelial growth and cancer spreading [7, 8].

This chapter aims to clarify the interconnection between polarization, metabolism, and consequent disease progression in macrophages. It presents all the classical and non-classical states of macrophage activation and molecular aspects of macrophage polarization and metabolism shifts associated with the polarization events. In addition, the chapter reflects on the present knowledge of the processes involved in macrophage polarization and its impact on inflammation, cancer, cardiovascular diseases, and other diseases and on the clinical implications of these findings.

2. Macrophage polarization

Macrophages belong to a group of immune cells classified as the myeloid lineage, which plays a critical role in several physiological and pathological conditions encompassing acute and chronic inflammation, pathogen recognition, host defense, and tissue reformation. Macrophages are culpable for phagocytosis, antigen presentation to adaptive immune cells, and secretion of immunoregulatory cytokines such as macrophage colony-stimulating factor (M-CSF) and macrophage migration inhibitory factor (MIF), and chemokines such as CCL5, CCL7, CCL20, and macrophage inflammatory protein 1a. Moreover, macrophages contribute to angiogenesis, tissue repair, and enhance inflammatory pathologies. During inflammation, macrophages promote lymphangiogenesis by transdifferentiation into lymphatic endothelial cells, and secreting various growth factors and proteases that contribute to lymphatic vessel formation which in turn leads to tumor metastasis. All macrophages, regardless of the origin are regulated by a class III, transmembrane tyrosine kinase receptor that is expressed on most mononuclear phagocytic cells known as macrophage colony-stimulating factor 1 receptor (CSF1R). Macrophages also express granulocyte–macrophage colony-stimulating factor (GM-CSF), and IL-3 acts as a macrophage growth factor in tissue culture.

There is a high degree of heterogeneity in tumor-associated macrophages (TAM), and the pattern of activation depends on the signal that macrophages will receive from the tumor microenvironment. These TAMs enhance tumor progression and invasion and are abundantly present in established tumors comprising 50% of the tumor mass [9, 10]. Activated macrophages can be polarized into two subsets M1 and M2. M1 phenotype is pro-inflammatory in nature and associated with the production of pro-inflammatory cytokines such as IL- β, IFN-γ, TNF- α, and IL-12. However, M2 phenotype is associated with the production and release of anti-inflammatory cytokines, including IL-6, IL-10, and TGF-β.

It has been found that TME predominantly polarizes TAMs toward the M2 phenotype and TAMs are usually referred as M2 macrophages [8]. It was found that in TME, to recruit more monocytes and M0 macrophages to the tumor site, malignant cells secrete M2-like cytokines such as CCL2, CXC12, IL-10, VEGF, and PDGF. Localization of TAMs within the TME was found to impact their ability regarding the regulation of tumor progression [1]. In tumors, crosstalk between endothelial cells and macrophages favors tumor progression. In TME, TAMs lead to endothelial cell activation and enable them toward promoting cancer cell intravasation and extravasation thereby favoring angiogenesis and tumor progression, an important step in cancer metastasis [11–15]. This crosstalk between these TAMs and activated endothelium can be exploited for the design of inhibitors and other therapeutic targets which in turn will prevent tumor progression [11, 15]. Here, we present the major factors that contribute to the formation of these specific M2 subsets, their implications in tumor progression, and discuss various therapeutic strategies to harness TAMs for cancer treatment.

Subsets of M2 phenotype have been found in TME. Subset M2a expresses cell surface markers CD206, CD209, and Dectin-1 and produces CCL17, CCL18, CCL22, and IL-10 [3, 6, 7, 16–20]. IL-4 and IL-13 polarize macrophages toward the M2a. M2b macrophages are anti-inflammatory in nature and regulates Th-1-Th2- cell response. These macrophages can shift toward Th2-cell response through IL-4 secretion, hence known as regulatory macrophages [16, 20–25]. The third subset M2c macrophages express CD163, Mer tyrosine kinase (MerTK), and Tie2 on the cell surface [16, 17, 19, 26]. M2c subset secrets pro-inflammatory cytokines TGF-β and IL-10 and chemokines such as CXCL13, CCL16, and CCL18 [27–30]. They also play an important role in immunoregulation, angiogenesis in tumors [28]. Last subset, M2d macrophages secrets high IL-10, CD14, CD163, TGF-β, CCL18 and low levels of CCL1, CCL17, CCL22, TNFα, and PTX3 [27–30].

2.1 Classical and alternative activation states

Monocyte-macrophage lineage cells are characterized by extensive diversity and plasticity. In tissues, surrounding environmental stimuli or signals (e.g., damaged cells, microbial products, activated lymphocytes) have a great impact on the polarization of macrophages and lead to their activation [9, 31]. Based on the expression of various markers and the production of specific factors these macrophages have been described in several forms in mice and humans [9, 31–33]. In response to stimulation by TLR ligands and IFN-γ, macrophages may be subjected to classical M1 activation. During inflammation, initial responders are M1 macrophages as part of the immune response, and their recruitment takes place shortly after an injury. They produce higher levels of pro-inflammatory cytokines and reactive oxygen species at the injury site, thereby magnifying local inflammation [16]. Cytokine profiles of M1 macrophages include high levels of IL-1α, IL-6, IL-12, IL-23, TNF-α, inducible nitric oxide synthase (iNOS), and IL-1β, etc. [17]. Chronic M1 macrophage activity may cause tissue damage and inflammation. Furthermore, M1 macrophages produce a cell proliferation inhibitor such as nitric oxide (NO). However, macrophages stimulated by IL-4/IL-13 subjected to alternative M2 activation and various stimuli can induce different subtypes of M2 macrophages 2 [18]. There are metabolic differences between M1/M2 macrophages, alternatively activated macrophages exhibit an increase in the arginine pathway producing ornithine [19]. Ornithine serves as a precursor for proline, enhances collagen synthesis, and stimulates cell proliferation, required for the repairing feature of M2 macrophages, and simultaneously inhibits iNOS activity. Phenotypic switch of macrophages from M1 to M2 during acute inflammatory conditions results in tissue repair, vascularization, and wound healing. In neoplastic tissues, M2 macrophages constitute the major inflammatory component thereby contributing to angiogenesis and cancer metastasis. Enzymatic cleavage of arginine by alternative methods produces ornithine and NO, both products inhibit the opposite catalytic process. Besides the cytokine and chemokine secretion, these M1 and M2 phenotypes exhibit different morphologies [16, 20]. Speculations are that in between M1/M2 macrophage phenotypes, there may be intermediate phenotypes among these opposite phenotypes [10]. According to the literature, transcriptome-based network analyses reveal that the phenotype of human macrophage activation is determined by the type of stimulus [34].

2.2 Molecular signaling pathways in macrophage polarization

It is known that the tissue microenvironment plays an outstanding role in macrophage polarization. The key ligand-receptor interactions involved in the polarization of both M1 and M2 macrophages are explored in this section.

2.2.1 Molecular signaling pathways in M1 polarization

M1 macrophage polarization is regulated by complex molecular signaling pathways that control a range of functions. These ligand-receptor interaction pathways contribute to M1 polarization and include:

2.2.1.1 The lipopolysaccharide (LPS) and toll-like receptor 4 (TLR4) pathway

As stated by Janeway, Toll-like receptors are essential pattern recognition receptors of our immune system that protect us from a wide range of pathogens. For macrophage polarization, TLR4 is the most important. TLRs are made up of a transmembrane type and an endosomal type of integral membrane glycoproteins. They belong to a larger IL-1 receptor superfamily due to significant homology in their cytoplasmic region [11].

When lipopolysaccharide (LPS), which is present in Gram-negative bacteria, binds to TLR4, it triggers dimerization of TLR/IL-1R, resulting in a structural change that is critical for the engagement of downstream pro-inflammatory signaling molecules. These molecules include the adapter protein myeloid differentiation primary-responsive protein 88 (MyD88), IL-1R-associated kinases (IRAK), TGF-β-activated kinase 1 (TAK1) and its binding partners TAK1-binding proteins 1 (TAB1) and 2 (TAB2), and TNF receptor-associated factor 6 (TRAF6) [12, 13]. TLR4 uses its own signaling mechanism in which various adapter proteins are involved. It recruits MyD88 via the MAL bridge adaptor and indirectly recruits the TIR domain-containing interferon-β-inducing adaptor (TRIF) via the TRAM bridge adaptor. As for TLR4, it is associated with the use of TRIF, TRAM, MyD88, and the MyD88 adapter-like protein (MAL/TIRAP). It has an organizational plan for both the TRIF and MyD88-dependent signaling routes by [14]. In the MyD88-dependent signaling pathway, MyD88 interacts directly with the TIR domain of TLR4 through its TIR domain activating a downstream kinase known as IRAK4 which in turn phosphorylates another molecule known as IRAK1 leading to its activation and kinase activity. Later on, IRAK1 binds to TRAF6 and ultimately results in K63-polyubiquitination of distinct targets including TRAF6 and the proteins IKKγ/NEMO and TAK1 kinase complex. This eventually leads to the assembling of the TAK1 complex that activates the INF-κB complex of IKKαβ and MAPK kinases in order to increase the intensity of typical M1 macrophage products, including pro-inflammatory cytokines [15]. This is achieved through the phosphorylation of mitogen-activated protein kinase kinases 4 and 7 and the activation of C-Jun N terminal kinases [35]. This makes a considerable contribution toward the morphology of the M1 macrophages. Moreover, TAK1 can be phosphorylated and activate MKK3 and MKK6, which in turn activate the p38α and the latter activate MK2. It also results in the synthesis of pro-inflammatory cytokines like IL-1β and TNF-α from the sequential activation. TAK1 can be activated by many signals such as by IL-1β, TNF-α, TLRs, and the B and T cell receptors [36].

There is conclusive evidence suggesting that the MEK/ERK pathway is induced by the TPL2 MAP3K. It is also reported that TPL2 is moved to the center by IKK-induced cleavage of the N-terminal part of the precursor protein of NF-κB p105 subunit and phosphorylation through IKKβ. These changes lead to the activation of the ERK signaling pathway signaling cascade These signaling changes result in activation of the ERK signaling cascade. In conjunction with Akt-NF-κB activation, this route upregulates the expression of "M1" responsive genes, including pro-inflammatory cytokines TNF-α, IL-1β, IL-6, and IL-12 [37]. The comprehensive map depicted above maps out all the interactions involved in the process through which LPS binds to TLR4 and sets off complex reactions that activate certain signaling molecules. This process reaches its peak in inflammation and results in an increase of pro-inflammatory cytokines as well as the M1 macrophage polarization. It is evident that this type of polarization plays a vital role in immune protection against pathogens (**Figure 1**).

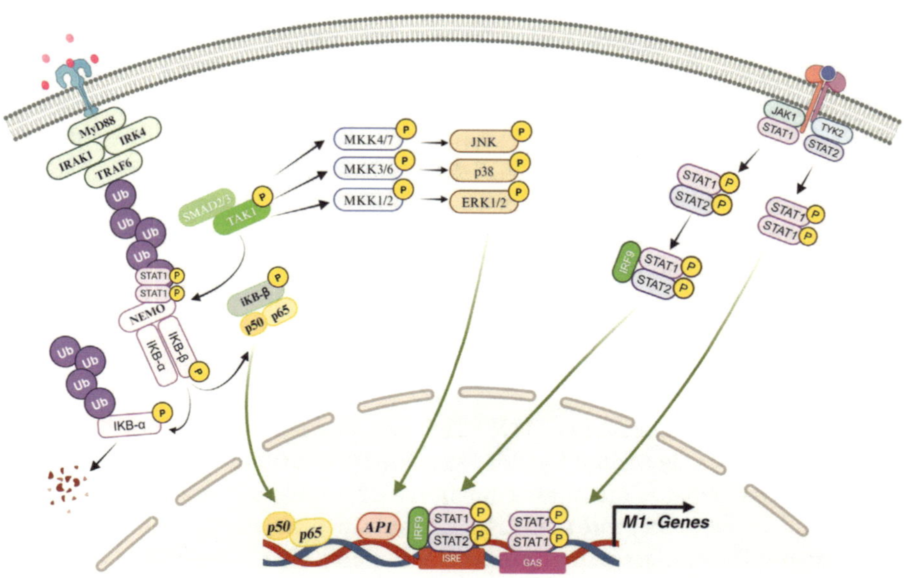

Figure 1.
Signaling pathways regulating M1-polarization (A) TLR/IL-1R, NF-κB, and MAPK Signaling pathways in M1 macrophages: TLR (toll-like receptors) and IL-1R (interleukin-1 receptor) signaling leads to the activation of NF-κB (nuclear factor kappa-light-chain-enhancer of activated B cells) and MAPK (mitogen-activated protein kinase) pathways, which are essential for the production of pro-inflammatory cytokines and mediators. (B) JAK-STAT pathway regulating Ml macrophages: The JAK (Janus kinase) family of tyrosine kinases and the STAT1/2 (Signal Transducer and Activator of Transcription) pathway play a pivotal role in regulating M1 macrophage polarization. Activation of this pathway is crucial for the transcription of genes involved in the inflammatory response and M1 macrophage functions.

2.2.1.2 Interferon-gamma (IFN-γ) and IFN-γ receptor pathway

Interferon-gamma (IFN-γ) and its receptor have been linked to immune response and inflammation in numerous scenarios. IFN-γ receptors include the IFN-γR1 and IFN-γR2 chains that are classified in group II cytokine receptors. As IFN-γ accesses the ligand binding domain of IFN-γR1, this recruits JAK1 and STAT1 to engage with IFN-γR1 at the intracellular domain. It is this interaction that triggers phosphorylation of the receptor and thus signal cascade transmission. Besides, the intracellular region of IFN-γR2 activation can recruit either JAK2 or the tyrosine kinase 2(TYK2) depending on the ligand to engage in signaling (**Figure 1**).

Upon ligand binding, key tyrosine kinases such as JAK1, JAK2, TYK2, and STAT1 are rapidly phosphorylated within 1 minute [38]. This phosphorylation cascade activates JAK2 and allows it to transphosphorylate JAK1, which then phosphorylates the Y440 residue of each IFN-γR1 chain. This phosphorylation generates docking sites for the latent SRC homology 2 (SH2) domain of STAT1 [25, 39]. Phosphorylation of the STAT1 pair occurs near the C-terminus at Y701, most likely by JAK2. This phosphorylation event leads to the dissociation of a STAT1 homodimer from the receptor [40]. After dissociation, the STAT1 homodimer translocates to the nucleus and binds to DNA at specific sequences known as GAS (gamma-activated sequences), characterized by the consensus sequence TTCNGAA [17, 41], which leads to the expression of various genes. Genes activated by STAT1 homodimers at GAS sites include iNOS, MIG (CXCL9), intercellular adhesion molecule 1 (ICAM-1), IRF1, and STAT1 itself. These gene products, such as ICAM-1, inhibit M2-related signaling pathways or activate pathways such as IRF1 and are closely linked to inflammation. They are preferentially expressed in the M1 phenotype of macrophages (**Figure 1**) [42].

In addition, STAT1 can form heterodimers with STAT2 when type I and III interferons (IFN-α and IFN-λ) bind to their respective receptors, IFNAR1 or IFNLR1. STAT2 is recruited after being activated at tyrosine 466 (Y466) of IFNAR1, which is phosphorylated by TYK2 [43]. STAT2 then recruits STAT1, which requires phosphorylation at Y701 for activation [43]. STAT1-STAT2 heterodimers, together with IRF9, form the transcription complex interferon-stimulated gene factor 3 (ISGF3). ISGF3 is able to recognize capable of recognizing IFN-stimulated response elements (ISRE) located within the promoter elements of genes that are specifically induced by IFNs in pro-inflammatory inflammatory tor 1α (HIF-1α) [44].

2.2.1.3 Tumor necrosis factor-alpha (TNF-α) and TNF receptor pathway

The TNF receptor superfamily (TNFRSF) encompasses 27 receptors that interact with over 20 structurally related ligands from the TNF superfamily (TNFSF). These TNFSF ligands can exist as membrane-anchored or soluble trimers, clustering their respective cell surface receptors to initiate signal transduction. TNFSF ligands and receptors possess unique structural properties that link them to cellular processes such as growth, survival, or death. Some molecules within this family can activate both inflammatory and cell death pathways, depending on the target cell type and external stimuli. TNF-α, a member of the TNFSF, serves as a positive regulator of M1 macrophage polarization through the NF-κB pathway. In this context, our focus will be on TNFR1 and TNFR2, which are subunits of the TNF-α receptor and are notably expressed at high levels in macrophages [45].

TNFR1 and TNFR2 are single-spanning type I transmembrane proteins with distinctive cysteine-rich domains (CRDs) in their extracellular regions. These CRDs play a role in their inactive self-association in the absence of ligands. The cytoplasmic domain of TNFR1 contains a death domain (DD) that enables interactions with cytoplasmic proteins also possessing a DD [46]. Upon TNF-α binding, TNFR1 recruits TNFR1-associated death domain (TRADD) and receptor-interacting serine/threonine-protein kinase 1 (RIPK1) through DD-DD interactions. This recruitment leads to the assembly of TRAF2 homotrimers and E3 ligases, activating classical NF-κB signaling. TRAF2 homodimers or TRAF3 form complexes with E3 ligases cIAP1 and cIAP2, which are then recruited to TRADD. RIPK1 undergoes modification with K63-linked ubiquitin chains, acting as docking sites for the LUBAC complex. This complex ubiquitinates NEMO, a component of the IKK complex. The IKK complex interacts with TRAF2 via its IKK2 subunit, while the TAK1-TAB2 complex binds to K63-ubiquitin-modified RIP1 through the TAB2 K63-ubiquitin binding subunit. Activated TAK1 phosphorylates IKK2, leading to the phosphorylation, ubiquitination, and subsequent degradation of IκBα. This process permits the p50/p65 NF-κB dimer to translocate to the nucleus, initiating the expression of pro-inflammatory genes (**Figure 1**) [47]. Upon internalization, the TNFR1 signaling complex releases molecules that can trigger apoptosis via caspase-8 activation or necroptosis through the formation of the RIPK3 complex. Apoptotic cells generate vesicles containing cellular material, which are subsequently cleared by macrophages during the resolution of inflammation. On the other hand, necroptosis leads to the release of intracellular damage-associated molecular patterns (DAMPs) and pro-inflammatory cytokines, thereby promoting inflammation [48].

TNFR2 activation indeed triggers classical NF-κB signaling by recruiting TRAF2 and cellular inhibitor of apoptosis proteins (cIAP1/2). However, this recruitment can lead to the depletion of these complexes in the cytoplasm, potentially affecting their functions. This depletion can then induce the alternative NF-κB pathway via the formation of the TRAF3: MAP3K NF-κB-inducing kinase (NIK) complex. Furthermore, cIAP1/2 is involved in the degradation of NIK, which in turn activates IKKα. This activation leads to the phosphorylation of p100, a component of NF-κB2, resulting in p100 degradation and the release of p52. Once released, p52 can bind to RelB, forming a complex that translocates to the nucleus to regulate gene transcription [49].

TNFR1 also activates MAPK cascades, including ERK, JNK, and P38 [50]. It triggers apoptosis-signaling kinase-1 (ASK-1) activation, which associates with TRAF2 in the TRADD-RIPK1-TRAF2 complex. This association leads to the activation of MAP2Ks, subsequently activating JNKs and P38 MAPK [51]. TNFRs also activate the ERK1/2 pathway via the TPL2-MAP2K1/2 pathways, often through NF-κB activation. This dual activation of MAPK cascades contributes to the diverse cellular responses triggered by TNFR1 activation [52]. TRAF2 plays a crucial role in initiating P38 activation by binding protein kinases such as GCK (germinal center kinase) and RIP (receptor-interacting protein). These kinases then signal upstream of JNKs and P38 MAPK, regulating pro-inflammatory responses and cytokine production in macrophages [53]. All these observations show that the TNFR family might play a major role in the production of inflammatory cytokines and chemokines, promoting M1 polarization. All together, these pathways coordinate to instigate M1-macrophage polarization depending on the inflammatory signals which participate in immune modulation in several pathological states.

2.2.2 Molecular signaling pathways in M2 polarization

Macrophage "class switching" process during M2 polarization operates through complex paracrine networks regulating tissue remodeling, inflammation resolution, immune regulation, and other processes in various diseases. Various key signaling pathways involved in M2 polarization include:

2.2.2.1 IL-4/IL-13-STAT6 pathway

There are two forms of IL-4 receptors; type I consists of the IL-4Rα and the γc chains, and type II consists of the IL-4Rα and the IL-13Rα1 chains. IL-4, a cytokine product of Th2 cells, specifically interacts with its receptor IL-4Rα; the receptor and cytokine come together to make up a ternary complex with either the gamma chain (γc) or IL-13Rα1. Receptor-associated kinases of cytokine receptors known as JAKs induce the phosphorylation of the cytoplasmic side of IL-4Rα through tyrosine residues thus recruiting other intracellular signaling molecules like STAT 6. JAKs are capable of phosphorylating STAT6 on tyrosine residues such that it steps down from the receptor where it intercalates with another STAT6 molecule at the phosphotyrosine 641 (Y641). STAT6 ligands then move into the nucleus which binds to particular DNA sequences at their target promoters where they activate the expression of M2-associated genes, including Arg1, Ym1, and Fizz1 (**Figure 2**) [54, 55].

Alternatively, IL-4 may signal by recruiting insulin receptor substrate (IRS) proteins to specific phosphotyrosine residues on IL-4Rα. IRS, mainly IRS2, can be phosphorylated and then recruit other signaling molecules such as the p85 subunit of PI3K. PI3K activation is a critical step in the activation of M2 macrophages in response to IL-4. Crosstalk between the STAT6 and PI3K pathways is essential for IL-4-induced M2 macrophage activation, especially in SHIP-deficient macrophages [56]. IRS

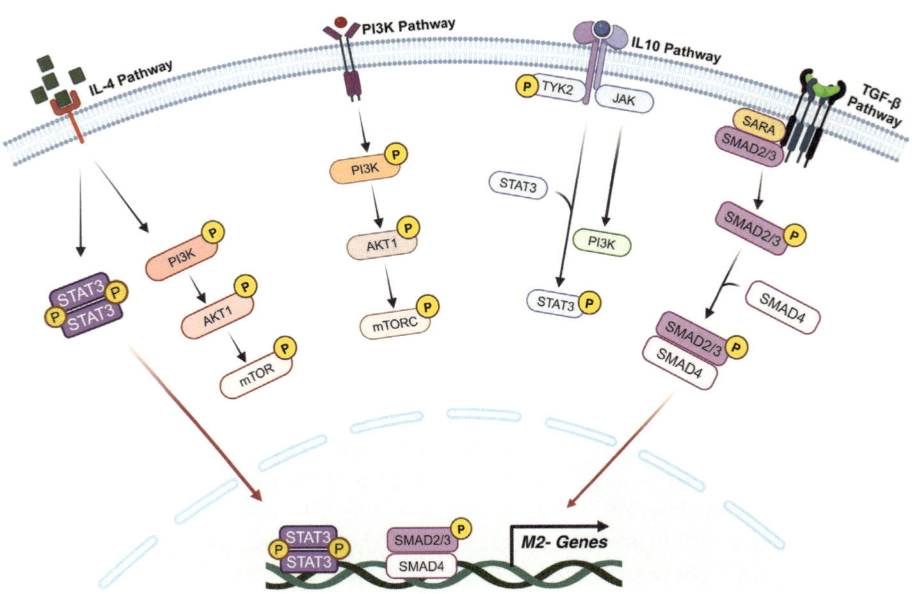

Figure 2.
Signaling pathways regulating M2-polarization. (A) IL-4 binding to its receptor leads to activation of phosphatidylinositol 3-kinase (PI3K) which can activate AKT, which potentially affects the phosphorylation of mTOR. Besides, it can also directly activate STAT6 by phosphorylating it. (B) Binding of growth factors or cytokines to their receptors activates the PI3K/AKT/mTOR axis, leading to polarization of macrophages to M2-phenotypee. (C) IL-10-mediated activation of TYK2 leads to STAT3 activation, while JAK1 activates PI3K, regulating M2- polarization. (D) Binding of TGFβ to its receptor activates SMAD2/3 which then binds to SMAD4, translocates to nucleus and regulate expression of M2-assiacted genes.

recruitment of PI3K leads to activation of the downstream protein serine/threonine kinase AKT/mTOR pathway. IRS can also interact with GRB2 in complex with SOS, leading to activation of Ras and downstream MAPK pathways.

2.2.2.2 PI3K-AKT pathway

The phosphoinositide 3-kinase (PI3K)-AKT pathway is activated by various growth factors and cytokines. When PI3K is phosphorylated or activated, it produces PIP3, which recruits and activates AKT. AKT is activated and then modulates several downstream targets to promote M2 gene expression. There are differences in the effect of kinase isoforms on phenotypic outcomes. Although it is known that PI3K activates AKT, how AKT isoform expression and activation are regulated in macrophages is unknown. The PI3K/AKT pathway is strongly associated with M2 polarization, but evidence suggests that its activation can lead to M1 (via PI3K/AKT2) or M2 (via PI3K/AKT1) polarization, depending on the AKT isoform [57]. In addition, different PI3K isoforms can exert opposing effects on macrophage polarization. In M2 macrophages, this pathway supports cell survival, proliferation, and metabolic changes required for M2 polarization (**Figure 2**) [21].

2.2.2.3 The IL-10-STAT3 pathway

The IL-10 receptor consists of at least two subunits, IL-10Rα and IL-10Rβ, two members of the interferon receptor (IFNR) family. IL-10R signaling is mainly mediated by the JAK/STAT pathway. IL-10Rα binds primarily to JAK1, whereas IL-10Rβ binds to TYK2 [22]. When IL-10 binds, this kinase phosphorylates STAT family transcription factors. STAT3, a downstream transcriptional regulator of IL-10 signaling, is an anti-inflammatory cytokine and plays an important role in the resolution of inflammation. Conditional genetic inactivation of STAT3 in murine macrophages has shown that STAT3 regulates inflammation, as these mice show decreased bacterial activity and increased production of pro-inflammatory cytokines (IL-12, IL-6, TNF-α, IL-1β, IFN-γ) in response to LPS and resistant to IL-10 treatment [23]. (CXCL10, ISG54, ICAM-1) in human monocytes by inhibiting IFN-induced STAT1 activation and tyrosine phosphorylation [24]. Levels of IL-6, IL-8, and TNF-α produced by LPS-stimulated primary human monocyte-macrophages are significantly reduced upon IL-10 treatment [23]. Furthermore, IL-10 induction in macrophages requires the activation of AKT [58], as well as p50, which promotes M2 polarization by inducing the activation of NF-κB, c-Maf, and STAT3 [59].

2.2.2.4 TGF-β-SMAD pathway

Transforming growth factor-beta (TGF-β) interacts with three isoforms of the TGF-β receptor (TβR): TβRI, TβRII, and TβRIII. TβRI and TβRII function as serine/threonine and tyrosine kinases, while TβRIII lacks kinase activity. The phosphorylation of TβRI/TβRII is essential for initiating canonical or non-canonical signaling pathways and modulating additional signaling pathways [60, 61]. The most studied downstream mediator of TGF-β signaling is the SMAD-dependent pathway. Upon TGF-β engagement, the TβRII subunit autophosphorylates and TβRI phosphorylates. The kinase domain of TβRI subsequently interacts with SMAD2 and SMAD3 through the SMAD anchor for receptor activation (SMARs) [62]. TβRI phosphorylates and activates SMAD2/3, which then binds to SMAD4. The SMAD2/3/4 complex translocates to the nucleus, where it induces the expression of ARG1 [63]. Additionally, TGF-β can induce the polarization of M2 macrophages by regulating the expression of SNAIL through the SMAD2/3 and PI3K/AKT signaling pathways [64]. Conversely, TGF-β signaling can also utilize a SMAD-independent pathway. TRAF6 can bind to the TGF-β receptor, leading to the activation of TAK1 and the subsequent induction of P38 MAPK, JNK, and an ERK-dependent M1 phenotype (**Figure 2**) [56, 60].

2.2.2.5 Notch signaling pathway

The Notch signaling pathway interacts with other signaling cascades to influence macrophage polarization. Activation of Notch receptors by ligands such as Jagged1 induces cleavage and release of the Notch intracellular domain (NICD). The NICD translocates to the nucleus and interacts with transcription factors to increase the expression of M2-related genes. Notch signaling also cooperates with the IL-4/STAT6 and TGF-β/SMAD pathways to promote M2 polarization [65].

The PPARγ pathway: Peroxisome proliferator-activated receptor gamma (PPARγ) is a nuclear receptor that regulates lipid metabolism and immune responses. Activation of PPARγ by ligands, such as prostaglandin D2 (PGD2), promotes M2 polarization. PPARγ forms a heterodimer with the retinoid X receptor (RXR) and binds to the PPAR response element (PPRE) in target gene promoters, leading to anti-inflammatory gene expression and tissue repair.

2.2.2.6 Hypoxia-inducible factor (HIF) pathway

In hypoxic conditions, HIF-2α is stabilized and translocates to the nucleus, where it induces the expression of genes that promote angiogenesis, tissue repair, and immunosuppression. HIF-2α interacts with the STAT3 and PPARγ signaling pathways to enhance M2 polarization [66]. This pathway promotes M2 macrophage polarization, tissue repair, immune regulation, and tumor resolution.

2.3 Metabolic reprogramming in macrophage polarization

The concept of metabolic reprogramming was developed and pioneered in the last century by Otto Warburg in his study of tumor cells [67]. Warburg discovered that in the presence of oxygen, cancer cells take up glucose and rapidly produce ATP through glycolysis, leading to an accumulation of lactic acid and a reduction in oxidative phosphorylation (OXPHOS). This phenomenon, known as the "Warburg effect," was also observed in macrophages in later studies [1, 26, 68]. In 1969, Hard [69] showed that activated macrophages increase glycolysis and reduce oxygen consumption.

Overall, the metabolic reprogramming of macrophages reflects a change in their functional activity, with a balance of phenotypic transitions explaining this process. This phenomenon causes changes in many metabolic pathways, including glycolysis, oxidative phosphorylation (OXPHOS), the tricarboxylic acid cycle (TCA), lipid metabolism, and amino acid metabolism [70]. Such metabolic shifts occur mainly in macrophages, which are classified according to the M1/M2 paradigm (**Figure 3**).

2.3.1 Glycolysis and the TCA cycle

Metabolic reprogramming accompanying macrophage polarization indicates functional adjustment to internal and external environmental changes. As immune

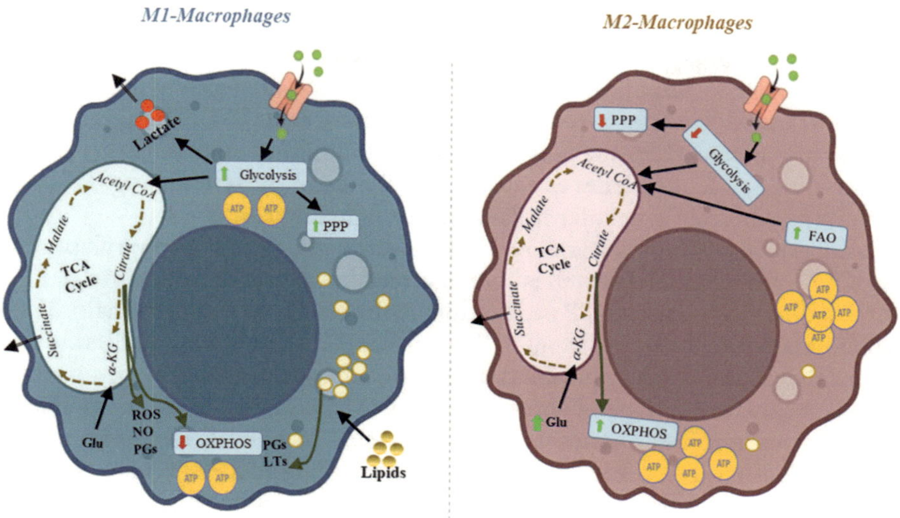

Figure 3.
Metabolic differences between Ml and M2 macrophages. Ml macrophages primarily rely on glycolysis for ATP production, which disrupts the TCA cycle and inhibits oxidative phosphorylation (OXPHOS). The increased flux of glycolytic intermediates feeds into the pentose phosphate pathway (PPP), resulting in heightened nucleotide and amino acid synthesis. This pathway also generates NADPH, which is crucial for producing reactive oxygen species (ROS) and nitric oxide (NO) via *NADPH oxidase and inducible nitric oxide synthase (iNOS), respectively. In contrast, M2 macrophages maintain an intact tricarboxylic acid cycle (TCA), enhanced oxidative phosphorylation, and fatty acid oxidation processes, all of which are accompanied by reduced glycolytic and PPP activity. Additionally, M2 macrophages exhibit increased glutamine metabolism, which contributes to the replenishment of the TCA cycle.*

cells, macrophages adapt their immune regulatory functions through metabolic reprogramming, which directly affects the uptake and utilization of energy substrates. This process is important for maintaining functional plasticity and sensitivity to environmental stimuli. In the 1970s, Hard et al. first conducted further research in this area and identified differences in the metabolic function of M1 macrophages. Immature macrophages rely primarily on glucose and fatty acid uptake for their metabolic pathways. It produces ATP by aerobic oxidation of glucose and β-oxidation of fatty acids using the well-developed cellular tricarboxylic acid cycle (TCA) and mitochondrial OXPHOS. However, in response to altered homeostasis, infiltration of pathological products, and exposure to exogenous substances, macrophages can activate different metabolic patterns to adapt to these changes. This change in metabolic pattern, known as metabolic reprogramming, allows macrophages to adapt to their environment. Macrophages show various metabolic changes when exposed to LPS or LPS in combination with interferon-gamma (IFN-γ). The rate of ATP production increases with the overuse of glycolysis [71, 72]. In this scenario, macrophages enter the M1 phase, where glucose is taken up at a high rate to enter the cell and undergo the glycolytic pathway to produce pyruvate. Due to the inhibition of isocitrate dehydrogenase (IDH) and succinate dehydrogenase (SDH) [71], the TCA cycle is disrupted, leading to the accumulation of citric and succinic acids. As a result, pyruvate is directly converted to lactate instead of acetyl coenzyme A, through its entry into the TCA cycle. In addition, nicotinamide adenine dinucleotide (NAD) depletion caused by TCA cycle inhibition attenuates OXPHOS activity. During pyruvate production in M1 macrophage glycolysis, the pentose phosphate pathway is activated and produces NADPH equivalents. Increased PPP activity increases the production of purines and pyrimidines, which can be used for biosynthesis in activated cells. It also provides NADPH for the enzyme NADPH oxidase, which produces ROS [73] which serves as a mechanism to kill bacteria [70]. These NADPH molecules, together with the accumulation of citric acid, contribute to the synthesis of fatty acids [74]. The synthesized fatty acids are then used for the production of inflammatory mediators such as prostaglandins and leukotrienes as well as for cell membrane remodeling. This process plays an important role in cellular inflammatory signaling (**Figure 3**).

In contrast, M2 macrophages show a shift toward oxidative phosphorylation (OXPHOS). This metabolic switch is characterized by increased mitochondrial activity leading to increased ATP production by the electron transport chain. These metabolic adaptations are consistent in line with anti-inflammatory and tissue repair functions that require energy production and mitochondrial function. In contrast, M2 macrophages do not depend entirely on aerobic glycolysis [75, 76]. It is evident that in M2 macrophages, the tricarboxylic acid cycle (TCA) cycle remains unaffected; fatty acid oxidation (FAO) and oxidative phosphorylation (OXPHOS) are regulated to support ATP production and energy supply. During the transition from M1 to M2 macrophages, the switch from glycolysis to oxidative phosphorylation represents a metabolic reprogramming consistent with their function.

2.3.2 Lipid metabolism

Lipids play an important role as the main source of energy for macrophages, contribute to the formation of cell membranes, and serve as precursors for bioactive lipids [77]. In addition, lipids are essential for the regulation of signal transduction during macrophage activation. The macrophage activation, or polarization, of macrophages, is controlled and driven by tissue-specific environmental stimuli that induce and direct them to perform actions. M1 macrophages show increased lipid uptake and intracellular lipid accumulation, leading to the formation of lipid droplets. These lipid reservoirs are used to produce lipid mediators such as prostaglandins and leukotrienes, which contribute to their inflammatory phenotype. M2 macrophages metabolize lipids in a different way differently, preferring OXPHOS and FAO pathways to generate and produce energy through the uptake of fatty acids acid, exhibit distinct functions as M2 macrophages rely on OXPHOS and FAO as key functional pathways to play a role in tissue breakdown resolution, and repair during functional recovery from injury [78]. Studies have shown that FAO can induce phenotypic changes in M2 macrophages, but whether this process is sufficient for M2 polarization remains unclear [79]. Despite these advances, the mechanistic relationship between fatty acid oxidation (FAO) and oxidative phosphorylation (OXPHOS) and the anti-inflammatory phenotype of M2 macrophages remains poorly understood. Understanding these metabolic changes is important to understand the complex mechanisms of macrophage polarization and to identify potential targets for therapeutic intervention in immune-related diseases.

2.3.3 Amino acid metabolism

In the 1980s and 1990s, thioglycollate-induced, LPS-stimulated, or zymosan-exposed macrophages exhibited a significant increase in cystine, the oxidized dimer form of cysteine, and released similar amounts of cysteine and glutathione [80]. However, recent studies have heightened interest in the regulation of redox homeostasis during inflammatory activation due to the elevated levels of reactive oxygen species (ROS) observed in M1 polarization. Glutathione, the primary antioxidant protecting cells from ROS, is synthesized by adding glycine to γ-glutamylcysteine, which is formed from glutamate and cysteine [81]. Although the exact mechanism is not fully understood, it is widely accepted that the transcription factor nuclear factor erythroid 2-related factor 2 (NRF2) is activated in response to oxidative stress, while NF-κB is activated in response to LPS, partly through the regulation of glutathione metabolism [82]. Inhibition of γ-glutamylcysteine synthetase with buthionine sulfoximine, a glutathione production inhibitor, has been shown to reduce serum IL-1β levels in endotoxemic mice [83, 84]. This indicates that despite the significant induction of ROS during M1 polarization, which regulates inflammatory cytokines, ROS levels must be kept below a certain threshold [85]. Excessive ROS production can disrupt the cellular redox balance and amplify the inflammatory response through NRF2 activation [86]. The serine synthetase pathway (SSP) has recently been implicated in an unexpected role in M1 polarization [80]. Glycolysis starts with the CNS branch and phosphoglycerate dehydrogenase (PHGDH) converts 3-phosphoglycerate to phosphopyruvate, phosphoserine, and finally serine [87]. Rodríguez et al. demonstrated that serine synthesized both environmentally and endogenously via the CNS is required for optimal LPS-induced Il1b mRNA expression [88]. Conversion of serine to glycine by hydroxymethyltransferase 1/2 provides carbon units for many reactions, including nucleotide synthesis and the formation of 5,10 methylenetetrahydrofolates from tetrahydrofolate [89]. However, formate, which provides a one-carbon unit, fails to rescue the reduced IL1b mRNA expression, indicating the importance of glycine production from serine for glutathione production, as exogenous glutathione restores Il1b mRNA expression in the absence of serine [88]. The importance of the CNS for the anti-LPS inflammatory response showed that injection of PHGDH inhibitors in a toxic shock model reduced mortality and circulating IL-1β levels, which was confirmed by another study [90].

A key question for future research is whether IL-1β reduction is dependent on extracellular serine in vitro but not de novo serine synthesis in vivo. Research has not clarified whether monocytes require PHGDH-dependent serine synthesis, despite the presence of serine and glycine in their environment. The exact mechanism by which the CNS affects IL-1β remains unclear. Other studies support the hypothesis that the CNS is essential for absorbing new ATP synthesis to drive the generation of S-adenosylmethionine (SAM) in inflammatory macrophages [91]. Isotope scavenging experiments with similarly labeled glucose or serine showed that LPS-activated macrophages increased carbon flux through the CNS and one-carbon exchange, and increased the SAM/S-adenosylhomocysteine ratio, which supported LPS-stimulated IL-1β production by promotion of H3K36. trimethylation required for transcription elongation and tumor gene splicing [92]. However, conflicting reports indicate that chemical inhibition of PHGDH increases IL-1β levels, suggesting the complexity of metabolic reprogramming during M1 polarization and the possible effect of time in these studies. In summary, the amino acids serine and glycine, their metabolic pathways—CNS and one-carbon metabolism—are influenced by inflammation, indicating an emerging theme in immunometabolism.

Arginine metabolism plays an important role in macrophage polarization. M1 macrophages express inducible nitric oxide synthase (iNOS), which catalyzes the conversion of arginine to nitric oxide (NO) and citrulline [93]. The NO product produced by iNOS is essential for its antimicrobial activity and anti-inflammatory effects in M1 macrophages. In contrast, M2 macrophages show high arginase-1 activity, which directs arginine metabolism to the production of ornithine and polyamines [93]. This metabolic pathway supports tissue repair, collagen synthesis, and immunoregulatory functions associated with M2 polarization.

2.4 Implications of macrophage polarization in disease

In Section 1 of this chapter, we have discussed the basic mechanism of macrophage polarization, its role, and very basic ideas regarding its role in disease. This section will discuss the negative impacts of macrophage polarization in various types of diseases. The liver and adipose tissues are central metabolic tissues regulating energy homeostasis; consequently, these tissues are infiltrated by many immune cells. These tissues and their metabolic products largely influence the activation of immune cells, reflecting the number and activation of immune cells in the animals. Among these immune cells, the liver and adipose cells dominantly influence the macrophages in context to their number and functions. The central key to the negative impacts of metabolic disorders lies in the impairment of glucose and lipid metabolism and its negative implications in terms of insulin resistance and atherosclerosis. The unregulated function of macrophages and their polarization is exhibited in various diseases such as inflammatory bowel disease, non-alcoholic steatohepatitis, and inflammatory bowel disease (**Table 1**). The current section is aimed to discuss macrophage polarization and its impacts on diseases.

2.4.1 Role of macrophage polarization in chronic inflammatory diseases

The immune system alteration possibly through endocrine responses, pathogen-induced and imbalance in nutrient intake may induce chronic inflammatory disease if untreated for a long time. Various metabolic implications are related to chronic inflammatory diseases such as type II diabetes mellitus, non-alcoholic steatohepatitis, atherosclerosis, and obesity.

2.4.2 The macrophage polarization and obesity

Obesity, a non-degenerative higher incidence disease is characterized by aggravated accumulation of adipose tissues in the human body influenced by dietary habits and abnormal/sedentary lifestyle [94]. Apart from the presence of adipocytes, adipose tissues also include cells such as pre-adipocytes, fibroblasts, endothelial cells, and immune cells like macrophages, NK cells, etc. [95]. It needs to be pointed out that a high-fat diet modifies the M1 (CD11c + CD301−) and M2 (CD11c − CD301+) distribution in visceral fat, in addition to an enhanced number of macrophages in adipose tissues.

The M1 macrophages are classically activated by lipopolysaccharide (LPS) or IFN-γ to phagocytize microbes and produce pro-inflammatory cytokines to initiate the avocation of the immune response. They produce reactive oxygen intermediates (ROI) or nitric oxide (NO) to protect host against the bacterial and viral infections and anti-tumoricidal action. Whereas, M2 macrophages also called alternatively activated macrophages (AAM) are primarily activated by cytokines such as IL-4, IL-10, or IL-13 to induce collagen production by producing proline or induce proliferation by producing polyamines. The M2 macrophages help in tissue repair, tissue remodeling, the wound healing process, and immunomodulatory function.

The hypertrophy of adipose tissues is triggered by high caloric intake and less expenditure of energy due to a sedentary lifestyle. Consequently, the adipocyte expansion primarily leads to deprivation of oxygen i.e., hypoxia, which in turn induces chemotaxis of macrophages. Later cells subsequently overexpress inflammatory cytokines and hence a serious imbalance in the homeostasis of the body. Additionally, the triggering of an angiogenic event will aid in the infiltration of immune cells, accumulation of extracellular matrix (ECM), and additional secretion of pro-inflammatory cytokines by infiltered

Macrophage type	The released cytokines	Mechanism of signaling/action	Functional impact of the animal system
M1	IL-1b, IL-6, IL-12, IL-23, TNF-a, CXCL1 ~ 3, CXCL8 ~ 10, CCL2 ~ 5, CCL11	TLR4/NF-kB, IRF5, JAK/STAT1, Notch	• Antigen presentation • Th1 immune reaction • pro-inflammatory response elimination of pathogens • To initiate anti-cancer processes
	IL-12 IL-23	—	• IL-12 induces the activation and clonal • expansion of Th17 cells which secrete high amounts of IL-17, and thus contribute to inflammation
	IL-1β, IL-6, IL-12, IL-23, IFN-β and TNF-α		• Drive Th1 responses • Triggers pro-inflammatory response
	IL-1β	IL-1R signaling	• Potent inhibition of insulin secretion • Islet destruction
	IFN-γ, LPS, GM-CSF, TNF-α	—	• Pro-inflammation, • Microbicidal effect, • Tumor resistance
M2	Arg1, IL-10, TGF-b, CCL17, CCL22	JAK/STAT6, c-Myc, IRF4	• Anti-inflammation, • Wound healing, • Th2 immune response, • Anaphylaxis, • Fibrosis
	PDGF, TGFβ, HGF, and bFGF	—	• Induces proliferation and metastasis of tumor cells.
Mox	IL-1b, VEGF	Nrf2, Keap1, TLR2	• Low chemotaxis • Phagocytosis
	IL1β and COX-2	TLR2	• Increases TLR2dependent mechanisms in response
M(Hb)	IL-10, IL-1R antagonist	PI3K/AKT, LXRa	• Cholesterol loading resistance, • ATP-binding cassette transporter up-regulation
M2b	LPS IC IL-1β	—	• Immunoregulation • Aids in promoting infection • Increases tumor progression

Table 1.
Showing the type of macrophage polarization, cytokine production, and their effects on the animal systems.

macrophages, further worsening the homeostatic balance of adipose tissues [96]. Experimental studies approved that obesity-induced inflammation and insulin resistance are due to macrophage polarization to it M1 state for inducing pro-inflammatory responses. The first consequence of adipose tissue hypertrophy leads to the induction of insulin resistance due to the activation of inhibitor of κ kinase (IKK) and c-jun-N-terminal kinase (JNK), both are responsible for the inactivation by the phosphorylation insulin receptor. The inflammation in adipose tissues is also facilitated by the production of pro-inflammatory cytokines by T lymphocytes, further aggravating the localized inflammation and its spread systemically. The surge of pro-inflammatory cytokines triggers macrophages to secrete macrophage-derived TNF-α, which later, in turn, binds to its receptors (TNF-α receptor) on adipocytes to stimulate lipolysis. The possible reason for lipolysis may be due to a reduction in the expression of perilipin (a protein that coats lipid droplets in adipocytes) by overexpression of proinflammatory cytokines such as TNF-α, which facilitates the lipases for converting the triglycerides to monoglycerides. The adipocytes release free fatty acids to initiate the NF-kB inflammatory pathway by binding to Toll-like receptor 4 (TLR4). The target of rapamycin complex 1 (mTORC1) plays a pivotal in macrophage polarization to regulate the metabolism of macrophages. The facilitation of LPS-based stimulation and activation of macrophages is mediated by elevated mTORC1 activity and downregulation of Akt signaling pathways. Moreover, the constitutive mTORC1 activity inhibits the M2 polarization through the decline in AKT activation in IL-4-induced polarization of macrophages [97].

2.4.3 Renal fibrosis and macrophage polarization

Chronic kidney disease (CKD) is a medical complication leading to the failure of kidneys and this disease is manifested by chronic inflammation and renal fibrosis. Wang Y and Harris DC (2011) reported the common feature of CKD is characterized by macrophage infiltration, the infiltration state largely depends on the extent of kidney damage and degree of invasion. Mounting pieces of evidence strongly suggest that renal fibrosis is considerably predisposed by alterations in macrophage phenotype. The scientific evidence attributed macrophage polarization as a key factor in regulating kidney injury, inflammation, and renal fibrosis [98, 99]. In particular, M1 macrophage infiltration is attributed to causing acute renal inflammation. Consequently, the development of renal fibrosis is reliable evidence for the progression of renal disease, which depends on the increased infiltration of macrophages. In addition, macrophages have a central role in the progression and development of diabetic kidney disease (DKD).

2.4.4 Macrophage polarization and skin diseases

Macrophage polarization is reported to be the major cause of a wide range of skin diseases such as scleroderma, dermatitis, psoriasis, and atopic. For instance, scleroderma is a chronic autoimmune disease of the skin, wherein, the skin and its underlying tissues are seriously damaged resulting in hardening and thickening of the skin due to the build-up of collagen fibers. Reports suggest that M2 macrophages play a crucial role in the progression and development of scleroderma by releasing cytokines, such as IL-13 and IL-4 in the presence of CD204, CD68, and CD163 aiding in the production and stimulation of collagen fibers. This excess of collagen production leads to the development of fibrotic tissues (**Figure 4**) [100]. Similarly, M1 macrophages also promote fibrosis by releasing PDGF and TGF-β, later factors

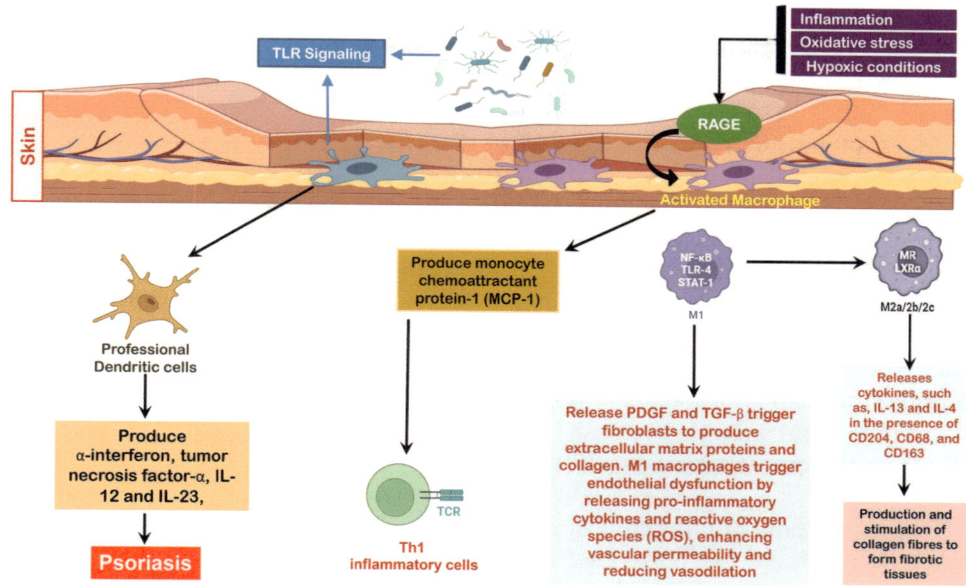

Figure 4.
Mechanisms and role of M1/M2 macrophages in the progression of skin diseases. Through the production of cytokines and triggering of pro-inflammatory and inflammatory cytokines to initiate skin diseases such as, scleroderma, dermatitis, psoriasis, and atopy.

trigger fibroblasts to produce extracellular matrix proteins and collagen. These M1 macrophages are also reported to trigger endothelial dysfunction by releasing pro-inflammatory cytokines and reactive oxygen species (ROS), enhancing vascular permeability and reducing vasodilation [101]. Additionally, M1 macrophages impair the functioning of regulatory T cells (Tregs), promoting inflammation and autoimmunity [102]. In line with this, reports suggest that M1 macrophages hamper the functioning and differentiation of Treg cells by producing IL-12 worsens the autoimmune responses in the case of scleroderma. Psoriasis is another skin disease characterized by chronic inflammation due to the uneven proliferation of keratinocytes and heavy infiltration of immune cells [103]. Among immune cells, M1 macrophages are found in the lesional skin of psoriasis patients to aggravate the production of pro-inflammatory chemokines and cytokines. In particular, the production of TNF-α by M1 macrophages is associated with psoriasis development during the initial stage when keratinocytes are damaged [104]. Additionally, it was found that in psoriasis lesional skin there was a drastic decrease in the infiltration of CD68 + CD163 + M2 macrophages and an increase in the infiltration of CD68 + iNOS + M1 macrophages [105]. Studies approved the role of M2 macrophages in resolving the clinical features of inflammation and also aided in tissue repair mechanism [106].

Other skin diseases, such as atopic dermatitis, characterized by pruritic eczematous lesions are induced by releases of inflammatory cytokines and chemokines by macrophages. The persistent M1 polarization leads to the progression and development of chronic skin inflammation in the case of atopic dermatitis [107]. Additionally, infiltration of Th2 lymphocytes and its release of cytokines such as IL-4, IL-5, IL-13, and IL-31 triggers the progression and development of AD lesions [108]. In conclusion, the pro-inflammatory mechanisms exhibited by M1 macrophage phenotypes via secretion of diverse types of cytokines play a central role in skin disorders, even in the development of skin cancers. Understanding the central players critical for the progression of diseases helps to easily devise proper and systematic therapies against underlying agents.

2.5 Macrophage polarization and immune disorders

Existing data suggests that several diseases are associated with altered balances of phenotypes of M1/M2 macrophages [109]. Autoimmune diseases such as Systemic lupus erythematosus (SLE), autoimmune myocarditis, inflammatory bowel diseases (IBD), autoimmune neuritis, and Sjögren syndrome are also found to be associated with the increased ratios of M1/M2 macrophages. The reduced frequency of M2 macrophages and activation of M1 macrophages are strongly speculated to develop injurious inflammation and hence progression of autoimmunity.

2.5.1 Systemic lupus erythematosus (SLE)

SLE is a systemic autoimmune disease, characterized by complications of various organs. It is believed that both genetic and environmental factors are responsible for the development of SLE pathogenesis. The hallmarks of this disease include the production of autoantibodies against self-antigens and also importantly chronic inflammation of various organs. The SLE pathogenesis is largely influenced by M1 macrophages, even though some reports suggest that M2 macrophages are also implied to the progression of SLE pathogenesis [110]. For instance, the recruitment of M1 macrophages into kidneys after injury promotes a pro-inflammatory response enabling the removal of damaged and apoptotic cells, important functions of M1 cells to maintain steady-state conditions (**Figure 5**). In contrast, the M2 macrophages suppress the inflammatory responses and induce repair and proliferation of cells.

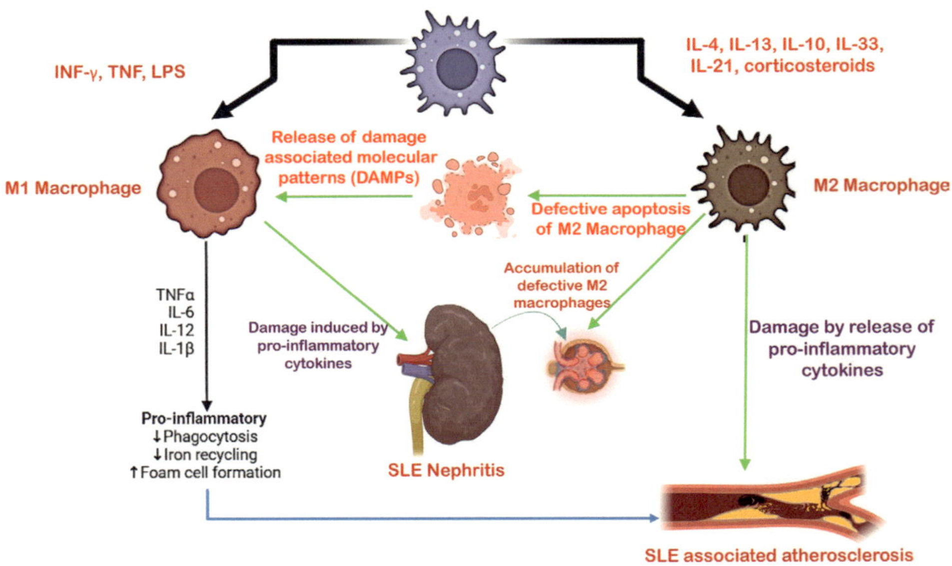

Figure 5.
Role of macrophage polarization in the progression of SLE-M1-like macrophage-derived cytokines like IL-6, IL-12 TNFα, and IFN-γ, which are pro-atherosclerotic reported in SLE patients. Moreover, M2 release of pro-inflammatory cytokines also induces atherosclerosis and nephritis.

Remarkably, Lee et al. [111] reported that IFN-γ induces the polarization of macrophages to M2 phenotype during the onset of kidney repair. For example, accumulated data shows that apoptotic or dying cells release S1P, which then activates EPO signaling in macrophages. EPO signaling then potentiates the clearance of apoptotic cells via upregulation of peroxisome proliferator-activated receptor-γ (PPARγ). The PPARγ is highly expressed in macrophages and this protein forms a heterodimer with its cognate receptors such as retinoid X receptors (RXRs). PPARγ/RXRα-based signaling helps to express the network of genes like Axl, CD36, C1q, and Mer critical for phagocytosis and a strong self-tolerance mechanism [112]. In PPARγ-deficient mice the macrophages were not able to carry out phagocytosis and were poor candidates to exhibit anti-inflammatory action after apoptosis. These mice models displayed the production of autoantibodies and developed a similar type of glomerulonephritis, as reported in SLE [112]. Similarly in NZB/W F1 mice, an SLE animal model, the remission of SLE symptoms was found upon treatment of mice with cyclophosphamide, which resulted in the presence of M2 macrophages (M2b subtype). On the other hand, M2c macrophages in treated SLE models also displayed upregulation of glucocorticoid and clearance of apoptotic cells.

The differentiation of monocyte-to-macrophage grossly contributes to SLE pathogenesis due to polarization toward the M1 activation. Additionally, it is reported that transplantation of M2 (but not M1 macrophages) improved the conditions of SLE diseases in clodronate- and activated lymphocyte-derived DNA-treated mice [113]. Further TNF-α-induced protein 8-like 2 (TIPE2), an immune-negative molecule is reported to be critical for homeostasis. The TIPE2 inhibits iNOS activity and NO production, thereby suppressing the inflammation. Experimental evidence found that TIPE2 alleviates the SLE induction via polarization of M2 macrophage [113, 114]. Other factors found to modulate macrophage polarization include C1q, leukocyte-associated Ig-like receptor-1, HMGB1, and RAGE to generate a multimolecular complex in membrane lipid rafts [113, 114].

2.5.2 Rheumatoid arthritis (RA) and macrophage polarization

RA is a systemic autoimmune disease found more frequently in elderly women than in males. The clinical features of diseases include synovitis in multiple joints, subsequent joint swelling, and other symptoms. The RA clinical features worsen to destruction of cartilage, necrotic joints, and disability if prolonged illness prevails [115]. Reports suggest that macrophages play a central role in the pathophysiology of RA. In particular, M1 macrophages are reported to produce cytokines such as IL-6, TNF-α, and other inflammatory ILs to maintain the inflammatory state of organs thereby aggravating the progression of RA [116]. The main manifestation of RA lies in the high expression of M1-like macrophages in peripheral blood and synovial tissues, where they express major histocompatibility complex (MHC) class II and surface markers like CD80, CD38, TNF-α, and IL-6. All these proteins help macrophages to present antigens to T lymphocytes. In particular, Th cells activated by these macrophages release cytokines to activate and differentiate B cells into antibody-producing plasma cells to thwart pathogen invasion and infection [117]. The M2 macrophages are central to RA remission due to their anti-inflammatory role indicating that treatment based on polarization of M2 macrophages is important for the treatment strategies of RA patients. Subsequently, therapies based on targeting macrophage polarization are still a preferable research area to explore possible therapeutics against RA.

Recent investigations have revealed the expression of some novel proteins and non-coding RNAs that influence macrophage polarization to control MS progression. For example, the intensification of MS illness was promoted by circRNA_0000518, a non-coding RNA by promoting the polarization of macrophages via the CaMKKβ/AMPK-PGC-1α pathway toward M1 macrophage [118].

2.6 The interconnectedness between macrophage polarization, immunometabolism, and disease progression

The metabolic reactions are the cells' central driving engines, and their changes play a pivotal role in cellular differentiation, activation, and other cellular morphologies. The last few decades have witnessed a close link between metabolic systems and the working dynamics of the immune system. For instance, since last decade mounting evidence suggests that macrophages are central to tissue homeostasis, host defense, and remodeling of tissues. This attribute of macrophages lies in their heterogeneous nature and adoption to various activated states. Central to all these magical workouts by macrophages depends on their modulation in metabolic networks. The current section aims to explore the metabolic pathways operating on macrophages to turn out these functions and more importantly regulator networks that control the macrophage metabolism.

In general, cells sense the environmental cues to reprogram the intracellular metabolism for structural and functional adjustments accordingly. To understand this metabolic adjustment, for example, in the presence of oxygen, the adenosine triphosphate (ATP) is produced by mitochondria by oxidative phosphorylation. The process requires NADH and FADH generally derived from the tricarboxylic acid cycle (TCA) or fatty acid oxidation. In contrast, under hypoxic conditions, cell shift their metabolism to glycolysis by activating hypoxia-inducible factor 1α (HIF1α) transcription factor to meet the ATP demands. Similarly, cells also sense nutrient levels and utilize these nutrient profiles to balance their metabolic networks. Reports reveal that certain metabolites are crucial for the regulation of immune cells such as macrophages, neutrophils, and T cells. O'Neill et al. [119] reported that metabolic reprogramming of immune cells is accomplished by stimulation of cytokine receptors, pattern recognition receptors, and antigen receptors. For instance, the mammalian target of rapamycin (mTOR), a protein kinase regulates several metabolic networks including autophagy, proliferation, cell migration, immune responses, and cellular homeostasis. Central to all these regulatory networks lies the activation of mTOR signaling that integrates nutritional information, like ATP and amino acid levels, to promote cell proliferation and cell activation. The mTOR is formed of two complexes viz., mTOR complexes 1 and 2, both these complexes are distinguished and formed by the presence of adaptors molecules, Raptor (in mTORC1) and Rictor (in mTORC2) [120]. The network of mTORC1/mTORC2 in macrophages is involved by many extracellular signaling cues such as TLR ligands, growth factors, and cytokines to mediate gene expression. For instance, Haloul [121] reported the role of mTORC1 in the polarization of macrophages to M1 phenotype, and the latter was found to induce the pathogenic fatal ehrlichiosis in the liver. In addition, the PI3K–mTOR pathway macrophages residing in bone marrow enhanced the polarization of M2 macrophages, whereas, on the other hand, inhibition of PI3K or mTOR stemmed in M1 macrophage, demonstrating the significance of PI3K or mTOR in macrophage polarization of macrophages [122]. Consequently, these reports suggest the central role of mTOR and other signaling cascades involved in macrophage polarization, and their dysregulation results in the progression of diseases such as atherosclerosis [123].

Reports suggest that macrophages have a central role in the development of acute lung injury (ALI)/acute respiratory distress syndrome (ARDS) by secreting pro-inflammatory cytokines and inducing the recruitment of neutrophils into the lungs to aggravate the progression of inflammation and injury to the lungs [124, 125]. Similarly, the development of pulmonary fibrosis also occurs when there is an overly dominant M2 polarization [125]. These studies show that depending on the regulation of macrophage phenotypes, the ALI/ARDS outcomes may greatly differ.

The molecular intermediates and modulation of immunometabolism receptors highly influence macrophage polarization. Described below are the effects on the different molecular targets of N5P inhibitor to result in the reduction of inflammation in ALI: N5P inhibitor suppresses the levels of genes such as ASIC1a, GLUT1, HIF-1α, HK2, IL-6, and IL-1β. Likewise, with the help of 2-deoxyglucose (2-DG), an inhibitor of glycolysis, a decrease in the severity of lung damage, low effect of oxidative stress, and less production of inflammatory cytokines were observed in the ALI mice models [126]. Likewise, when macrophages were treated with 1,2,3-benzentricarboxylic acid (BTA) there was decreased mitochondrial citrate carrier (CIC/SLC25a1) activity that consequently reduced the citrate accumulation in cytosol of activated macrophages causing a reduction in NO production. Contraceptive methods included investor, receptor only MA, and prostaglandin [127]. The present study reinforced the earlier findings by demonstrating that the intraperitoneal administration of α-KG in mice reduced inflamed cytokines and suppressed the genes of IL-1β, TNF-α, and IL −6 and increased Arg1 levels to reduce lung injury [128]. Therefore, one can say that the more moderate disease severity depends mainly on adjusting the macrophage polarization by means of immunometabolism.

3. Conclusions

In conclusion, macrophages, as the cells that play essential roles in the innate immune system, display great functional heterogeneity and tissue plasticity, enabling them to respond to numerous physiological and pathological processes. They have the capacity to switch between M1 and M2, so that macrophages are instrumental in causing inflammation and also in healing tissue injury. The M1 macrophages are particularly involved in protective host defense and acute inflammatory events due to the synthesis of pro-inflammatory cytokines and ROS. However, the recruitment and activation of M1 is not beneficial for a long time, as it leads to tissue damage and sustained inflammation. Conversely, M2 macrophage moniker originate from IL-4/IL-13 signals, they are involved in inflammation resolution, tissue remodeling as well as in processes that support angiogenic and cancer-promoting functions.

IR insightful, we continue to learn that macrophage polarization is a dynamic and highly integrated process whereby molecular signaling pathways and metabolic reprogramming mediate macrophage states and functions and the interdependence of immunological signaling and metabolic pathways. Knowledge of these processes is useful in the elucidation of pathophysiological processes of numerous diseases such as chronic/acute inflammation, cancer, and other diseases. This knowledge also reveals possible paths toward creating more specific anti-inflammatory treatments for diseases through the manipulation of macrophages to restoration of proper function and more.

Thus, the current chapter offers a concise and detailed understanding of the processes described in the context of macrophage polarization in correlation with health and disease. This highlights the importance of understanding and characterizing multi-lineage cells such as macrophages in disease processes and the development of novel strategies to modulate the potential clinical application of macrophage-oriented regimens.

Acknowledgements

We want to acknowledge the Department of Biotechnology (DBT), Ministry of Science and Technology, New Delhi for supported Nissar Ahmad Wani with RamalingaSwami Fellowship (Grant No. BT/HRD/35/02/2006).

Conflict of interest

The authors declare no conflict of interest.

Author details

Rakeeb Ahmad Mir[1], Owais M. Bhat[1], Abid Hamid Dar[1], Mohammad Muzamil Shah[2] and Nissar Ahmad Wani[1*]

1 Department of Biotechnology, School of Life Sciences, Central University of Kashmir, Ganderbal, Jammu and Kashmir, India

2 Department of Physical Education, Central University of Kashmir, Ganderbal, Jammu and Kashmir, India

*Address all correspondence to: waninh@cukashmir.ac.in

IntechOpen

© 2024 The Author(s). Licensee IntechOpen. This chapter is distributed under the terms of the Creative Commons Attribution License (http://creativecommons.org/licenses/by/3.0), which permits unrestricted use, distribution, and reproduction in any medium, provided the original work is properly cited. (cc) BY

References

[1] Arora S, Dev K, Agarwal B, et al. Macrophages: Their role, activation and polarization in pulmonary diseases. Immunobiology. 2018;**223**:4-5. DOI: 10.1016/j.imbio.2017.11.001

[2] Bajgar A, Krejčová G. On the origin of the functional versatility of macrophages. Frontiers in Physiology. 2023;**14**(1128984). DOI: 10.3389/fphys.2023.1128984

[3] Atri C, Guerfali FZ, Laouini D. Role of human macrophage polarization in inflammation during infectious diseases. International Journal of Molecular Sciences. 2018;**19**(6):1801. DOI: 10.3390/ijms19061801

[4] Chen S, Saeed AFUH, Liu Q, et al. Macrophages in immunoregulation and therapeutics. Signal Transduction and Targeted Therapy. 2023;**8**(1):207. DOI: 10.1038/s41392-023-01452-1

[5] Harada D, Nagamachi S, Aso K, et al. Oral administration of L-ornithine increases the content of both collagen constituting amino acids and polyamines in mouse skin. Biochemical and Biophysical Research Communications. 2019;**512**(4):712-715. DOI: 10.1016/j.bbrc.2019.03.147

[6] Kotwal GJ, Chien S. Macrophage differentiation in normal and accelerated wound healing. In: Results and Problems in Cell Differentiation. 2017;**62**:353-364. DOI: 10.1007/978-3-319-54090-0_14

[7] Mehraj U, Dar AH, Wani NA, et al. Tumor microenvironment promotes breast cancer chemoresistance. Cancer Chemotherapy and Pharmacology. 2021;**87**(2):147-158. DOI: 10.1007/s00280-020-04222-w

[8] Mehraj U, Mushtaq U, Mir MA, et al. Chemokines in triple-negative breast cancer heterogeneity: New challenges for clinical implications. Seminars in Cancer Biology. 2022;**86**(2):769-783. DOI: 10.1016/j.semcancer.2022.03.008

[9] Mosser DM, Edwards JP. Exploring the full spectrum of macrophage activation. Nature Reviews Immunology. 2008;**8**(12):958-969. DOI: 10.1038/nri2448

[10] Martinez FO, Gordon S. The M1 and M2 paradigm of macrophage activation: Time for reassessment. Faculty of 1000 Prime Reports. 2014;**6**(13). DOI: 10.12703/P6-13

[11] Lu YC, Yeh WC, Ohashi PS. LPS/TLR4 signal transduction pathway. Cytokine. 2008;**42**(2):145-151. DOI: 10.1016/j.cyto.2008.01.006

[12] Vidyarthi A, Khan N, Agnihotri T, et al. TLR-3 stimulation skews M2 macrophages to M1 through IFN-αβ signaling and restricts tumor progression. Frontiers in Immunology. 2018;**9**(1650). DOI: 10.3389/fimmu.2018.01650

[13] Takeda K, Kaisho T, Akira S. Toll-like receptors. Annual Review of Immunology. 2001;**21**:335-376. DOI: 10.1146/annurev.immunol.21.120601.141126

[14] Ullah MO, Sweet MJ, Mansell A, et al. TRIF-dependent TLR signaling, its functions in host defense and inflammation, and its potential as a therapeutic target. Journal of Leukocyte Biology. 2016;**100**(1):27-45. DOI: 10.1189/jlb.2ri1115-531r

[15] Deguine J, Barton GM. MyD88: A central player in innate immune

signaling. Faculty of 1000 Prime Reports. 2014;**4**(6):97. DOI: 10.12703/P6-97

[16] Vannella KM, Wynn TA. Mechanisms of organ injury and repair by macrophages. Annual Review of Physiology. 2017;**10**(79):593-617. DOI: 10.1146/annurev-physiol-022516-034356

[17] Shapouri-Moghaddam A, Mohammadian S, Vazini H, et al. Macrophage plasticity, polarization, and function in health and disease. Journal of Cellular Physiology. 2018;**233**(9):6425-6440. DOI: 10.1002/jcp.26429

[18] Hibbs JB, Vavrin Z, Taintor RR. L-arginine is required for expression of the activated macrophage effector mechanism causing selective metabolic inhibition in target cells. Journal of Immunology. 1987;**138**(2):550-565. DOI: 10.4049/jimmunol.138.2.550

[19] Biswas SK, Mantovani A. Macrophage plasticity and interaction with lymphocyte subsets: Cancer as a paradigm. Nature Immunology. 2010;**11**(10):889-896. DOI: 10.1038/ni.1937

[20] Wynn TA, Vannella KM. Macrophages in tissue repair, regeneration, and fibrosis. Immunity. 2016;**44**(3):450-462. DOI: 10.1016/j.immuni.2016.02.015

[21] Vergadi E, Ieronymaki E, Lyroni K, et al. Akt Signaling pathway in macrophage activation and M1/M2 polarization. Journal of Immunology. 2017;**198**(3):1006-1014. DOI: 10.4049/jimmunol.1601515

[22] Kotenko SV, Krause CD, Izotova LS, et al. Identification and functional characterization of a second chain of the interleukin-10 receptor complex. The EMBO Journal. 1997;**16**(19):5894-5903. DOI: 10.1093/emboj/16.19.5894

[23] Saxton RA, Tsutsumi N, Su LL, et al. Structure-based decoupling of the pro- and anti-inflammatory functions of interleukin-10. Science. 2021;**371**(6535):8433. DOI: 10.1126/science.abc8433

[24] Ito S, Ansari P, Sakatsume M, et al. Interleukin-10 inhibits expression of both interferon α– and interferon γ–induced genes by suppressing tyrosine phosphorylation of STAT1. Blood. 1999;**93**(5):1456-1463. DOI: 10.1182/blood.v93.5.1456

[25] Briscoe J, Rogers NC, Witthuhn BA, et al. Kinase-negative mutants of JAK1 can sustain interferon-γ-inducible gene expression but not an antiviral state. The EMBO Journal. 1996;**15**(4):799-809. DOI: 10.1002/j.1460-2075.1996.tb00415.x

[26] Guo C, Islam R, Zhang S, et al. Metabolic reprogramming of macrophages and its involvement in inflammatory diseases. EXCLI Journal. 2021;**20**:628-641. DOI: 10.17179/excli2020-3053

[27] Cheng H, Wang Z, Fu L, et al. Macrophage polarization in the development and progression of ovarian cancers: An overview. Frontiers in Oncology. 2019;**9**:421. DOI: 10.3389/fonc.2019.00421

[28] Yunna C, Mengru H, Lei W, et al. Macrophage M1/M2 polarization. European Journal of Pharmacology. 2020;**15**:877. DOI: 10.1016/j.ejphar.2020.173090

[29] Boutilier AJ, Elsawa SF. Macrophage polarization states in the tumor microenvironment. International Journal of Molecular Sciences. 2021;**22**(13). DOI: 10.3390/ijms22136995

[30] Curren Smith EW. Macrophage polarization and its role in cancer. Journal

of Clinical & Cellular Immunology. 2015;**6**(4):10.4172/2155-9899.1000338

[31] Murray PJ. Macrophage polarization. Annual Review of Physiology. 2017;**79**:541-566. DOI: 10.1146/annurev-physiol-022516-034339

[32] Mantovani A, Sica A, Sozzani S, et al. The chemokine system in diverse forms of macrophage activation and polarization. Trends in Immunology. 2004;**25**(12):677-686. DOI: 10.1016/j.it.2004.09.015

[33] Chinetti-Gbaguidi G, Colin S, Staels B. Macrophage subsets in atherosclerosis. Nature Reviews Cardiology. 2015;**12**(1):10-17. DOI: 10.1038/nrcardio.2014.173

[34] Xue J, Schmidt SV, Sander J, et al. Transcriptome-based network analysis reveals a spectrum model of human macrophage activation. Immunity. 2014;**40**(2):274-288. DOI: 10.1016/j.immuni.2014.01.006

[35] Repici M, Mare L, Colombo A, et al. c-Jun N-terminal kinase binding domain-dependent phosphorylation of mitogen-activated protein kinase kinase 4 and mitogen-activated protein kinase kinase 7 and balancing cross-talk between c-Jun N-terminal kinase and extracellular signal-regulated kinase. Neuroscience. 2009;**159**(1):94-103. DOI: 10.1016/j.neuroscience.2008.11.049

[36] Dai L, Aye Thu C, Liu XY, et al. TAK1, more than just innate immunity. IUBMB Life. 2012;**64**(10):825-834. DOI: 10.1002/iub.1078

[37] Rousseau S, Papoutsopoulou M, Symons A, et al. TPL2-mediated activation of ERK1 and ERK2 regulates the processing of pre-TNFα in LPS-stimulated macrophages. Journal of Cell Science. 2008;**121**(2):149-154. DOI: 10.1242/jcs.018671

[38] Igarashi KI, Garotta G, Ozmen L, et al. Interferon-γ induces tyrosine phosphorylation of interferon-γ receptor and regulated association of protein tyrosine kinases, Jak1 and Jak2, with its receptor. The Journal of Biological Chemistry. 1994;**269**(20):14333-14336. DOI: 10.1016/s0021-9258(17)36621-8

[39] Heim MH, Kerr Lan M, Stark GR, et al. Contribution of STAT SH2 groups to specific interferon signaling by the Jak-STAT pathway. Science. 1995;**267**:1347-1349. DOI: 10.1126/science.7871432

[40] Greenlund AC, Morales MO, Viviano BL, et al. Stat recruitment by tyrosine-phosphorylated cytokine receptors: An ordered reversible affinity-driven process. Immunity. 1995;**2**(6):677-687. DOI: 10.1016/1074-7613(95)90012-8

[41] Cassetta L, Cassol E, Poli G. Macrophage polarization in health and disease. Scientific World Journal. 2011;**11**:2391-2402. DOI: 10.1100/2011/213962

[42] Yang M, Liu J, Piao C, et al. ICAM-1 suppresses tumor metastasis by inhibiting macrophage M2 polarization through blockade of efferocytosis. Cell Death & Disease. 2015;**6**(6):1780. DOI: 10.1038/cddis.2015.144

[43] Mogensen KE, Lewerenz M, Reboul J, et al. The type I interferon receptor: Structure, function, and evolution of a family business. Journal of Interferon and Cytokine Research. 1999;**19**(10):1069-1098. DOI: 10.1089/107999099313019

[44] Cheon H, Holvey-Bates EG, Schoggins JW, et al. IFNβ-dependent increases in STAT1, STAT2, and IRF9 mediate resistance to viruses and DNA damage. The EMBO Journal. 2013;**32**(20):2751-2763. DOI: 10.1038/emboj.2013.203

[45] Kratochvill F, Neale G, Haverkamp JM, et al. TNF counterbalances the emergence of M2 tumor macrophages. Cell Reports. 2015;**12**(11):1902-1914. DOI: 10.1016/j.celrep.2015.08.033

[46] Hyun HP, Lo YC, Lin SC, et al. The death domain superfamily in intracellular signaling of apoptosis and inflammation. Annual Review of Immunology. 2007;**25**:561-586. DOI: 10.1146/annurev.immunol.25.022106.141656

[47] Wajant H, Scheurich P. TNFR1-induced activation of the classical NF-κB pathway. FEBS Journal. 2011;**278**(6):862-876. DOI: 10.1111/j.1742-4658.2011.08015.x

[48] Kearney CJ, Martin SJ. An inflammatory perspective on necroptosis. Molecular Cell. 2017;**65**(6):965-973. DOI: 10.1016/j.molcel.2017.02.024

[49] Sun SC. The non-canonical NF-κB pathway in immunity and inflammation. Nature Reviews Immunology. 2017;**17**(9):545-558. DOI: 10.1038/nri.2017.52

[50] Natoli G, Costanzo A, Ianni A, et al. Activation of SAPK/JNK by TNF receptor 1 through a noncytotoxic TRAF2- dependent pathway. Science. 1997;**275**:200-203. DOI: 10.1126/science.275.5297.200

[51] Dérijard B, Raingeaud J, Barrett T, et al. Independent human MAP kinase signal transduction pathways defined by MEK and MKK isoforms. Science. 1995;**267**(5198):682-685. DOI: 10.1126/science.7839144

[52] Dasi S, Choi J, Lambertz I, et al. Tpl2/cot signals activate ERK, JNK, and NF-κB in a cell-type and stimulus-specific manner. The Journal of Biological Chemistry. 2005;**280**(25):23748-23757. DOI: 10.1074/jbc.M412837200

[53] Jin J, Xiao Y, Hu H, et al. Proinflammatory TLR signalling is regulated by a TRAF2-dependent proteolysis mechanism in macrophages. Nature Communications. 2015;7(6):5930. DOI: 10.1038/ncomms6930

[54] Khaled WT, Read EKC, Nicholson SE, et al. The IL-4/IL-13/stat6 signalling pathway promotes luminal mammary epithelial cell development. Development. 2007;**134**(15):2739-2750. DOI: 10.1242/dev.003194

[55] Symowski C, Voehringer D. Th2 cell-derived IL-4/IL-13 promote ILC2 accumulation in the lung by ILC2-intrinsic STAT6 signaling in mice. European Journal of Immunology. 2019;**49**(9):1421-1432. DOI: 10.1002/eji.201948161

[56] Zhou C, Lu C, Pu H, et al. TRAF6 promotes IL-4-induced M2 macrophage activation by stabilizing STAT6. Molecular Immunology. 2020;**127**:223-229. DOI: 10.1016/j.molimm.2020.09.001

[57] Arranz A, Doxaki C, Vergadi E, et al. Akt1 and Akt2 protein kinases differentially contribute to macrophage polarization. Proceedings of the National Academy of Sciences of the United States of America. 2012;**109**(24):9517-9522. DOI: 10.1073/pnas.1119038109

[58] Pengal RA, Ganesan LP, Wei G, et al. Lipopolysaccharide-induced production of interleukin-10 is promoted by the serine/threonine kinase Akt. Molecular Immunology. 2006;**43**(10):1557-1564. DOI: 10.1016/j.molimm.2005.09.022

[59] Ambade A, Satishchandran A, Saha B, et al. Hepatocellular carcinoma is accelerated by NASH involving M2 macrophage polarization mediated by hif-1αinduced IL-10. Oncoimmunology. 2016;**5**(10):e1221557. DOI: 10.1080/2162402X.2016.1221557

[60] Valluru M, Staton CA, Reed MWR, et al. Transforming growth factor-β and endoglin signaling orchestrate wound healing. Frontiers in Physiology. 2011;**2**:89. DOI: 10.3389/fphys.2011.00089

[61] Derynck R, Zhang YE. Smad-dependent and Smad-independent pathways in TGF-β family signalling. Nature. 2003;**425**(6958):577-584. DOI: 10.1038/nature02006

[62] Massagué J, Seoane J, Wotton D. Smad transcription factors. Genes and Development. 2005;**19**(23):2783-2810. DOI: 10.1101/gad.1350705

[63] Raes G, Brys L, Dahal BK, et al. Macrophage galactose-type C-type lectins as novel markers for alternatively activated macrophages elicited by parasitic infections and allergic airway inflammation. Journal of Leukocyte Biology. 2004;**77**(3):321-327. DOI: 10.1189/jlb.0304212

[64] Zhang F, Wang H, Wang X, et al. TGF-β induces M2-like macrophage polarization via SNAIL mediated suppression of a pro-inflammatory phenotype. Oncotarget. 2016;**7**(32):52294-52306. DOI: 10.18632/oncotarget.10561

[65] Palaga T, Wongchana W, Kueanjinda P. Notch signaling in macrophages in the context of cancer immunity. Frontiers in Immunology. 2018;**9**:652. DOI: 10.3389/fimmu.2018.00652

[66] Zhang Z, Tang J, Cui X, et al. New insights and novel therapeutic potentials for macrophages in myocardial infarction. Inflammation. 2021;**44**(5):1696-1712. DOI: 10.1007/s10753-021-01467-2

[67] Li AM, Ye J. Deciphering the Warburg effect: Metabolic reprogramming, epigenetic remodeling, and cell dedifferentiation. Annual Review of Cancer Biology. 2024;**8**:35-58. DOI: 10.1146/annurev-cancerbio-062822-120857

[68] Kasmi EL, KC, Stenmark KR. Contribution of metabolic reprogramming to macrophage plasticity and function. Seminars in Immunology. 2015;**27**(4):267-275. DOI: 10.1016/j.smim.2015.09.001

[69] Hard GC. Some biochemical aspects of the immune macrophage. British Journal of Experimental Pathology. 1970;**51**(1):97-105

[70] West AP, Brodsky IE, Rahner C, et al. TLR signalling augments macrophage bactericidal activity through mitochondrial ROS. Nature. 2011;**472**(7344):476-480. DOI: 10.1038/nature09973

[71] Drapier JC, Hibbs JB. Differentiation of murine macrophages to express nonspecific cytotoxicity for tumor cells results in L-arginine-dependent inhibition of mitochondrial iron-sulfur enzymes in the macrophage effector cells. Journal of Immunology. 1988;**140**(8):2829-2838. DOI: 10.4049/jimmunol.140.8.2829

[72] Palsson-Mcdermott EM, O'Neill LAJ. The Warburg effect then and now: From cancer to inflammatory diseases. BioEssays. 2013;**35**(11):965-973. DOI: 10.1002/bies.201300084

[73] Bedard K, Krause KH. The NOX family of ROS-generating NADPH oxidases: Physiology and pathophysiology. Physiological Reviews. 2007;**87**(1):245-313. DOI: 10.1152/physrev.00044.2005

[74] Clementi E, Brown GC, Feelisch M, et al. Persistent inhibition of

cell respiration by nitric oxide: Crucial role of S-nitrosylation of mitochondrial complex I and protective action of glutathione. Proceedings of the National Academy of Sciences of the United States of America. 1998;**95**(13):7631-7636. DOI: 10.1073/pnas.95.13.7631

[75] Erratum: Enhanced fatty acid oxidation in adipocytes and macrophages reduces lipid-induced triglyceride accumulation and inflammation (Am J Physiol Endocrinol Metab, (2015) 308, (E756-E769), 10.1152/ajpendo.00362.2014). American Journal of Physiology - Endocrinology and Metabolism. 2016;**308**(9):E756-E769. DOI: 10.1152/ajpendo.zh1-7562-corr.2011

[76] Huang SCC, Smith AM, Everts B, et al. Metabolic reprogramming mediated by the mTORC2-IRF4 signaling axis is essential for macrophage alternative activation. Immunity. 2016;**45**(4):817-830. DOI: 10.1016/j.immuni.2016.09.016

[77] Florance I, Ramasubbu S. Current understanding on the role of lipids in macrophages and associated diseases. International Journal of Molecular Sciences. 2023;**24**(1):589. DOI: 10.3390/ijms24010589

[78] Van den Bossche J, O'Neill LA, Menon D. Macrophage immunometabolism: Where are we (going)? Trends in Immunology. 2017;**38**(6):395-406. DOI: 10.1016/j.it.2017.03.001

[79] Rosa Neto JC, Calder PC, Curi R, et al. The immunometabolic roles of various fatty acids in macrophages and lymphocytes. International Journal of Molecular Sciences. 2021;**22**(16):8460. DOI: 10.3390/ijms22168460

[80] Kieler M, Hofmann M, Schabbauer G. More than just protein building blocks: How amino acids and related metabolic pathways fuel macrophage polarization. FEBS Journal. 2021;**288**(12):3694-3714. DOI: 10.1111/febs.15715

[81] Liu J, Han X, Zhang T, et al. Reactive oxygen species (ROS) scavenging biomaterials for anti-inflammatory diseases: From mechanism to therapy. Journal of Hematology and Oncology. 2023;**16**(1):116. DOI: 10.1186/s13045-023-01512-7

[82] Ma Q. Role of Nrf2 in oxidative stress and toxicity. Annual Review of Pharmacology and Toxicology. 2013;**53**:401-426. DOI: 10.1146/annurev-pharmtox-011112-140320

[83] Griffith OW, Meister A. Potent and specific inhibition of glutathione synthesis by buthionine sulfoximine (S-n-butyl homocysteine sulfoximine). The Journal of Biological Chemistry. 1979;**254**(16):7558-7560. DOI: 10.1016/s0021-9258(18)35980-5

[84] Griffith OW. Mechanism of action, metabolism, and toxicity of buthionine sulfoximine and its higher homologs, potent inhibitors of glutathione synthesis. The Journal of Biological Chemistry;**257**(22):13704-13712. DOI: 10.1016/s0021-9258(18)33504-x

[85] Tan HY, Wang N, Li S, et al. The reactive oxygen species in macrophage polarization: Reflecting its dual role in progression and treatment of human diseases. Oxidative Medicine and Cellular Longevity. 2016:2795090. DOI: 10.1155/2016/2795090

[86] Schieber M, Chandel NS. ROS function in redox signaling and oxidative stress. Current Biology. 2014;**24**(10):R453-R462. DOI: 10.1016/j.cub.2014.03.034

[87] Shin E, Koo JS. Glucose metabolism and glucose transporters in breast cancer.

Frontiers in Cell and Developmental Biology. 2021;**9**:728759. DOI: 10.3389/fcell.2021.728759

[88] Rodriguez AE, Ducker GS, Billingham LK, et al. Serine metabolism supports macrophage IL-1β production. Cell Metabolism. 2019;**29**(4):1003-1011. DOI: 10.1016/j.cmet.2019.01.014

[89] Labrie V, Roder JC. The involvement of the NMDA receptor d-serine/glycine site in the pathophysiology and treatment of schizophrenia. Neuroscience and Biobehavioral Reviews. 2010;**34**(3):351-372. DOI: 10.1016/j.neubiorev.2009.08.002

[90] Yücel G, Zhao Z, El-Battrawy I, et al. Lipopolysaccharides induced inflammatory responses and electrophysiological dysfunctions in human-induced pluripotent stem cell derived cardiomyocytes. Scientific Reports. 2017;**7**(1):2935. DOI: 10.1038/s41598-017-03147-4

[91] Yu W, Wang Z, Zhang K, et al. One-carbon metabolism supports S-Adenosylmethionine and histone methylation to drive inflammatory macrophages. Molecular Cell. 2019;**75**(6):1147-1160. DOI: 10.1016/j.molcel.2019.06.039

[92] Puchalska P, Huang X, Martin SE, et al. Isotope tracing untargeted metabolomics reveals macrophage polarization-state-specific metabolic coordination across intracellular compartments. iScience. 2018;**9**:298-313. DOI: 10.1016/j.isci.2018.10.029

[93] Rath M, Müller I, Kropf P, et al. Metabolism via arginase or nitric oxide synthase: Two competing arginine pathways in macrophages. Frontiers in Immunology. 2014;**5**:532. DOI: 10.3389/fimmu.2014.00532

[94] Haidar YM, Cosman BC. Obesity epidemiology. Clinics in Colon and Rectal Surgery. 2011;**24**(4):205-210. DOI: 10.1055/s-0031-1295684

[95] Ouchi N, Parker JL, Lugus JJ, et al. Adipokines in inflammation and metabolic disease. Nature Reviews Immunology. 2011;**11**(2):85-97. DOI: 10.1038/nri2921

[96] Lumeng CN. Innate immune activation in obesity. Molecular Aspects of Medicine. 2013;**34**(1):12-29. DOI: 10.1016/j.mam.2012.10.002

[97] Byles V, Covarrubias AJ, Ben-Sahra I, et al. The TSC-mTOR pathway regulates macrophage polarization. Nature Communications. 2013;**4**:2834. DOI: 10.1038/ncomms3834

[98] Cao Q, Wang Y, Wang XM, et al. Renal F4/80+CD11c+ mononuclear phagocytes display phenotypic and functional characteristics of macrophages in health and in Adriamycin nephropathy. Journal of the American Society of Nephrology : JASN. 2015;**26**(2):349-363. DOI: 10.1681/ASN.2013121336

[99] Tang PMK, Nikolic-Paterson DJ, Lan HY. Macrophages: Versatile players in renal inflammation and fibrosis. Nature Reviews Nephrology. 2019;**15**(3):144-158. DOI: 10.1038/s41581-019-0110-2

[100] Braga TT, Agudelo JSH, Camara NOS. Macrophages during the fibrotic process: M2 as friend and foe. Frontiers in Immunology. 2015;**6**:602. DOI: 10.3389/fimmu.2015.00602

[101] Toledo DM, Pioli PA. Macrophages in systemic sclerosis: Novel insights and therapeutic implications. Current Rheumatology Reports. 2019;**21**(7):31. DOI: 10.1007/s11926-019-0831-z

[102] Zhao X, Di Q, Liu H, et al. MEF2C promotes M1 macrophage polarization and Th1 responses. Cellular & Molecular Immunology. 2022;**19**(4):540-553. DOI: 10.1038/s41423-022-00841-w

[103] Ni X, Lai Y. Keratinocyte: A trigger or an executor of psoriasis? Journal of Leukocyte Biology. 2020;**108**(2):485-491. DOI: 10.1002/JLB.5MR0120-439R

[104] Kamata M, Tada Y. Dendritic cells and macrophages in the pathogenesis of psoriasis. Frontiers in Immunology. 2022;**13**:941071. DOI: 10.3389/fimmu.2022.941071

[105] Kim HJ, Jang J, Lee EH, et al. Decreased expression of response gene to complement 32 in psoriasis and its association with reduced M2 macrophage polarization. Journal of Dermatology. 2019;**46**(2):166-168. DOI: 10.1111/1346-8138.14733

[106] Locati M, Mantovani A, Sica A. Macrophage activation and polarization as an adaptive component of innate immunity. In: Advances in Immunology. 2013;**2013**(120):163-184. DOI: 10.1016/B978-0-12-417028-5.00006-5

[107] Ay E. Atopic dermatitis. In: Chronic Disease Follow-Ups for Adults in Primary Care. 2022;**39**(3):145-155. DOI: 10.55041/ijsrem28482

[108] Homey B, Steinhoff M, Ruzicka T, et al. Cytokines and chemokines orchestrate atopic skin inflammation. Journal of Allergy and Clinical Immunology. 2006;**118**(1):178-189. DOI: 10.1016/j.jaci.2006.03.047

[109] Liu YC, Zou XB, Chai YF, et al. Macrophage polarization in inflammatory diseases. International Journal of Biological Sciences. 2014;**10**(5):520-529. DOI: 10.7150/ijbs.8879

[110] Orme J, Mohan C. Macrophage subpopulations in systemic lupus erythematosus. Discovery Medicine. 2012;**13**(69):151-158

[111] Lee S, Huen S, Nishio H, et al. Distinct macrophage phenotypes contribute to kidney injury and repair. Journal of the American Society of Nephrology: JASN. 2011;**22**(2):317-326. DOI: 10.1681/ASN.2009060615

[112] Rőszer T, Menéndez-Gutiérrez MP, Lefterova MI, et al. Autoimmune kidney disease and impaired engulfment of apoptotic cells in mice with macrophage peroxisome proliferator-activated receptor γ or retinoid X receptor α deficiency. Journal of Immunology. 2011;**186**(1):621-631. DOI: 10.4049/jimmunol.1002230

[113] Li F, Yang Y, Zhu X, et al. Macrophage polarization modulates development of systemic lupus erythematosus. Cellular Physiology and Biochemistry. 2015;**37**(4):1279-1288. DOI: 10.1159/000430251

[114] Ma C, Xia Y, Yang Q, et al. The contribution of macrophages to systemic lupus erythematosus. Clinical Immunology. 2019;**207**:1-9. DOI: 10.1016/j.clim.2019.06.009

[115] Yang Y, Guo L, Wang Z, et al. Targeted silver nanoparticles for rheumatoid arthritis therapy via macrophage apoptosis and Re-polarization. Biomaterials. 2021;**264**:120390. DOI: 10.1016/j.biomaterials.2020.120390

[116] Udalova IA, Mantovani A, Feldmann M. Macrophage heterogeneity in the context of rheumatoid arthritis. Nature Reviews Rheumatology. 2016;**12**(8):472-485. DOI: 10.1038/nrrheum.2016.91

[117] Duque GA, Descoteaux A. Macrophage cytokines: Involvement in immunity and infectious diseases. Frontiers in Immunology. 2014;**5**:491. DOI: 10.3389/fimmu.2014.00491

[118] Jiang F, Liu X, Cui X, et al. Circ_0000518 promotes macrophage/microglia M1 polarization via the FUS/CaMKKβ/AMPK pathway to aggravate multiple sclerosis. Neuroscience. 2022;**490**:131-143. DOI: 10.1016/j.neuroscience.2021.12.012

[119] O'Neill LAJ, Kishton RJ, Rathmell J. A guide to immunometabolism for immunologists. Nature Reviews Immunology. 2016;**16**(9):553-565. DOI: 10.1038/nri.2016.70

[120] Weichhart T, Hengstschläger M, Linke M. Regulation of innate immune cell function by mTOR. Nature Reviews Immunology. 2015;**15**(10):599-614. DOI: 10.1038/nri3901

[121] Haloul M, Oliveira ERA, Kader M, et al. mTORC1-mediated polarization of M1 macrophages and their accumulation in the liver correlate with immunopathology in fatal ehrlichiosis. Scientific Reports. 2019;**9**(1):14050. DOI: 10.1038/s41598-019-50320-y

[122] Rocher C, Singla DK. SMAD-PI3K-Akt-mTOR pathway mediates BMP-7 polarization of monocytes into M2 macrophages. PLoS One. 2013;**8**(12):e84009. DOI: 10.1371/journal.pone.0084009

[123] Tian F, Yu BL, Hu JR. MTOR mediates the cross-talk of macrophage polarization and autophagy in atherosclerosis. International Journal of Cardiology. 2014;**177**(1):144-145. DOI: 10.1016/j.ijcard.2014.09.035

[124] Chen X, Tang J, Shuai W, et al. Macrophage polarization and its role in the pathogenesis of acute lung injury/acute respiratory distress syndrome. Inflammation Research. 2020;**69**(9):883-895. DOI: 10.1007/s00011-020-01378-2

[125] Cheng P, Li S, Chen H. Macrophages in lung injury, repair and fibrosis. Cells. 2021;**10**(2):436. DOI: 10.3390/cells10020436

[126] Zhong WJ, Yang HH, Guan XX, et al. Inhibition of glycolysis alleviates lipopolysaccharide-induced acute lung injury in a mouse model. Journal of Cellular Physiology. 2019;**234**(4):4641-4654. DOI: 10.1002/jcp.27261

[127] Infantino V, Convertini P, Cucci L, et al. The mitochondrial citrate carrier: A new player in inflammation. The Biochemical Journal. 2011;**438**(3):433-436. DOI: 10.1042/BJ20111275

[128] Liu M, Chen Y, Wang S, et al. α-Ketoglutarate modulates macrophage polarization through regulation of PPARγ transcription and mTORC1/p70S6K pathway to ameliorate ALI/ARDS. Shock. 2020;**53**(1):103-113. DOI: 10.1097/SHK.0000000000001333

Chapter 2

The Impact of Glucose Intermediates, Lactate and Amino Acids on Macrophage Metabolism and Function

Najia Jeroundi, Léa Paolini and Pascale Jeannin

Abstract

Macrophages (Mφs) are long-lived innate immune cells present in almost all tissues. In addition to phagocytic properties, Mφs are characterized by their plasticity. They are involved in tissue homeostasis, anti-infectious, pro- and anti-inflammatory responses depending on the needs of the tissue. Mφ functional phenotypes are tightly tied to their metabolic pathways. Glucose-related metabolic pathways including glycolysis, pentose phosphate pathway and glycogen metabolism have been associated with the control of inflammatory response. On the contrary, Krebs cycle activity fueled with glutamine or lactate has been associated with Mφs harboring repair properties. For some metabolites, their fate is directly dependent on Mφ phenotype as exemplified with arginase in murine Mφs: proinflammatory Mφs express nitric oxide synthase synthesizing NO while trophic Mφs express arginase-producing L-ornithine and urea. In this chapter, we propose an overview of the metabolic requirement for Mφs function with an emphasis on the differences between human and murine Mφs.

Keywords: glucose, Krebs cycle metabolites, phagocytosis, inflammation, macrophage polarization, metabolic plasticity

1. Introduction

Macrophages (Mφ) are myeloid cells of innate immunity present in most tissues which control crucial physiological processes such as antimicrobial and inflammatory responses as well as tissue homeostasis and repair. Tissue-resident Mφs (TRMs) exhibit tissue-specific functions and maintain tissue homeostasis [1, 2]. For example, alveolar Mφs are located in alveoli and eliminate debris, surfactant and apoptotic cells while osteoclasts are located in the bone where they orchestrate bone remodeling. During infection or inflammation, when TRMs are overwhelmed, blood monocytes are recruited and differentiate locally into Mφ (hereafter called recruited Mφ) [3] (**Figure 1a**). Murine embryos with defects in Mφs development are not viable in both human and mice, genetic defects in Mφ lead to several pathologies including

IntechOpen

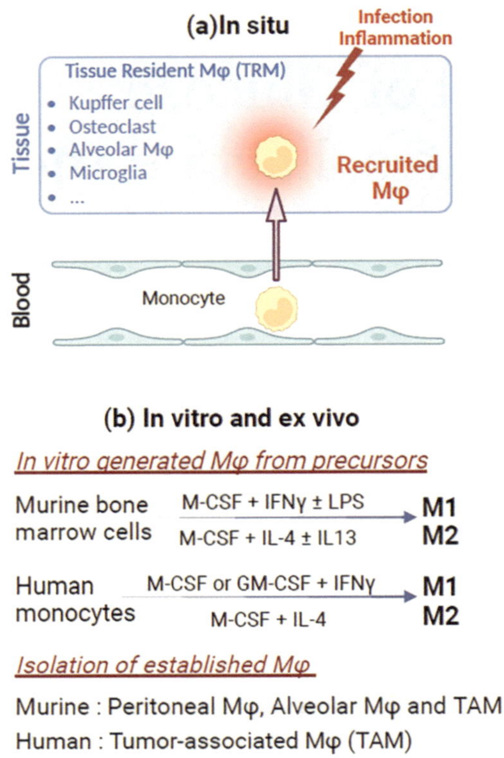

Figure 1.
A simplified view of Mφ subsets. (a) In situ Mφ includes TRM and newly recruited Mφ. (b) Human and murine Mφ subsets commonly used for in vitro and ex vivo assays.

neurodevelopmental defects, bone deformities, multiorgan dysfunctions [4] which emphasize the importance of these immune cells.

Mφs are long-lived cells that continuously sense their environment (pH, O2, cytokines, metabolites) and adapt their functions to tissue demands, a process called functional plasticity [3, 5, 6]. Mφs acquire proinflammatory, trophic or immunoregulatory properties. Based on the classification of CD4+ T lymphocytes as Th1 vs. Th2, a classification of Mφs differentiated in vitro from myeloid precursors has been proposed. It opposed proinflammatory Mφs called M1 with reparative and immunoregulatory Mφs called M2 [7].

The M1/M2 classification is imperfect because it is reductive since these two states represent the ends of a functional polarization continuum [8] exemplified by the multiple intermediary's phenotypes that have been observed [9–17]. Although imperfect, the classification based on M1 and M2 Mφs remains commonly used (**Figure 1b**) [18]. Since the phenotypic and metabolic characteristics of human and murine macrophages (Mφs) differ on many points, a parallel analysis of the two models is required, and results obtained from one model should not be transposed to the other.

In mice, both tissue-resident Mφs and bone marrow-derived Mφs (BMDM) are studied [19]. In human, monocytes-derived Mφs are easily generated in vitro while obtaining access to tissue-resident Mφs is obviously limited [20]. Macrophages (Mφs) rely on three growth factors for their differentiation and survival: M-CSF and IL-34 [21] which signal through their receptor CD115, and GM-CSF, an inflammatory cytokine produced at sites of inflammation that signals through CD116 [22]. It should be noted that in mice, bone marrow precursors exposed to GM-CSF differentiate into both dendritic cells and Mφs in vitro [23] while M-CSF induces the generation of a more homogeneous population of Mφs after a 7-days differentiation protocol [24]. Multiple factors polarize Mφs: Interferon-γ (IFN-γ), interleukin-1β (IL-1β), lipopolysaccharide (LPS) trigger the generation of murine and human M1 Mφs that produce IL-12 and inflammatory cytokines (including TNFα, IL-1β, IL-6) but are weak producer of IL-10 [8]. M2 Mφs are generated in the presence of the polarizing cytokines IL-10, IL-4 and IL-13 and they produce growth factors, immunosuppressive cytokines including IL-10, thereby promoting resolution of inflammation and tissue repair [25]. Of note, human Mφs present in inflammatory and tumor sites usually exhibit a mixed M1/M2 phenotype [9–17, 26]. An important mechanism by which Mφs polarize toward pro-(M1) and anti-inflammatory (M2) phenotypes is via changes in metabolism, also called metabolic reprogramming, to sustain the cell's function [27]. Distinct phenotypes of Mφs are associated with the pathophysiology of different disorders: M1 cells are involved in the inflammatory processes associated with diabetes and autoimmune diseases while M2 cells contribute to tumor growth and fibrosis [28].

This issue is complicated by variations between species. Murine and human Mφs differ in the way they are generated in vitro and in their phenotypes [8, 19, 29]. Murine Mφs are usually generated from bone marrow cells while human Mφs from monocytes [19]. Importantly, human inflammatory Mφ can be generated with GM-CSF while GM-CSF switches human myeloid precursor to murine DC [23]. Moreover, human Mφs need LPS activation to reveal their phenotype while for murine Mφs, LPS is a polarizing factor. Finally, in the murine in vitro model, Mφs from distinct strains do not respond equivalently to PRR activation [29] as some murine strains (e.g., C57BL/6) are more prone to inflammation compared to others (BALB/c). Differences between metabolism have been also highlighted [30]. Murine M1 cells polarization enhanced glycolysis, pentose phosphate pathway and displays a broken tricarboxylic acid cycle (TCA), and this permits M1 polarized Mφs to rapidly trigger microbicide activity and to cope with a hypoxic tissue microenvironment, thus meeting their energy needs [31, 32]. In human Mφs, M1 glycolytic Mφs do not harbor a broken Krebs cycle (personal data). M2 cells uptake fatty acids to fuel OXPHOS over glycolysis, contributing to tissue remodeling, repair and wound healing [25, 32, 33]. Another example of the metabolic differences between human and mice is observed regarding nitric oxide. Murine proinflammatory Mφs activated by PRR secrete nitric oxide which is toxic for bacteria and intracellular parasites. They express an inducible form of nitric oxide synthase named iNOS that, once induced, is stable for several hours, thus enabling the production of NO at the micromolar range [34]. In contrast, human Mφs do not secrete NO as the transcription of Nos2, the gene encoding iNOS, is methylated and thus limited [35].

2. Overview of metabolic pathways and technical analysis

The aim of cellular metabolism is to generate ATP, NADPH and FADH2 molecules and, in several immune cells including Mφs, metabolic pathways also support the acquisition of functional phenotypes [36]. In addition to their involvement in energy production and redox regulation, some metabolites are involved in chromatin remodeling and thus directly contribute to the regulation of gene expression (**Figure 2**) [37, 38]. α-Ketoglutarate (α-KG), succinate and fumarate regulate the activities of enzymes involved in histone methylation and DNA methylation [37].

Glycolysis is the metabolic pathway that relies on glucose utilization, leading to the formation of pyruvate, a 3-carbon entity and ATP. At the organism level, glucose homeostasis is tightly regulated and for most tissues is the major pathway in producing ATP [39]. Glycolysis generates ATP faster than mitochondrial oxidative phosphorylation and is thus often a primary metabolic fuel. Glucose metabolism involves multiple interconnected pathways including glycolysis, the pentose phosphate pathway (PPP), glycogenesis, gluconeogenesis and glycogenolysis [40]. Within the cells, free glucose is immediately phosphorylated by hexokinase producing glucose-6-phosphate (G6P), thereby preventing its diffusion out of the cell [41]. G6P is at a crossroads of several metabolic pathways (**Figure 2**). G6P can be processed in glycolysis that drives the generation of 2 molecules of pyruvate, 2 molecules of ATP and antioxidant power via NADPH. In Mφs, NADPH is required for NADPH oxidase (NOX), a key player in pathogen defense [40]. Pyruvate can be metabolized by lactate dehydrogenase (LDH), leading to the formation of lactate, which is exported out of the cell via monocarboxylate transporters (MCT) along with a proton, enabling the reoxidation of NADH to NAD+. If G6P is oxidized by glucose 6-phosphate dehydrogenase (G6PD), it enters the PPP. The conversion of G6P to glucose 1-phosphate (G1P) by phosphoglucomutase (PGM) supports glycogen synthesis (glycogenesis), a critical intracellular reservoir of carbons. In the liver, glycogen can also be synthesized by non-carbohydrate precursors such as lactate (transported from peripheral tissues) and glycerol (released from lipolysis), a metabolic process called gluconeogenesis, which is responsible for the generation of glucose as a fuel for other tissues. We have recently observed that some human M1 cells are capable of gluconeogenesis (unpublished results). Synthesized glycogen is stored in the cytoplasm or enters glycogenolysis for degradation (glycogenolysis), eliciting G6P (**Figure 3**) [42].

The pyruvate produced from glycolysis can also be imported into the mitochondria matrix, converted to acetyl-CoA by pyruvate dehydrogenase complex, and incorporated into the TCA cycle (also named Krebs cycle) in conjunction with oxaloacetate. This cycle that mediates the catabolism of acetyl-CoA from the oxidative decarboxylation of pyruvate is linked to the electron transport chain (ETC), a set of multi-protein complexes (complexes 1–4) located in the mitochondrial inner membrane. The respiratory chain creates a proton gradient across the mitochondrial membrane that enables ATP synthase (complex V) to function, resulting in the generation of 38 ATP, whereas glycolysis alone produces 2 ATP. O2 is the terminal electron acceptor of the respiratory chain, so its function is impaired under hypoxia. The Krebs cycle can also be supplied by fatty acids and amino acids including glutamine or ketone bodies (**Figure 2**).

To assess Mφ metabolism, multiple techniques are available that do not overlap as they gave different information regarding the pathways and nutrients used [43]. First of all, the analysis of transcripts, notably by single-cell technologies, assesses the expression of enzymes or transcription factors involved in energy production [43]. Regarding glycolysis, enzymatic assays can be used to assess the activity of an enzyme (e.g., LDH) or to quantify in cell culture supernatant glucose and lactate concentrations. Enzymatic activities have also been realized on tissue, thus highlighting metabolic networks in situ [44]. The gold standard to analyze both glycolysis and OXPHOS required an extracellular flux analyzer that generated data in real time (for example, Seahorse® technology by Agilent). Glycolytic flux is assessed by the acidification of cell culture supernatant as lactate export is accompanied with the export of a proton (ECAR, extracellular acidification rate) and OXPHOS is monitored by the consumption of O2 in cell culture. Flow cytometry can also be used to assess the expression of

DOI: http://dx.doi.org/10.5772/intechopen.1005523

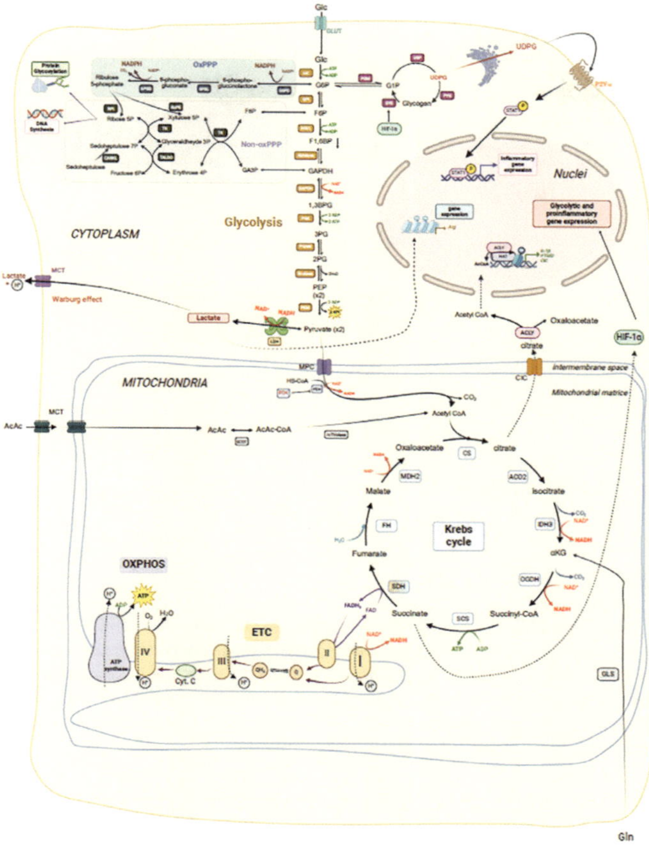

Figure 2.

Interconnection between metabolic pathways and macrophage's phenotype and function. Macrophages rely on multiple metabolic pathways to produce energy and cofactors in order to survive and to perform their key functions (efferocytosis, cytokine production). As a central metabolite, G6P can be channeled in different directions: being oxidized to pyruvate along glycolysis, to ribose-5 phosphate (R5P) pr xululose-5P (X5P) via pentose phosphate pathway (PPP), or to glycogen via glucose-1P (G1P). Pyruvate has two fates in macrophages: it can be metabolized by lactate dehydrogenase (LDH) generating lactate which is exported out of the cell with a proton. Pyruvate can be transported into the mitochondria via the mitochondrial pyruvate carrier and then be metabolized into acetyl-CoA. This initiates the tricarboxylic acid cycle or Krebs cycle. A complete cycle generates three NADH and one FADH2 cofactors, which transfer their electrons to the respiratory chain that is localized in the intermembrane space of the mitochondria. In the respiratory chain, electrons are transferred between the four multi-protein complexes (complexes I, II, III and IV), and the complexes I, III and IV pump protons from the matrix across the inner mitochondrial membrane. A proton gradient is then established on which depends ATP synthase (also named complex V) to produce ATP from ADP, a process designated as oxidative phosphorylation. PPP generates abundant NADPH and R5P, respectively, to ensure high levels of reduced glutathione for inflammatory macrophage survival as well as DNA synthesis and protein glycosylation. Glycogen metabolism also activates UDPG/P2Y14 signaling pathway to upregulate the inflammatory gene expression via STAT1activation. Multiple metabolites of the TCA (citrate, acetyl-CoA, succinate) and lactate participate in the regulation of gene expression. HK, hexokinase; GPI, phosphoglucose isomerase; PFK, phosphofructokinase; GAPDH, glyceraldehyde 3-phosphate dehydrogenase; PGK, phosphoglycerate kinase; PGAM, phosphoglycerate mutase; PKM, pyruvate kinase; LDH, lactate dehydrogenase; G6PD, glucose-6-phosphate dehydrogenase; 6PGL, 6-phosphogluconolactonase; 6PGD, 6-phosphogluconate dehydrogenase; PGM1, phosphoglucomutase; GYS, glycogen synthase; UGP, UDP-glucose pyrophosphorylase; UDPG, UDP-glucose; PDH, pyruvate dehydrogenase; CIC, mitochondrial citrate carrier; SCOT, succinyl-CoA:3-ketoacid coenzyme A transferase; PDH, pyruvate dehydrogenase; PDK, pyruvate dehydrogenase kinase; CS, citrate synthase; ACO2, aconitase 2; IDH3, isocitrate dehydrogenase 3; OGHD, 2-oxoglutarate dehydrogenase; SCS, succinyl-coenzyme A synthetase; SDH, succinate dehydrogenase; FH, fumarate hydratase; MDH2, malate dehydrogenase 2; ACLY, ATP-citrate lyase; HAT, histone acetyl transferase; STAT, signal transducers and activators of transcription; P2Y14, purinergic 14 receptor; Cyt C, cytochrome c; PE, ribulose-phosphate 3-epimerase; RPI, ribose-5-phosphate isomerase; FBPase, fructose 1,6-bisphophatase; ALDO, fructose-bisphosphate aldolase.

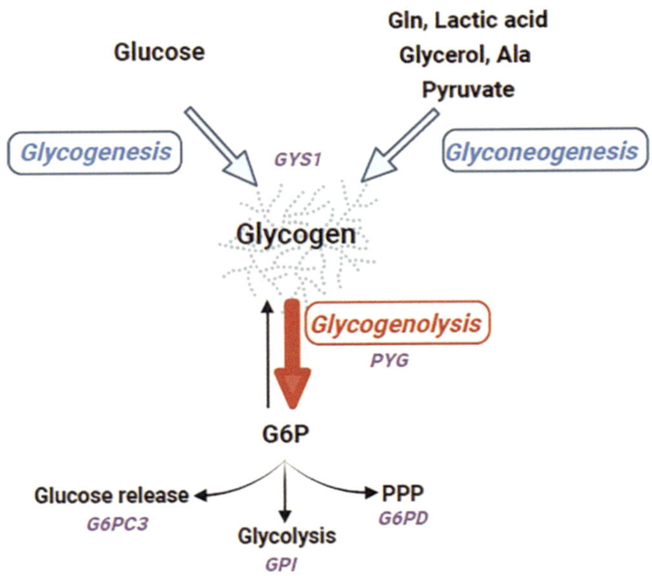

Figure 3.
Simplified view of glycogen metabolism. Glycogen can be synthesized from Glc (glycogenesis) or from non-carbohydrate substrates (glyconeogenesis). Glycogen degradation (glycogenolysis) gives rise to glucose-6-phosphate (G6P) which supplies three different pathways: glucose release, glycolysis or the pentose phosphate pathway. The enzymes mentioned in the proposal are in purple. Ala, alanine; Gln, glutamine; G6P, glucose-6 phosphate; GYS, glycogen synthase; PYG, glycogen phosphorylase; G6PC3, glucose-6 phosphatase catalytic subunit 3; GPI, phosphoglucose isomerase; G6PD, glucose 6-phosphate dehydrogenase.

metabolism-related protein expression or to assess the uptake of probes that reflect nutrient uptake or mitochondrial mass for example [45]. Metabolites from both glycolysis and OXHOS can be measured by liquid or gas chromatography-mass spectrometry [43], eventually with heavy isotope-labeled nutrients (e.g., stable isotope 13C-labeled glucose) to do isotope tracing [46].

3. Glucose metabolism

3.1 Glucose metabolism in proinflammatory Mφs

The first studies demonstrating the need for Mφs to use glycolysis date back to the 1960s. The increased use of the glycolysis pathway by Mφs for phagocytosis or cytokine production in a proinflammatory context has been demonstrated both in vitro and in vivo [47–49]. The M1 cell polarization is associated with increased glycolytic activity, compared to IL-4-exposed Mφs (M2 cells) [31, 50]. Moreover, GM-CSF (that induces inflammatory Mφs) increases human Mφ glycolytic activity more than M-CSF, while M-CSF increases OXPHOS utilization more than GM-CSF [33]. The cell surface expression of the glucose transporter GLUT1 (encoded by slc2a1) is upregulated in M1 inflammatory cells and is associated with increased glycolysis [51] and ROS production [52, 53]. Regarding Mφ stimulation, LPS stabilizes the transcription factor HIF1a [54] and upregulates the expression of several glycolysis enzymes (**Figure 2**) [55, 56]. Accordingly, LPS-stimulated monocytes harbor an increased ECAR as monitored by Seahorse analysis, thus indicating an upregulation of glycolytic metabolism [57].

Metabolic shifts are associated with profound transcriptional regulation of gene expression, and several studies have identified different glycolytic enzymes as being crucial to Mφ biology. Hexokinase acts as a glucose sensor and phosphorylates glucose for subsequent utilization (**Figure 2**). The isoform 2 of hexokinase behaves as a pattern recognition receptor as it binds N-acetylglucosamine, leading to NLRP3 inflammasome activation [58, 59], thus linking innate immunity to glycolysis.

The first rate-limiting enzyme in glycolysis is 6-phosphofructo-2-kinase/fructose-2,6-bisphosphatase (PFK-2/FBPase, PFK), which catalyzes the conversion of fructose-6-phosphate to fructose-2,6-bisphosphate, a rate-limiting step in glycolysis [60]. Mφ activation induces a switch in the expression of PFKFB2 isoform, from the liver type-PFK2 (L-PFKFB 2) to the more active ubiquitous PFK2 (u-PFKFB2) isoenzymes through HIF-1α independent mechanism [31]. This enzyme is a potent driver of glycolysis because its overwhelming activity leads to the production of fructose-2,6-biphosphate, which activates PFKFB1 [61, 62]. The isozymes encoded by Pfkfb3 and Pfkfb4 are implicated in Mφ glycolysis at transcriptional levels upon stimulation with IFN-γ and LPS, and silencing Pfkfb3 has been shown to lower glycolysis in inflammatory Mφs [63–65]. Recently, Chen and colleagues [65] have shown that PFKFB3-mediated glycolysis promotes IFN-γ-induced M1 polarization through the JAK2/STAT1 signaling pathway [65].

GAPDH catalyzes the conversion of glyceraldehyde-3-phosphate into D-glycerate 1,3-bisphosphate (**Figure 2**). When glycolysis activity is low, GAPDH binds to TNF-α mRNA and inhibits its transcription, thus decreasing its translation [66]. This is specially the case in endotoxin tolerant monocytes that have been previously exposed to LPS [66]. The RNA-binding property of GAPDH is decreased by its malonylation [67], which consists in the addition of a malonyl-CoA group which is synthetized in the cytosol from acetyl-CoA by acetyl-CoA carboxylase (ACC). GAPDH capacity to behave as a transcriptional repressor is inversely proportional to its activity in glycolysis.

PRR-mediated Mφ activation drives inflammation that is dependent on the glycolytic pathway. This could be explained by the fact that glycolysis is faster than OXPHOS if substrates are available [68]. The production of lactate from glycolysis-derived pyruvate enables the regeneration of NAD+ in cell cytosol. In addition, pyruvate kinase M2 (PKM2), an enzyme from the glycolysis that converts phosphoenol pyruvate (PEP) into pyruvate, is dimerized in LPS-treated Mφs and gets acetylated [69], thus slowing glycolysis and allowing flux of glycolysis intermediates into biosynthetic pathways [70]. PKM2 is a key molecular determinant in the enhancement of proinflammatory response of Mφs, through the HIF-1α-dependent mechanism, leading to IL-1β induction by directly binding to its promoter [70, 71]. Recently, Dong and colleagues have shown that increased production of IL-1β by glycolysis was mediated through enhanced H3K9 acetylation in activated murine M1 cells [72]. The acetylation level increased resulting in the opening of IL-1β gene binding chromatin structures leading to HIF1α/PKM2 fixation [72]. Two of the most important signaling pathways for M1 cell activation, NF-κB and Akt/mTOR, converge to stabilize HIF-1α, which increases the expression of several glycolytic genes [73]. In addition to the modulation of inflammatory response, PKM2 seems to be responsible for increased expression of PD-L1 in TAM from hepatocellular carcinoma [74]; PKM2 binds to hypoxia response elements in Mφs and dendritic cells and, in combination with HIF1α, upregulate PD-L1 transcription [75]. In addition to a crucial role in proinflammatory activation, glycolysis also supports pyroptosis [76] in activated Mφs.

Another key feature of the metabolic reprogramming of M1 phenotype upon activation is the upregulation of the PPP (**Figure 2**). G6P from glycolysis supplies the PPP, resulting in the production of two major products: nicotinamide adenine dinucleotide phosphate (NADPH), that is crucial for preventing ROS production, and ribose-5-phosphate, essential for nucleic acid synthesis [77]. The glucose 6 phosphate dehydrogenase (G6PD) is the first and rate-limiting enzyme of the PPP [40, 77, 78]. Overexpression of G6PD in murine Mφ cell line enhanced the activation of NF-κB and p38-MAPK signaling pathways and potentiated the expression of inflammatory cytokines (such as IL-6, IL-1β, MCP-1 and TNF-α) as well as ROS production [79]. Moreover, Haschemi and colleagues have identified by kinase screening, CARKL, as a novel regulator of human and murine Mφ activation [80]. CARKL catalyzes the formation of sedoheptulose (S7P), an intermediate of the PPP, whose expression rapidly decreased upon M1-polarized Mφ activation. Inflammatory cytokines and intracellular superoxide production rates were blunted upon CARKL overexpression, an effect mediated by sustained S7P production, suggesting that CARKL downregulation is critical for proper M1 polarization [80].

In addition to glycolysis and PPP, Mφs utilize other glucose-related metabolic pathways to drive their inflammatory phenotype. Recently, the role of glycogen metabolism on metabolic reprogramming has become a recognized feature of some myeloid cells under stress conditions such as hypoxia and glucose deprivation [61, 81–83]. Glycogen present an important reservoir form of glucose in cells which is essential for energy supply and glucose homeostasis [84]. Glycogen can be generated from glucose (direct pathway, **Figure 3**) or by using non-carbohydrate substrates, a process called gluconeogenesis that occurs mainly in the liver (indirect pathway) [42]. Glycogen metabolism is regulated by glycogen synthesis (glycogenesis) and degradation (glycogenolysis) requiring a coordination action of two key enzymes, glycogen synthesis (GYS) and glycogen phosphorylase (PYG), respectively. Glycogenolysis-derived G6P can fuel different metabolic pathways (**Figure 3**). Two studies have revealed a direct association of glycogen metabolism and inflammation in murine Mφs. Ma et al. [81] have reported that, unlike IL-4 stimulation, IFNy/LPS treatment stimulates glycogenesis and glycogenolysis in murine M1 Mφs, by upregulating the enzymes involved in glycogen metabolism (including GYS1, PGM1, UGP2 and PYG). The study demonstrated that glycogen metabolism has a central function in controlling inflammatory murine Mφs by two related mechanisms: (i) M1 Mφ uses G6P-derived glycogenolysis which is channeled through the PPP to produce large amounts of NADPH required for inflammatory Mφ survival, (ii) UDPG-derived glycogenesis binds to P2Y14 receptors to induce inflammatory Mφs, and cytokines such as TNF, IL-6 Il-1b were subsequently upregulated in an autocrine fashion via UDPG/P2Y14/STAT1 signaling transduction [81]. Recently Qian et al. [85] studied the importance of UDPG/P2Y14 signaling pathway in a model of inflammation. The authors showed that HIF-1α directly regulates glycogen synthase 1 (GYS1), thus promoting glycogen synthesis. Knock-down of HIF-1α gene interfered with GYS1 both at the mRNA and protein level, suggesting that GYS1 is a downstream target gene of HIF1a. Moreover, LPS stimulation of murine and human M1 Mφs increases UGPG and P2Y14 secretion, while HIF-1α stabilizer (MK8617) treatment exerts an anti-inflammatory effect by inhibiting UDPG and P2Y14 production, leading to the release of inflammatory mediators in M1 Mφs. This study proposed a novel specific regulatory mechanism to prevent inflammation by which MK8617 prevents intracellular HIF-1α degradation through GYS1/UDPG/P2Y14 pathway, thereby attenuating M1 Mφ inflammation (**Figure 2**) [85].

The mechanisms of inflammatory metabolic reprogramming have mostly been studied using LPS treatment in vitro or in vivo [10, 86–89]. Recently, Murugina et al. [90] have shown that metabolic reprogramming from oxidative phosphorylation to aerobic glycolysis in human monocyte-derived Mφs and in mouse peritoneal Mφs was also induced by agonists of NOD1 and NOD2 receptors similar to TLR4 agonist lipopolysaccharide. But the rewiring of metabolism toward glycolysis is not strictly conserved for all PRR as TLR2 ligation in monocytes activated bot glycolysis and OXHPOS, a requirement for phagocytic activity and cytokine production [57].

3.2 Glucose-related metabolism in M2 Mφs

Prototypic or alternative M2 cells are generated in the presence of M-CSF, IL-4 or IL-13, and harbor a trophic/wound healing and immunoregulatory phenotype [22]. In contrast to murine M1 cells, alternatively activated M2 cells possess a fully intact TCA cycle and obtain much of their energy from fatty acid oxidation (FAO) and oxidative metabolism, to execute cellular functions [91]. Furthermore, aerobic and anaerobic glucose metabolism also fuel phagocytosis, which is an energy-demanding process and a key property of M2-polarized Mφs [25]; of note human M1 cells (GM-CSF + IFNγ) do not exhibit phagocytic properties.

Lactate is a signaling metabolite that affects both the phenotype and metabolism of Mφs. Lactic acid (LA), produced by glycolysis from pyruvate by LDH, accumulates in the microenvironment in case of injury, bacterial infection or tumors [92]. In a landmark study in 2014, Ruslan Medzitov and collaborators identified LA as a local factor driving murine M2 cell polarization [93]. Lactate is imported by MCT of the Scl16a family [94] with a proton. Lactate-mediated stabilization of HIF1α was required to increase several M2-specific genes including Arg1 and Vegf (**Figure 2**). Lactate was oxidized by murine tumor-associated Mφs (TAM) as highlighted in tracing experiments.

We and others have shown that LA triggers inflammatory gene expression in human monocytes [95] and in monocytes-derived Mφs [17, 96]. More precisely, human Mφs generated in the presence of GM-CSF and lactic acid acquired a mixed profile associating M2 and M1 phenotype. Lactic acid driven M2 phenotype included CD163 membrane expression, growth factors secretion and the expression of several M-CSF dependent genes [17]. We identified HIF1α as a factor that unlocked the consumption of M-CSF, while increasing the proinflammatory secretory profile (IL-1b, IL-6, TNF-a). Lactate internalization by Mφs was necessary for the acquisition of the phenotype and our study contributed to explain how human Mφs can harbor both proinflammatory and trophic properties. It has been recently published that lactate induces histone lactylation [97]. In addition to its role once internalized in the cell, lactate is a ligand for the protein-coupled receptor (GPCR) 132 whose activation triggers chemokine synthesis by TAM [74].

It has been demonstrated several years later in murine Mφs that pyruvate generated from glucose or lactate is taken up in the mitochondria and incorporated in TCA cycle. A portion of citrate is imported outside the mitochondria and cleaved by ACLY into acetyl-coenzyme A (acetyl-CoA), thus regulating histone acetylation on M2-specific promoters [98]. The function of ACLY in the regulation of the M2 phenotype of murine Mφs has also been studied in the context of LPS stimulation by Shi et al. [99]. The authors realized transposase-accessible chromatin with high-throughput sequencing (ATAC-seq) and identified numerous genomic sequences whose accessibility was reduced by LA, including proinflammatory genes coding for IL-1β and TNF-α. However, these results are not fully transposable to human Mφs, whose biology differs from murine Mφs notably regarding the phenotype as discussed previously [19, 96].

Following M2 polarization, the Pfkb1 gene is expressed instead of Pfkb3, resulting in higher levels of the liver isoform of PFKB2 and lower levels of fructose-2,6-biphosphate [31]. The downregulation of the glycolytic pathway is compensated with a massive augmentation of an oxidative metabolic program, ranging from fatty acid uptake and oxidation to oxidative phosphorylation and mitochondrial respiration. The molecular pathway that directly links mitochondrial oxidative metabolism to the anti-inflammatory program is upregulated by STAT6-PGC-1 following IL-4 activation [100]. Active STAT6 induces the coactivator protein peroxisome proliferator-activated receptor (PPAR) gamma-coactivator 1 (PGC-1), which in turn induces mitochondrial function to promote murine M2 cell polarization [101, 102]. Indeed, transgenic expression of PGC-1 primes Mφs for alternative activation and strongly inhibits inflammatory cytokine production, whereas inhibition of oxidative metabolism or RNAi-mediated knock-down of PGC-1 attenuates this immune response [103, 104]. Thus, PGC is considered as the key player responsible for the metabolic switch in M2 Mφs.

Even though they consume glucose modestly, human or/and murine M2 cells also rely on glycolysis to maintain their phenotype [30, 105, 106]. Glucose oxidation, but not that of fatty acids, plays a critical role in the early differentiation of M2 Mφs via pyruvate dehydrogenase kinase 1 (PDK1). PDK1 knock-down remarkably enhanced the expression of M2 markers and augmented mitochondrial oxidative phosphorylation at the early time point in IL-4-stimulated Mφs. This study suggests that PDK1 regulates M2 Mφ differentiation via controlling glucose oxidation during the early differentiation of M2 Mφs [107]. Moreover, it has been shown that glucose uptake increases over time in Mφs activated by IL-4 [105]. The implied mechanistic link between glycolysis and M2 Mφ activation is the generation of pyruvate by glycolysis, which then feeds into the TCA cycle to promote Ac-CoA synthesis and histone acetylation by ACLY enzyme [105] or mitochondrial OXPHOS [106]. Efferocytosis is one of Mφ's key functions as it prevents leakage of intracellular contents into tissue, its malfunction driving pathologies including atherosclerosis [60]. Interestingly, phagocytosis of dead cells by Mφs induces an early and transient increase in glycolysis, with glycolysis rate returning to basal activity after 24 h [59]. This metabolic activity is therefore quite distinct from the increase in glycolysis as part of the inflammatory response, whose action is prolonged over time. It has been shown that this transient glycolysis allows the expression of membrane receptors and also activates one of the pH-sensitive receptors, GPR132, which augments Myc expression and thus drives murine Mφ proliferation [61]. In murine Mφs, the Akt-mTORC1 pathway is responsible for increasing glucose consumption in M2 Mφs following IL-4 stimulation. Thus, increasing ACLY enzymatic activity and histone acetylation and, subsequently, M2 gene induction (including chemokine production and gene regulating cellular proliferation) [105]. In human Mφs, although ACLY inhibition attenuated IL-4-induced gene expression, it failed to alter cellular Acetyl-CoA levels and histone acetylation, suggesting that IL-4-induced gene expression occurred independently of ACLY [108]. Those studies noticed considerable differences in metabolic requirements of human vs. murine Mφs toward IL-4-induced polarization. Finally, polarization of Mφs in M2 phenotype induced CARKL upregulation, enhancing the non-oxidative steps of PPP, leading to ribose-5P production, necessary for nucleotide and UDP-GlcNAC synthesis (**Figure 2**) [80]. UDP-GlcNAC is required for N-glycosylation of different cell surface proteins (i.e., CD206) abundantly expressed in M2 Mφs [10].

4. Krebs cycle and respiratory metabolism

4.1 Oxidative metabolism in inflammatory Mφs

As discussed previously, glycolysis is upregulated in M1 cells in murine M1 cells, the TCA cycle is truncated after the generation of citrate and succinate with accumulation of TCA cycle intermediaries, such as α-ketoglutarate and fumarate. However, it is important to note that the data on TCA cycle disruption in M1 Mφs come from murine Mφs, and a body of evidence suggests that the metabolism of human and murine Mφs differs fundamentally [30, 33].

Succinate stabilizes HIF1α, thus increasing Il-1b transcription (**Figure 2**). Moreover, the oxidation of succinate in inflammatory Mφs by the succinate dehydrogenase enzyme (SDH) produces ROS [109], required for the acquisition of inflammatory phenotype [110]. SDH belongs to the electron transfer chain, whose assembly dictates Mφ's inflammatory response [111].

In addition to its plethora of regulatory roles in cell metabolism, citrate sustains inflammatory Mφ response. LPS stimulation of murine M1 cells induces a downregulation of isocitrate dehydrogenase (IDH), which catalyzes the conversion of citrate to isocitrate [10], and upregulation of CIC [112], leading to citrate accumulation and its exportation from the mitochondria to cytosol, which is essential for NO, ROS and prostaglandin production [113, 114]. Pharmacological or genetic targeting of CIC in human Mφs decreases these inflammatory mediators [112]. ATP citrate lyase (ACLY) catalyzes the conversion of cytosolic citrate to acetyl-CoA and plays a critical role in supporting the inflammatory response through its regulation of many inflammatory gene expressions [115, 116]. In activated human Mφs, ACLY activates NF-κB acetylation, enhancing the transcription of several inflammatory genes such as IL-1β and PTGS2, as well as the mitochondrial citrate carrier (CIC) (**Figure 2**) [117]. These studies demonstrate how Mφ metabolism is not simply needed for providing the energy but can play a pivotal role at transcriptional regulation of the immune response.

In TLR-stimulated murine M1 Mφs, glycolysis upregulation also leads to an upregulation of glutamine consumption, and to an increase of succinate levels [56] explained by glutamine-dependent anaplerosis or the GABA shunt. Although some discrepancy exists in the literature [10], glutamine also contributes to (murine) M1 cell polarization.

Strategies aimed at switching TAM (M1/M2) into antitumor inflammatory Mφs are in demand in oncology as TAMs are the major infiltrate in solid tumors and they harbor multiple protumor properties [118]. CD40 is highly expressed by Mφs and TAM and an agonistic anti-CD40-antibody reverts TAM phenotype into antitumor cells, improves antitumor response and mice survival [119]. On the metabolic level, we would expect this reversion to be associated with a transition from an oxidative metabolism into a more glycolytic metabolism. Intriguingly, agonistic CD40-antibody hugely increases mitochondrial activity. In addition, in Cpt1-deficient Mφs, the phenotypic reversion was inhibited showing that FAO was unexpectedly associated with M2 to M1 phenotype switch [120]. Moreover, glutamine degradation enabled the production of pyruvate that was metabolized to lactate and this process was required for the maintenance of NAD+/NADH ratio and OXPHOS activity. Finally, the upregulation of inflammatory mediators was mediated by epigenetic regulation that required FAO-derived acetyl-CoA [120]. Thus, phenotypic reversion of murine TAM into M1 cells appears supported by mitochondrial metabolism, not glycolysis.

A similar phenomenon was observed in murine Mφs treated with oxidized lipids and LPS that acquired a hyperinflammatory phenotype [121]. While LPS augmented glycolysis as previously shown, oxidized lipids increased glutamine-mediated oxidative metabolism. This led to the export of citrate generated in the TCA cycle from the mitochondria to the cytoplasm where it was converted into oxaloacetate which stabilized HIF1a, as previously reported [122] and thus increasing IL-1b production.

4.2 Oxidative metabolism in M2-alternative activated Mφs

Even though glycolysis is also functioning in M2 cells, M2 polarization has been associated with mitochondrial oxidative metabolism since 2006 [103]. It was observed that murine Mφs exposed to IL-4 exhibited an upregulation of the mRNA expression of acyl-CoA dehydrogenases and enoyl-CoA hydratases, two enzymes involved in mitochondrial FAO [103]. They also identified PGC-1β as an important coactivator for the M2 phenotype. The knock-down of PGC1β, or the use of an inhibitor of ETC, embedded M2 polarization and led to an inflammatory phenotype, even in the presence of Il-4.

Several years later, triacylglycerol was identified as the main FA supporting the acquisition of M2 properties in IL-4-generated murine Mφs. The role of the scavenger receptor CD36, which enables FA internalization and lipolysis by lysosomal acid lipase (LAL), thus promoting TCA utilization in both murine and human M2 cells, was highlighted [123]. CD36 expression is now considered as an M2 marker for both murine and human Mφs [124]. Of note, inhibition of FAO with etomoxir might exert a confounder effect. Depending on its concentrations, etomoxir might lead to the generation of etomoxiryl-CoA that depletes CoA and thus disturbs cellular CoA metabolism [125]. Moreover, the role of FAO regarding human Mφ polarization is debated [112]. The importance of FAO for murine M2-like polarization has been described by multiple labs [103, 126] and multiple substrates fueling FAO permit the acquisition of the M2 phenotype including glycolysis-derived pyruvate [126]. More generally, mitochondrial fitness appears as a key event for murine M2 polarization [107].

Glutamine, a non-essential amino acid, is produced from glutamate and NH3 by glutamine synthetase and is converted by glutaminase into glutamate, thus liberating NH4. It is a substrate for Mφs and lymphocytes [47]. Glutamine fuels TCA by a branching to 2-oxoglutarate [127]. Glutaminolysis is required for proper efferocytosis in vitro and in vivo, as evidenced by LysM-Cre × Gls1fl/fl knock-out mice that do not phagocytose apoptotic cells correctly [128]. When realizing efferocytosis, IL-4-Mφ's upregulation of glutamine uptake increases the formation of glutamate through Gls1-mediated transamination. Glutamate is then metabolized into TCA, thus providing energy and redox buffering for M2 murine Mφs. Reinforcing its importance for M2-dependent polarization, the inhibition of Kir2.1, a potassium channel that senses extracellular K+ concentrations, embedded glutamine uptake by TAM and was therefore accompanied by their polarization into antitumor M1 Mφs [129]. The metabolization of glutamine, a requirement for the acquisition of IL-4-dependent markers, permits the increase of intracellular a-KG, a Krebs cycle intermediary that is also a co-stimulator factor for Jmjd3, a demethylase that decreases the trimethylation of histone H3 K27 [130] on the promoters of genes encoding for M2-like markers including Arg1 and Mrc1. Glutamine induces M2 cell polarization through the glutamine-UDP-N-acetylglucosamine pathway [10, 130].

Other mitochondrial substrates can be used by Mφs, for example, the ketone body acetoacetate (AcAc) (**Figure 2**). Two ketone bodies are potent energetic substrates for cells to produce ATP [131], AcAc and D-β-hydroxybutyrate (D-βOHB) but only AcAc can be metabolized by murine and human Mφs due to the absence of expression of the mitochondrial enzyme D-βOHB dehydrogenase (BDH1) [132, 133]. AcAc is produced by hepatocytes and is shuttled in Kupffer cells, the resident Mφs of the liver. The importance of this metabolic connection is observed in Mφs which do not express succinyl-CoA:3-oxoacid-CoA transferase (SCOT, encoded by oxct1). This deletion resulted in an increase of fibrosis in mice exposed to high-fat diet, AcAc is thus a key metabolite to preserve Kupffer cell function [132] and AcAc metabolization imprints Mφ's phenotype. We recently demonstrated that the oxidation of AcAc alleviates the capacity of human Mφs to survive to lactic acidosis [133]. Human Mφs exposed to lactic acidosis harbor depolarized mitochondria, decrease transiently their mitochondrial mass through mitophagy and stop consuming nutrients. AcAc constitutes an alternative fuel that prevents mitochondrial integrity and nutrient consumption. We also identified AcAc as a metabolite that increases VEGF secretion by both murine and human Mφs (unpublished personal data).

In addition to their action as substrates, KB are seen as signaling molecules that activate GPCR [134]. Moreover, D-βOHB (and not AcAc) is an inhibitor of NRLP3 inflammasome assembly. NLRP3 is a multi-protein complex whose activation triggers the activation of caspase-1 and the subsequent cleavage of its substrates including the pro-form of IL-1β and IL-18. Once cleaved, these inflammatory cytokines are secreted in their active form. Monocytes treated with D-βOHB secreted less IL-1β and IL-18 [135] in vitro; in vivo the administration of D-βOHB in a model of gout decreased inflammation.

Most studies characterizing the proinflammatory M1 phenotype associated with glycolysis and oxidative phosphorylation (OXPHOS) in contrast to the trophic/M2 phenotype relying on oxidative phosphorylation have been conducted in vitro using bone marrow-derived macrophages (BMDM) or monocyte-derived macrophages (Mφs). However, it appears that resident macrophages exhibit unique metabolic profiles, likely reflecting the distinct availability of metabolites depending on the tissue context [136, 137]. For example, peritoneum is a glutamate-rich environment and peritoneal Mφs rely on its use to fuel oxphos via glutaminolysis [136]. Peritoneal Mφs's oxidative burst relies on glutamine metabolism, as opposed to neutrophil and this does not depend on TLR engagement, this study shows that the environment dictates Mφ metabolism. Not all resident Mφs are equivalently affected by OXPHOS defect as assessed by Wculek collaborators [138] who showed that alveolar Mφs, Langherans cells, Kupffer cells and peritoneal Mφs are partially depleted upon deletion of TFAM expression, a transcription factor involved in the expression of several ETC proteins. Heterogeneity of Mφ metabolism has also been described at the organ level, more specifically in the lung that contains two subsets of resident Mφs: alveolar Mφs and interstitial Mφs [139]. Alveolar Mφs harbor reduced ECAR rates compared to interstitial Mφs [140]. Transcriptomic studies have also shown that the metabolic discrepancy exists between alveolar and interstitial Mφs [139, 140]. To sustain their activity, alveolar Mφs rely on fatty acid oxidation [139]. In the muscle, glutamine use can restrain the activity of satellite cells and this decreases tissue regeneration. The inhibition of glutamate dehydrogenase 1 (GLUD1) in Mφs increases the production and export of glutamine in the extracellular environment, that became available for satellite cells [141]. Glutamine has also been identified as the mediator of a crosstalk between Mφs and ovarian tumor cells, with the secretion of glutamine by TAM improving tumor cell aggressivity [142]. Finally, recent data from the Rathmell lab using positron emission tomography tracers indicate that TAMs are the main glucose consumers in the tumor microenvironment and that glucose consumption is not tied to its local concentration but rather to Mφs' propensity toward glutamine metabolism [143]. This landmark study shows that, contrary to what was previously thought, in tumor microenvironment, the consumption of nutrients such as glucose or glutamine is not dictated by a restricted environment in terms of concentration, but by the cells' preference for a metabolic substrate. This notion could be further challenged by the coexistence of multiple Mφ subsets that vary in terms of phenotype [9] and metabolism [144] eventually over time [145]. Metabolic and phenotypic data obtained over time will certainly be very informative since Mφs survive in tissues for a long time.

5. Conclusion

In severe or chronic diseases, Mφs accumulate in damaged tissues where they exhibit inadequate responses and participate in the chronicity of the pathology. Metabolic reprogramming of Mφs has been proposed as a promising therapeutic target to combat inflammatory disorders [30, 36]. Moreover, tumor-associated Mφs (TAMs) promote tumor progression and metastasis whereas Mφ in atherosclerosis exacerbates inflammation [146]. Different strategies to reprogram or eliminate Mφ are currently being evaluated in clinical trials, including novel approaches targeting their metabolism [26]. However, it must be kept in mind that these approaches must target Mφ present at inflammatory sites that are characterized by a nutrient-poor and lactic acid-enriched environment [92]. To date, the metabolic adaptations that allow Mφ to survive and function under these harsh conditions remain largely unknown [133]. Their identification remains a major challenge and is required to propose strategies specifically targeting the metabolism of inflammatory Mφ.

Acknowledgements

This work was supported by institutional fundings from Angers and Sorbonne Paris Nord universities.

Authors contribution

NJ and LP wrote the manuscript. PJ revised the manuscript. All authors contributed to the article and approved the submitted version.

Author details

Najia Jeroundi[1*†], Léa Paolini[2,3,†] and Pascale Jeannin[1,4]

1 Univ Angers, Nantes Université, Inserm, CNRS, CRCI2NA, SFR ICAT, LabEx IGO, Angers, France

2 Inserm UMR-1125, Bobigny, France

3 Sorbonne Paris Nord University, Bobigny, France

4 Immunology and Allergology laboratory, University Hospital, Angers, France

*Address all correspondence to: najia.jeroundi@univ-angers.fr

†These authors contributed equally to this work.

IntechOpen

© 2024 The Author(s). Licensee IntechOpen. This chapter is distributed under the terms of the Creative Commons Attribution License (http://creativecommons.org/licenses/by/3.0), which permits unrestricted use, distribution, and reproduction in any medium, provided the original work is properly cited.

References

[1] Lazarov T, Juarez-Carreño S, Cox N, Geissmann F. Physiology and diseases of tissue-resident macrophages. Nature. 2023;**618**:698-707. DOI: 10.1038/s41586-023-06002-x

[2] Mass E, Nimmerjahn F, Kierdorf K, Schlitzer A. Tissue-specific macrophages: How they develop and choreograph tissue biology. Nature Reviews. Immunology. 2023;**23**:563-579. DOI: 10.1038/s41577-023-00848-y

[3] Okabe Y, Medzhitov R. Tissue biology perspective on macrophages. Nature Immunology. 2016;**17**:9-17. DOI: 10.1038/ni.3320

[4] Cox N, Pokrovskii M, Vicario R, Geissmann F. Origins, biology, and diseases of tissue macrophages. Annual Review of Immunology. 2021;**39**:313-344. DOI: 10.1146/annurev-immunol-093019-111748

[5] Xue J, Schmidt SV, Sander J, Draffehn A, Krebs W, Quester I, et al. Transcriptome-based network analysis reveals a spectrum model of human macrophage activation. Immunity. 2014;**40**:274-288. DOI: 10.1016/j.immuni.2014.01.006

[6] Gosselin D, Link VM, Romanoski CE, Fonseca GJ, Eichenfield DZ, Spann NJ, et al. Environment drives selection and function of enhancers controlling tissue-specific macrophage identities. Cell. 2014;**159**:1327-1340. DOI: 10.1016/j.cell.2014.11.023

[7] Mosser DM, Edwards JP. Exploring the full spectrum of macrophage activation. Nature Reviews. Immunology. 2008;**8**:958-969. DOI: 10.1038/nri2448

[8] Murray PJ, Wynn TA. Obstacles and opportunities for understanding macrophage polarization. Journal of Leukocyte Biology. 2011;**89**:557-563. DOI: 10.1189/jlb.0710409

[9] Chevrier S, Levine JH, Zanotelli VRT, Silina K, Schulz D, Bacac M, et al. An immune atlas of clear cell renal cell carcinoma. Cell. 2017;**169**:736-749.e18. DOI: 10.1016/j.cell.2017.04.016

[10] Jha AK, Huang SC-C, Sergushichev A, Lampropoulou V, Ivanova Y, Loginicheva E, et al. Network integration of parallel metabolic and transcriptional data reveals metabolic modules that regulate macrophage polarization. Immunity. 2015;**42**:419-430. DOI: 10.1016/j.immuni.2015.02.005

[11] Azizi E, Carr AJ, Plitas G, Cornish AE, Konopacki C, Prabhakaran S, et al. Single-cell map of diverse immune phenotypes in the breast tumor microenvironment. Cell. 2018;**174**:1293-1308.e36. DOI: 10.1016/j.cell.2018.05.060

[12] Müller S, Kohanbash G, Liu SJ, Alvarado B, Carrera D, Bhaduri A, et al. Single-cell profiling of human gliomas reveals macrophage ontogeny as a basis for regional differences in macrophage activation in the tumor microenvironment. Genome Biology. 2017;**18**:234. DOI: 10.1186/s13059-017-1362-4

[13] Reinartz S, Schumann T, Finkernagel F, Wortmann A, Jansen JM, Meissner W, et al. Mixed-polarization phenotype of ascites-associated macrophages in human ovarian carcinoma: Correlation of CD163 expression, cytokine levels and early relapse. International Journal of Cancer. 2014;**134**:32-42. DOI: 10.1002/ijc.28335

[14] Biswas SK. A distinct and unique transcriptional program expressed

by tumor-associated macrophages (defective NF-B and enhanced IRF-3/STAT1 activation). Blood. 2006;**107**:2112-2122. DOI: 10.1182/blood-2005-01-0428

[15] Moganti K, Li F, Schmuttermaier C, Riemann S, Klüter H, Gratchev A, et al. Hyperglycemia induces mixed M1/M2 cytokine profile in primary human monocyte-derived macrophages. Immunobiology. 2017;**222**:952-959. DOI: 10.1016/j.imbio.2016.07.006

[16] Mitsi E, Kamng'ona R, Rylance J, Solórzano C, Reiné JJ, Mwandumba HC, et al. Human alveolar macrophages predominately express combined classical M1 and M2 surface markers in steady state. Respiratory Research. 2018;**19**:66. DOI: 10.1186/s12931-018-0777-0

[17] Paolini L, Adam C, Beauvillain C, Preisser L, Blanchard S, Pignon P, et al. Lactic acidosis together with GM-CSF and M-CSF induces human macrophages toward an inflammatory protumor phenotype. Cancer Immunology Research. 2020;**8**:383-395. DOI: 10.1158/2326-6066.CIR-18-0749

[18] Locati M, Curtale G, Mantovani A. Diversity, mechanisms, and significance of macrophage plasticity. Annual Review of Pathology: Mechanisms of Disease. 2020;**15**:123-147. DOI: 10.1146/annurev-pathmechdis-012418-012718

[19] Monnier M, Paolini L, Vinatier E, Mantovani A, Delneste Y, Jeannin P. Antitumor strategies targeting macrophages: The importance of considering the differences in differentiation/polarization processes between human and mouse macrophages. Journal for Immunotherapy of Cancer. 2022;**10**:e005560. DOI: 10.1136/jitc-2022-005560

[20] Bao Y, Wang G, Li H. Approaches for studying human macrophages. Trends in Immunology. 2024;**45**:237-247. DOI: 10.1016/j.it.2024.02.007

[21] Stanley ER, Guilbert LJ, Tushinski RJ, Bartelmez SH. CSF-1—A mononuclear phagocyte lineage-specific hemopoietic growth factor. Journal of Cellular Biochemistry. 1983;**21**:151-159. DOI: 10.1002/jcb.240210206

[22] Jeannin P, Paolini L, Adam C, Delneste Y. The roles of CSFs on the functional polarization of tumor-associated macrophages. The FEBS Journal. 2018;**285**:680-699. DOI: 10.1111/febs.14343

[23] Helft J, Böttcher J, Chakravarty P, Zelenay S, Huotari J, Schraml BU, et al. GM-CSF mouse bone marrow cultures comprise a heterogeneous population of CD11c(+)MHCII(+) macrophages and dendritic cells. Immunity. 2015;**42**:1197-1211. DOI: 10.1016/j.immuni.2015.05.018

[24] Gonçalves R, Kaliff Teófilo Murta G, Aparecida de Souza I, Mosser DM. Isolation and culture of bone marrow-derived macrophages from mice. Journal of Visualized Experiments. 2023;**196**:e64566. DOI: 10.3791/64566

[25] Biswas SK, Mantovani A. Macrophage plasticity and interaction with lymphocyte subsets: Cancer as a paradigm. Nature Immunology. 2010;**11**:889-896. DOI: 10.1038/ni.1937

[26] Mantovani A, Sozzani S, Locati M, Allavena P, Sica A. Macrophage polarization: Tumor-associated macrophages as a paradigm for polarized M2 mononuclear phagocytes. Trends in Immunology. 2002;**23**:549-555. DOI: 10.1016/S1471-4906(02)02302-5

[27] Van Den Bossche J, O'Neill LA, Menon D. Macrophage immunometabolism: Where are we (going)? Trends in Immunology.

2017;**38**:395-406. DOI: 10.1016/j.it.2017.03.001

[28] Sica A, Mantovani A. Macrophage plasticity and polarization: In vivo veritas. The Journal of Clinical Investigation. 2012;**122**:787-795. DOI: 10.1172/JCI59643

[29] Mills CD, Kincaid K, Alt JM, Heilman MJ, Hill AM. M-1/M-2 macrophages and the Th1/Th2 paradigm. Journal of Immunology. 2000;**164**:6166-6173. DOI: 10.4049/jimmunol.164.12.6166

[30] Van den Bossche J, Baardman J, Otto NA, van der Velden S, Neele AE, van den Berg SM, et al. Mitochondrial dysfunction prevents repolarization of inflammatory macrophages. Cell Reports. 2016;**17**:684-696. DOI: 10.1016/j.celrep.2016.09.008

[31] Rodríguez-Prados J-C, Través PG, Cuenca J, Rico D, Aragonés J, Martín-Sanz P, et al. Substrate fate in activated macrophages: A comparison between innate, classic, and alternative activation. Journal of Immunology. 2010;**185**:605-614. DOI: 10.4049/jimmunol.0901698

[32] Viola A, Munari F, Sánchez-Rodríguez R, Scolaro T, Castegna A. The metabolic signature of macrophage responses. Frontiers in Immunology. 2019;**10**:1462. DOI: 10.3389/fimmu.2019.01462

[33] Izquierdo E, Cuevas VD, Fernández-Arroyo S, Riera-Borrull M, Orta-Zavalza E, Joven J, et al. Reshaping of human macrophage polarization through modulation of glucose catabolic pathways. Journal of Immunology. 2015;**195**:2442-2451. DOI: 10.4049/jimmunol.1403045

[34] Cinelli MA, Do HT, Miley GP, Silverman RB. Inducible nitric oxide synthase: Regulation, structure, and inhibition. Medicinal Research Reviews. 2020;**40**:158-189. DOI: 10.1002/med.21599

[35] Gross TJ, Kremens K, Powers LS, Brink B, Knutson T, Domann FE, et al. Epigenetic silencing of the human NOS2 gene: Rethinking the role of nitric oxide in human macrophage inflammatory responses. Journal of Immunology. 2014;**192**:2326-2338. DOI: 10.4049/jimmunol.1301758

[36] O'Neill LAJ, Pearce EJ. Immunometabolism governs dendritic cell and macrophage function. The Journal of Experimental Medicine. 2016;**213**:15-23. DOI: 10.1084/jem.20151570

[37] Arnold PK, Finley LWS. Regulation and function of the mammalian tricarboxylic acid cycle. The Journal of Biological Chemistry. 2023;**299**:102838. DOI: 10.1016/j.jbc.2022.102838

[38] Martínez-Reyes I, Chandel NS. Mitochondrial TCA cycle metabolites control physiology and disease. Nature Communications. 2020;**11**:102. DOI: 10.1038/s41467-019-13668-3

[39] Han H-S, Kang G, Kim JS, Choi BH, Koo S-H. Regulation of glucose metabolism from a liver-centric perspective. Experimental & Molecular Medicine. 2016;**48**:e218-e218. DOI: 10.1038/emm.2015.122

[40] TeSlaa T, Ralser M, Fan J, Rabinowitz JD. The pentose phosphate pathway in health and disease. Nature Metabolism. 2023;**5**:1275-1289. DOI: 10.1038/s42255-023-00863-2

[41] Rajas F, Gautier-Stein A, Mithieux G. Glucose-6 phosphate, a central hub for liver carbohydrate metabolism. Metabolites. 2019;**9**:282. DOI: 10.3390/metabo9120282

[42] Adeva-Andany MM, González-Lucán M, Donapetry-García C, Fernández-Fernández C, Ameneiros-Rodríguez E. Glycogen metabolism in humans. BBA Clinical. 2016;**5**:85-100. DOI: 10.1016/j.bbacli.2016.02.001

[43] Artyomov MN, Van den Bossche J. Immunometabolism in the single-cell era. Cell Metabolism. 2020;**32**:710-725. DOI: 10.1016/j.cmet.2020.09.013

[44] Miller A, Nagy C, Knapp B, Laengle J, Ponweiser E, Groeger M, et al. Exploring metabolic configurations of single cells within complex tissue microenvironments. Cell Metabolism. 2017;**26**:788-800.e6. DOI: 10.1016/j.cmet.2017.08.014

[45] Verberk SGS, de Goede KE, Gorki FS, van Dierendonck XAMH, Argüello RJ, Van den Bossche J. An integrated toolbox to profile macrophage immunometabolism. Cell Reports Methods. 2022;**2**:100192. DOI: 10.1016/j.crmeth.2022.100192

[46] Bartman CR, Faubert B, Rabinowitz JD, DeBerardinis RJ. Metabolic pathway analysis using stable isotopes in patients with cancer. Nature Reviews. Cancer. 2023;**23**:863-878. DOI: 10.1038/s41568-023-00632-z

[47] Newsholme P, Curi R, Gordon S, Newsholme EA. Metabolism of glucose, glutamine, long-chain fatty acids and ketone bodies by murine macrophages. The Biochemical Journal. 1986;**239**:121-125. DOI: 10.1042/bj2390121

[48] Michl J, Ohlbaum DJ, Silverstein SC. 2-Deoxyglucose selectively inhibits Fc and complement receptor-mediated phagocytosis in mouse peritoneal macrophages. I. Description of the inhibitory effect. The Journal of Experimental Medicine. 1976;**144**:1465-1483. DOI: 10.1084/jem.144.6.1465

[49] Hamilton JA, Vairo G, Lingelbach SR. CSF-1 stimulates glucose uptake in murine bone marrow-derived macrophages. Biochemical and Biophysical Research Communications. 1986;**138**:445-454. DOI: 10.1016/0006-291x(86)90301-3

[50] Van den Bossche J, Baardman J, de Winther MPJ. Metabolic characterization of polarized M1 and M2 bone marrow-derived macrophages using real-time extracellular flux analysis. Journal of Visualized Experiments. 2015;**105**:e53424. DOI: 10.3791/53424

[51] Fukuzumi M, Shinomiya H, Shimizu Y, Ohishi K, Utsumi S. Endotoxin-induced enhancement of glucose influx into murine peritoneal macrophages via GLUT1. Infection and Immunity. 1996;**64**:108-112. DOI: 10.1128/iai.64.1.108-112.1996

[52] Freemerman AJ, Johnson AR, Sacks GN, Milner JJ, Kirk EL, Troester MA, et al. Metabolic reprogramming of macrophages: Glucose transporter 1 (GLUT1)-mediated glucose metabolism drives a proinflammatory phenotype. The Journal of Biological Chemistry. 2014;**289**:7884-7896. DOI: 10.1074/jbc.M113.522037

[53] Nishizawa T, Kanter JE, Kramer F, Barnhart S, Shen X, Vivekanandan-Giri A, et al. Testing the role of myeloid cell glucose flux in inflammation and atherosclerosis. Cell Reports. 2014;**7**:356-365. DOI: 10.1016/j.celrep.2014.03.028

[54] Liu L, Lu Y, Martinez J, Bi Y, Lian G, Wang T, et al. Proinflammatory signal suppresses proliferation and shifts macrophage metabolism from Myc-dependent to HIF1α-dependent. Proceedings of the National Academy of Sciences of the United States of America. 2016;**113**:1564-1569. DOI: 10.1073/pnas.1518000113

[55] Wang T, Liu H, Lian G, Zhang S-Y, Wang X, Jiang C. HIF1α-induced glycolysis metabolism is essential to the activation of inflammatory macrophages. Mediators of Inflammation. 2017;**2017**:9029327. DOI: 10.1155/2017/9029327

[56] Tannahill GM, Curtis AM, Adamik J, Palsson-McDermott EM, McGettrick AF, Goel G, et al. Succinate is an inflammatory signal that induces IL-1β through HIF-1α. Nature. 2013;**496**:238-242. DOI: 10.1038/nature11986

[57] Lachmandas E, Boutens L, Ratter JM, Hijmans A, Hooiveld GJ, Joosten LAB, et al. Microbial stimulation of different toll-like receptor signalling pathways induces diverse metabolic programmes in human monocytes. Nature Microbiology. 2016;**2**:16246. DOI: 10.1038/nmicrobiol.2016.246

[58] Wolf AJ, Reyes CN, Liang W, Becker C, Shimada K, Wheeler ML, et al. Hexokinase is an innate immune receptor for the detection of bacterial peptidoglycan. Cell. 2016;**166**:624-636. DOI: 10.1016/j.cell.2016.05.076

[59] Baik SH, Ramanujan VK, Becker C, Fett S, Underhill DM, Wolf AJ. Hexokinase dissociation from mitochondria promotes oligomerization of VDAC that facilitates NLRP3 inflammasome assembly and activation. Science Immunology. 2023;**8**:eade7652. DOI: 10.1126/sciimmunol.ade7652

[60] Mor I, Cheung EC, Vousden KH. Control of glycolysis through regulation of PFK1: Old friends and recent additions. Cold Spring Harbor Symposia on Quantitative Biology. 2011;**76**:211-216. DOI: 10.1101/sqb.2011.76.010868

[61] Sadiku P, Willson JA, Ryan EM, Sammut D, Coelho P, Watts ER, et al. Neutrophils fuel effective immune responses through gluconeogenesis and glycogenesis. Cell Metabolism. 2021;**33**:411-423.e4. DOI: 10.1016/j.cmet.2020.11.016

[62] Boscá L, González-Ramos S, Prieto P, Fernández-Velasco M, Mojena M, Martín-Sanz P, et al. Metabolic signatures linked to macrophage polarization: From glucose metabolism to oxidative phosphorylation. Biochemical Society Transactions. 2015;**43**:740-744. DOI: 10.1042/BST20150107

[63] Finucane OM, Sugrue J, Rubio-Araiz A, Guillot-Sestier M-V, Lynch MA. The NLRP3 inflammasome modulates glycolysis by increasing PFKFB3 in an IL-1β-dependent manner in macrophages. Scientific Reports. 2019;**9**:4034. DOI: 10.1038/s41598-019-40619-1

[64] Tawakol A, Singh P, Mojena M, Pimentel-Santillana M, Emami H, MacNabb M, et al. HIF-1α and PFKFB3 mediate a tight relationship between proinflammatory activation and anerobic metabolism in atherosclerotic macrophages. ATVB. 2015;**35**:1463-1471. DOI: 10.1161/ATVBAHA.115.305551

[65] Ngai D, Schilperoort M, Tabas I. Efferocytosis-induced lactate enables the proliferation of pro-resolving macrophages to mediate tissue repair. Nature Metabolism. 2023;**5**:2206-2219. DOI: 10.1038/s42255-023-00921-9

[66] Millet P, Vachharajani V, McPhail L, Yoza B, McCall CE. GAPDH binding to TNF-α mRNA contributes to posttranscriptional repression in monocytes: A novel mechanism of communication between inflammation and metabolism. Journal of Immunology. 2016;**196**:2541-2551. DOI: 10.4049/jimmunol.1501345

[67] Galván-Peña S, Carroll RG, Newman C, Hinchy EC, Palsson-McDermott E, Robinson EK, et al. Malonylation of GAPDH is an inflammatory signal in macrophages. Nature Communications. 2019;**10**:338. DOI: 10.1038/s41467-018-08187-6

[68] O'Neill LAJ, Kishton RJ, Rathmell J. A guide to immunometabolism for immunologists. Nature Reviews. Immunology. 2016;**16**:553-565. DOI: 10.1038/nri.2016.70

[69] Das Gupta K, Shakespear MR, Curson JEB, Murthy AMV, Iyer A, Hodson MP, et al. Class IIa histone deacetylases drive toll-like receptor-inducible glycolysis and macrophage inflammatory responses via pyruvate kinase M2. Cell Reports. 2020;**30**:2712-2728.e8. DOI: 10.1016/j.celrep.2020.02.007

[70] Palsson-McDermott EM, Curtis AM, Goel G, Lauterbach MAR, Sheedy FJ, Gleeson LE, et al. Pyruvate kinase M2 regulates Hif-1α activity and IL-1β induction and is a critical determinant of the Warburg effect in LPS-activated macrophages. Cell Metabolism. 2015;**21**:65-80. DOI: 10.1016/j.cmet.2014.12.005

[71] Xie M, Yu Y, Kang R, Zhu S, Yang L, Zeng L, et al. PKM2-dependent glycolysis promotes NLRP3 and AIM2 inflammasome activation. Nature Communications. 2016;7:13280. DOI: 10.1038/ncomms13280

[72] Dong Z, Li R, Xu L, Xin K, Xu Y, Shi H, et al. Histone hyperacetylation mediates enhanced IL-1β production in LPS/IFN-γ-stimulated macrophages. Immunology. 2020;**160**:183-197. DOI: 10.1111/imm.13183

[73] Soto-Heredero G, Heras MMGDL, Gabandé-Rodríguez E, Oller J, Mittelbrunn M. Glycolysis—A key player in the inflammatory response. The FEBS Journal. 2020;**287**:3350-3369. DOI: 10.1111/febs.15327

[74] Lu L-G, Zhou Z-L, Wang X-Y, Liu B-Y, Lu J-Y, Liu S, et al. PD-L1 blockade liberates intrinsic antitumourigenic properties of glycolytic macrophages in hepatocellular carcinoma. Gut. 2022;**71**:2551-2560. DOI: 10.1136/gutjnl-2021-326350

[75] Palsson-McDermott EM, Dyck L, Zasłona Z, Menon D, McGettrick AF, Mills KHG, et al. Pyruvate kinase M2 is required for the expression of the immune checkpoint PD-L1 in immune cells and tumors. Frontiers in Immunology. 2017;**8**:1300. DOI: 10.3389/fimmu.2017.01300

[76] Aki T, Funakoshi T, Noritake K, Unuma K, Uemura K. Extracellular glucose is crucially involved in the fate decision of LPS-stimulated RAW264.7 murine macrophage cells. Scientific Reports. 2020;**10**:10581. DOI: 10.1038/s41598-020-67396-6

[77] Stanton RC. Glucose-6-phosphate dehydrogenase, NADPH, and cell survival. IUBMB Life. 2012;**64**:362-369. DOI: 10.1002/iub.1017

[78] Ge T, Yang J, Zhou S, Wang Y, Li Y, Tong X. The role of the pentose phosphate pathway in diabetes and cancer. Frontiers in Endocrinology. 2020;**11**:365. DOI: 10.3389/fendo.2020.00365

[79] Ham M, Lee J-W, Choi AH, Jang H, Choi G, Park J, et al. Macrophage glucose-6-phosphate dehydrogenase stimulates proinflammatory responses with oxidative stress. Molecular and Cellular Biology. 2013;**33**:2425-2435. DOI: 10.1128/MCB.01260-12

[80] Haschemi A, Kosma P, Gille L, Evans CR, Burant CF, Starkl P, et al. The sedoheptulose kinase CARKL directs macrophage polarization through control of glucose metabolism. Cell Metabolism. 2012;**15**:813-826. DOI: 10.1016/j.cmet.2012.04.023

[81] Ma J, Wei K, Liu J, Tang K, Zhang H, Zhu L, et al. Glycogen metabolism regulates macrophage-mediated acute inflammatory responses. Nature Communications. 2020;**11**:1769. DOI: 10.1038/s41467-020-15636-8

[82] Ma R, Ji T, Zhang H, Dong W, Chen X, Xu P, et al. A Pck1-directed glycogen metabolic program regulates formation and maintenance of memory CD8+ T cells. Nature Cell Biology. 2018;**20**:21-27. DOI: 10.1038/s41556-017-0002-2

[83] Thwe PM, Amiel E. The role of nitric oxide in metabolic regulation of dendritic cell immune function. Cancer Letters. 2018;**412**:236-242. DOI: 10.1016/j.canlet.2017.10.032

[84] Zois CE, Harris AL. Glycogen metabolism has a key role in the cancer microenvironment and provides new targets for cancer therapy. Journal of Molecular Medicine. 2016;**94**:137-154. DOI: 10.1007/s00109-015-1377-9

[85] Qian L, Chen X-Q, Kong D, Wang G, Cao Y, Xiao Y, et al. MK8617 inhibits M1 macrophage polarization and inflammation via the HIF-1α/GYS1/UDPG/P2Y14 pathway. PeerJ. 2023;**11**:e15591. DOI: 10.7717/peerj.15591

[86] Everts B, Amiel E, Huang SC-C, Smith AM, Chang C-H, Lam WY, et al. TLR-driven early glycolytic reprogramming via the kinases TBK1-IKKε supports the anabolic demands of dendritic cell activation. Nature Immunology. 2014;**15**:323-332. DOI: 10.1038/ni.2833

[87] Krawczyk CM, Holowka T, Sun J, Blagih J, Amiel E, DeBerardinis RJ, et al. Toll-like receptor–induced changes in glycolytic metabolism regulate dendritic cell activation. Blood. 2010;**115**:4742-4749. DOI: 10.1182/blood-2009-10-249540

[88] Meiser J, Krämer L, Sapcariu SC, Battello N, Ghelfi J, D'Herouel AF, et al. Pro-inflammatory macrophages sustain pyruvate oxidation through pyruvate dehydrogenase for the synthesis of itaconate and to enable cytokine expression. Journal of Biological Chemistry. 2016;**291**:3932-3946. DOI: 10.1074/jbc.M115.676817

[89] Lampropoulou V, Sergushichev A, Bambouskova M, Nair S, Vincent EE, Loginicheva E, et al. Itaconate links inhibition of succinate dehydrogenase with macrophage metabolic remodeling and regulation of inflammation. Cell Metabolism. 2016;**24**:158-166. DOI: 10.1016/j.cmet.2016.06.004

[90] Murugina NE, Budikhina AS, Dagil YA, Maximchik PV, Balyasova LS, Murugin VV, et al. Glycolytic reprogramming of macrophages activated by NOD1 and TLR4 agonists: No association with proinflammatory cytokine production in normoxia. Journal of Biological Chemistry. 2020;**295**:3099-3114. DOI: 10.1074/jbc.RA119.010589

[91] Zhang Q, Wang J, Yadav DK, Bai X, Liang T. Glucose metabolism: The metabolic signature of tumor associated macrophage. Frontiers in Immunology. 2021;**12**:702580. DOI: 10.3389/fimmu.2021.702580

[92] Sun S, Li H, Chen J, Qian Q. Lactic acid: No longer an inert and end-product

of glycolysis. Physiology (Bethesda). 2017;**32**:453-463. DOI: 10.1152/physiol.00016.2017

[93] Colegio OR, Chu N-Q, Szabo AL, Chu T, Rhebergen AM, Jairam V, et al. Functional polarization of tumour-associated macrophages by tumour-derived lactic acid. Nature. 2014;**513**:559-563. DOI: 10.1038/nature13490

[94] Halestrap AP. The SLC16 gene family—Structure, role and regulation in health and disease. Molecular Aspects of Medicine. 2013;**34**:337-349. DOI: 10.1016/j.mam.2012.05.003

[95] Arts RJW, Plantinga TS, Tuit S, Ulas T, Heinhuis B, Tesselaar M, et al. Transcriptional and metabolic reprogramming induce an inflammatory phenotype in non-medullary thyroid carcinoma-induced macrophages. Oncoimmunology. 2016;**5**:e1229725. DOI: 10.1080/2162402X.2016.1229725

[96] Samuvel DJ, Sundararaj KP, Nareika A, Lopes-Virella MF, Huang Y. Lactate boosts TLR4 signaling and NF-kappaB pathway-mediated gene transcription in macrophages via monocarboxylate transporters and MD-2 up-regulation. Journal of Immunology. 2009;**182**:2476-2484. DOI: 10.4049/jimmunol.0802059

[97] Zhang D, Tang Z, Huang H, Zhou G, Cui C, Weng Y, et al. Metabolic regulation of gene expression by histone lactylation. Nature. 2019;**574**:575-580. DOI: 10.1038/s41586-019-1678-1

[98] Noe JT, Rendon BE, Geller AE, Conroy LR, Morrissey SM, Young LEA, et al. Lactate supports a metabolic-epigenetic link in macrophage polarization. Science Advances. 2021;**7**:eabi8602. DOI: 10.1126/sciadv.abi8602

[99] Shi W, Cassmann TJ, Bhagwate AV, Hitosugi T, Ip WKE. Lactic acid induces transcriptional repression of macrophage inflammatory response via histone acetylation. Cell Reports. 2024;**43**:113746. DOI: 10.1016/j.celrep.2024.113746

[100] Galván-Peña S, O'Neill LAJ. Metabolic reprograming in macrophage polarization. Frontiers in Immunology. 2014;**5**:420. DOI: 10.3389/fimmu.2014.00420

[101] Cheng C-F, Ku H-C, Lin H. PGC-1α as a pivotal factor in lipid and metabolic regulation. International Journal of Molecular Sciences. 2018;**19**:3447. DOI: 10.3390/ijms19113447

[102] Chen L, Qin Y, Liu B, Gao M, Li A, Li X, et al. PGC-1α-mediated mitochondrial quality control: Molecular mechanisms and implications for heart failure. Frontiers in Cell and Development Biology. 2022;**10**:871357. DOI: 10.3389/fcell.2022.871357

[103] Vats D, Mukundan L, Odegaard JI, Zhang L, Smith KL, Morel CR, et al. Oxidative metabolism and PGC-1beta attenuate macrophage-mediated inflammation. Cell Metabolism. 2006;**4**:13-24. DOI: 10.1016/j.cmet.2006.05.011

[104] Tang J, Dong W, Wang D, Deng Q, Guo H, Xiao G. Upregulation of PGC-1α expression by pioglitazone mediates prevention of sepsis-induced acute lung injury. Brazilian Journal of Medical and Biological Research. 2024;**57**:e13235. DOI: 10.1590/1414-431x2024e13235

[105] Covarrubias AJ, Aksoylar HI, Yu J, Snyder NW, Worth AJ, Iyer SS, et al. Akt-mTORC1 signaling regulates Acly to integrate metabolic input to control of macrophage activation. eLife. 2016;**5**:e11612. DOI: 10.7554/eLife.11612

[106] Hung SSC, Van Bergen NJ, Jackson S, Liang H, Mackey DAA, Hernández D, et al. Study of mitochondrial respiratory defects on reprogramming to human induced pluripotent stem cells. Aging. 2016;**8**: 945-957. DOI: 10.18632/aging.100950

[107] Tan Z, Xie N, Cui H, Moellering DR, Abraham E, Thannickal VJ, et al. Pyruvate dehydrogenase kinase 1 participates in macrophage polarization via regulating glucose metabolism. The Journal of Immunology. 2015;**194**:6082-6089. DOI: 10.4049/jimmunol.1402469

[108] Namgaladze D, Zukunft S, Schnütgen F, Kurrle N, Fleming I, Fuhrmann D, et al. Polarization of human macrophages by interleukin-4 does not require ATP-citrate lyase. Frontiers in Immunology. 2018;**9**:2858. DOI: 10.3389/fimmu.2018.02858

[109] Mills EL, Kelly B, Logan A, Costa ASH, Varma M, Bryant CE, et al. Succinate dehydrogenase supports metabolic repurposing of mitochondria to drive inflammatory macrophages. Cell. 2016;**167**:457-470.e13. DOI: 10.1016/j.cell.2016.08.064

[110] West AP, Brodsky IE, Rahner C, Woo DK, Erdjument-Bromage H, Tempst P, et al. TLR signalling augments macrophage bactericidal activity through mitochondrial ROS. Nature. 2011;**472**:476-480. DOI: 10.1038/nature09973

[111] Garaude J, Acín-Pérez R, Martínez-Cano S, Enamorado M, Ugolini M, Nistal-Villán E, et al. Mitochondrial respiratory-chain adaptations in macrophages contribute to antibacterial host defense. Nature Immunology. 2016;**17**:1037-1045. DOI: 10.1038/ni.3509

[112] Infantino V, Convertini P, Cucci L, Panaro MA, Di Noia MA, Calvello R, et al. The mitochondrial citrate carrier: A new player in inflammation. Biochemical Journal. 2011;**438**:433-436. DOI: 10.1042/BJ20111275

[113] Infantino V, Iacobazzi V, Palmieri F, Menga A. ATP-citrate lyase is essential for macrophage inflammatory response. Biochemical and Biophysical Research Communications. 2013;**440**:105-111. DOI: 10.1016/j.bbrc.2013.09.037

[114] Infantino V, Iacobazzi V, Menga A, Avantaggiati ML, Palmieri F. A key role of the mitochondrial citrate carrier (SLC25A1) in TNFα- and IFNγ-triggered inflammation. Biochimica et Biophysica Acta (BBA) - Gene Regulatory Mechanisms. 2014;**1839**:1217-1225. DOI: 10.1016/j.bbagrm.2014.07.013

[115] Lauterbach MA, Hanke JE, Serefidou M, Mangan MSJ, Kolbe C-C, Hess T, et al. Toll-like receptor signaling rewires macrophage metabolism and promotes histone acetylation via ATP-citrate lyase. Immunity. 2019;**51**:997-1011.e7. DOI: 10.1016/j.immuni.2019.11.009

[116] Verberk SGS, Van Der Zande HJP, Baardman J, De Goede KE, Harber KJ, Keuning ED, et al. Myeloid ATP citrate lyase regulates macrophage inflammatory responses In vitro without altering inflammatory disease outcomes. Frontiers in Immunology. 2021;**12**:669920. DOI: 10.3389/fimmu.2021.669920

[117] Santarsiero A, Convertini P, Todisco S, Pierri CL, De Grassi A, Williams NC, et al. ACLY nuclear translocation in human macrophages drives proinflammatory gene expression by NF-κB acetylation. Cells. 2021;**10**:2962. DOI: 10.3390/cells10112962

[118] Christofides A, Strauss L, Yeo A, Cao C, Charest A, Boussiotis VA. The complex role of tumor-infiltrating

macrophages. Nature Immunology. 2022;**23**:1148-1156. DOI: 10.1038/s41590-022-01267-2

[119] Beatty GL, Chiorean EG, Fishman MP, Saboury B, Teitelbaum UR, Sun W, et al. CD40 agonists alter tumor stroma and show efficacy against pancreatic carcinoma in mice and humans. Science. 2011;**331**:1612-1616. DOI: 10.1126/science.1198443

[120] Liu P-S, Chen Y-T, Li X, Hsueh P-C, Tzeng S-F, Chen H, et al. Author correction: CD40 signal rewires fatty acid and glutamine metabolism for stimulating macrophage anti-tumorigenic functions. Nature Immunology. 2023;**24**:1591. DOI: 10.1038/s41590-023-01611-0

[121] Di Gioia M, Spreafico R, Springstead JR, Mendelson MM, Joehanes R, Levy D, et al. Endogenous oxidized phospholipids reprogram cellular metabolism and boost hyperinflammation. Nature Immunology. 2020;**21**:42-53. DOI: 10.1038/s41590-019-0539-2

[122] Koivunen P, Hirsilä M, Remes AM, Hassinen IE, Kivirikko KI, Myllyharju J. Inhibition of hypoxia-inducible factor (HIF) hydroxylases by citric acid cycle intermediates. Journal of Biological Chemistry. 2007;**282**:4524-4532. DOI: 10.1074/jbc.M610415200

[123] Huang SC-C, Everts B, Ivanova Y, O'Sullivan D, Nascimento M, Smith AM, et al. Cell-intrinsic lysosomal lipolysis is essential for alternative activation of macrophages. Nature Immunology. 2014;**15**:846-855. DOI: 10.1038/ni.2956

[124] Martinez FO, Gordon S, Locati M, Mantovani A. Transcriptional profiling of the human monocyte-to-macrophage differentiation and polarization: New molecules and patterns of gene expression. Journal of Immunology. 2006;**177**:7303-7311. DOI: 10.4049/jimmunol.177.10.7303

[125] Divakaruni AS, Hsieh WY, Minarrieta L, Duong TN, Kim KKO, Desousa BR, et al. Etomoxir inhibits macrophage polarization by disrupting CoA homeostasis. Cell Metabolism. 2018;**28**:490-503.e7. DOI: 10.1016/j.cmet.2018.06.001

[126] Huang SC-C, Smith AM, Everts B, Colonna M, Pearce EL, Schilling JD, et al. Metabolic reprogramming mediated by the mTORC2-IRF4 signaling Axis is essential for macrophage alternative activation. Immunity. 2016;**45**:817-830. DOI: 10.1016/j.immuni.2016.09.016

[127] Curi R, Newsholme P, Marzuca-Nassr GN, Takahashi HK, Hirabara SM, Cruzat V, et al. Regulatory principles in metabolism-then and now. The Biochemical Journal. 2016;**473**:1845-1857. DOI: 10.1042/BCJ20160103

[128] Merlin J, Ivanov S, Dumont A, Sergushichev A, Gall J, Stunault M, et al. Non-canonical glutamine transamination sustains efferocytosis by coupling redox buffering to oxidative phosphorylation. Nature Metabolism. 2021;**3**:1313-1326. DOI: 10.1038/s42255-021-00471-y

[129] Chen S, Cui W, Chi Z, Xiao Q, Hu T, Ye Q, et al. Tumor-associated macrophages are shaped by intratumoral high potassium via Kir2.1. Cell Metabolism. 2022;**34**:1843-1859.e11. DOI: 10.1016/j.cmet.2022.08.016

[130] Liu P-S, Wang H, Li X, Chao T, Teav T, Christen S, et al. α-Ketoglutarate orchestrates macrophage activation through metabolic and epigenetic reprogramming. Nature Immunology. 2017;**18**:985-994. DOI: 10.1038/ni.3796

[131] Puchalska P, Crawford PA. Metabolic and signaling roles of ketone bodies in

health and disease. Annual Review of Nutrition. 2021;**41**:49-77. DOI: 10.1146/annurev-nutr-111120-111518

[132] Puchalska P, Martin SE, Huang X, Lengfeld JE, Daniel B, Graham MJ, et al. Hepatocyte-macrophage acetoacetate shuttle protects against tissue fibrosis. Cell Metabolism. 2019;**29**:383-398.e7. DOI: 10.1016/j.cmet.2018.10.015

[133] Adam C, Paolini L, Gueguen N, Mabilleau G, Preisser L, Blanchard S, et al. Acetoacetate protects macrophages from lactic acidosis-induced mitochondrial dysfunction by metabolic reprograming. Nature Communications. 2021;**12**:7115. DOI: 10.1038/s41467-021-27426-x

[134] Nelson AB, Queathem ED, Puchalska P, Crawford PA. Metabolic messengers: Ketone bodies. Nature Metabolism. 2023;**5**:2062-2074. DOI: 10.1038/s42255-023-00935-3

[135] Youm Y-H, Nguyen KY, Grant RW, Goldberg EL, Bodogai M, Kim D, et al. The ketone metabolite β-hydroxybutyrate blocks NLRP3 inflammasome-mediated inflammatory disease. Nature Medicine. 2015;**21**:263-269. DOI: 10.1038/nm.3804

[136] Davies LC, Rice CM, Palmieri EM, Taylor PR, Kuhns DB, McVicar DW. Peritoneal tissue-resident macrophages are metabolically poised to engage microbes using tissue-niche fuels. Nature Communications. 2017;**8**:2074. DOI: 10.1038/s41467-017-02092-0

[137] Heieis GA, Patente TA, Almeida L, Vrieling F, Tak T, Perona-Wright G, et al. Metabolic heterogeneity of tissue-resident macrophages in homeostasis and during helminth infection. Nature Communications. 2023;**14**:5627. DOI: 10.1038/s41467-023-41353-z

[138] Wculek SK, Heras-Murillo I, Mastrangelo A, Mañanes D, Galán M, Miguel V, et al. Oxidative phosphorylation selectively orchestrates tissue macrophage homeostasis. Immunity. 2023;**56**:516-530.e9. DOI: 10.1016/j.immuni.2023.01.011

[139] Svedberg FR, Brown SL, Krauss MZ, Campbell L, Sharpe C, Clausen M, et al. The lung environment controls alveolar macrophage metabolism and responsiveness in type 2 inflammation. Nature Immunology. 2019;**20**:571-580. DOI: 10.1038/s41590-019-0352-y

[140] Huang L, Nazarova EV, Tan S, Liu Y, Russell DG. Growth of *Mycobacterium tuberculosis* in vivo segregates with host macrophage metabolism and ontogeny. The Journal of Experimental Medicine. 2018;**215**:1135-1152. DOI: 10.1084/jem.20172020

[141] Shang M, Cappellesso F, Amorim R, Serneels J, Virga F, Eelen G, et al. Macrophage-derived glutamine boosts satellite cells and muscle regeneration. Nature. 2020;**587**:626-631. DOI: 10.1038/s41586-020-2857-9

[142] Menga A, Favia M, Spera I, Vegliante MC, Gissi R, De Grassi A, et al. N-acetylaspartate release by glutaminolytic ovarian cancer cells sustains protumoral macrophages. EMBO Reports. 2021;**22**:e51981. DOI: 10.15252/embr.202051981

[143] Reinfeld BI, Madden MZ, Wolf MM, Chytil A, Bader JE, Patterson AR, et al. Cell-programmed nutrient partitioning in the tumour microenvironment. Nature. 2021;**593**:282-288. DOI: 10.1038/s41586-021-03442-1

[144] Geeraerts X, Fernández-Garcia J, Hartmann FJ, de Goede KE, Martens L, Elkrim Y, et al. Macrophages are metabolically heterogeneous within

the tumor microenvironment. Cell Reports. 2021;**37**:110171. DOI: 10.1016/j.celrep.2021.110171

[145] Willenborg S, Sanin DE, Jais A, Ding X, Ulas T, Nüchel J, et al. Mitochondrial metabolism coordinates stage-specific repair processes in macrophages during wound healing. Cell Metabolism. 2021;**33**:2398-2414.e9. DOI: 10.1016/j.cmet.2021.10.004

[146] Sheu KM, Hoffmann A. Functional hallmarks of healthy macrophage responses: Their regulatory basis and disease relevance. Annual Review of Immunology. 2022;**40**:295-321. DOI: 10.1146/annurev-immunol-101320-031555

Section 2

Macrophages Functions in Cancer

Chapter 3

Macrophages and Myeloid-Derived Suppressor Cells in the Tumor Microenvironment: Unraveling Molecular Pathways, Immunometabolic Processes, and Their Significance in Immunotherapy for Hepatocellular Carcinoma (HCC)

Chia-Sheng Chu and Li-Ling Wu

Abstract

Hepatocellular carcinoma (HCC) is a major global health concern, and understanding the complex interplay of immune cells within the tumor microenvironment is crucial. This review explores the roles of myeloid-derived suppressor cells (MDSCs) and macrophages in HCC, focusing on their molecular pathways, immunometabolic processes, and implications for immunotherapy. We begin by elucidating the origin, expansion, and immunosuppressive mechanisms of MDSCs, emphasizing the importance of molecular pathways and immunometabolism in regulating their functions. In parallel, we delve into the dual nature of tumor-associated macrophages (TAMs) and discuss the molecular and metabolic cues governing their plasticity. Tumor metabolism is a central theme, with a comprehensive overview of altered metabolic processes in cancer cells and their impact on immune cells in the tumor microenvironment. We examine the metabolic crosstalk between tumor cells, MDSCs, and macrophages, shedding light on how tumor metabolism contributes to immune evasion. Furthermore, we discuss the challenges and limitations faced in the clinical application of immunotherapy in HCC. In conclusion, this review highlights the intricate web of molecular pathways and immunometabolic processes shaping the functions of MDSCs and macrophages in HCC. Understanding these dynamics is essential for the innovative immunotherapeutic interventions in HCC, improving outcomes of this devastating disease.

Keywords: macrophages, myeloid-derived suppressor cells (MDSCs), tumor microenvironment, hepatocellular carcinoma (HCC), immunotherapy, immunometabolism, tumor-associated macrophages (TAMs), metabolic crosstalk, immunotherapy

1. Introduction

Hepatocellular carcinoma (HCC) stands as a formidable global health challenge, representing the most prevalent type of liver cancer and posing a substantial burden on public health systems worldwide [1, 2]. Its formidable nature arises from its insidious progression, often remaining asymptomatic until reaching an advanced stage, limiting therapeutic options and yielding a high mortality rate [3–5]. Therefore, it is imperative to unravel the intricacies of HCC pathogenesis and discover innovative therapeutic strategies.

The tumor microenvironment (TME) constitutes an indispensable player in the context of HCC progression [6, 7]. Beyond the tumor cells themselves, the TME is an intricate ecosystem comprising a multitude of cell types, extracellular matrix components, and signaling molecules. This dynamic milieu serves as a critical regulator of disease evolution, influencing tumor growth, metastasis, and the response to therapy [8].

Within the TME, two key players come into focus: myeloid-derived suppressor cells (MDSCs) and macrophages. These immune cell populations, although integral components of the immune system, paradoxically wield immunosuppressive capabilities that can be harnessed by HCC to its advantage. Their recruitment, activation, and subsequent functions within the TME significantly contribute to the evasion of immune surveillance and immune-mediated tumor destruction.

Myeloid-derived suppressor cells, a heterogeneous population of immature myeloid cells, expand in response to chronic inflammation and are potent inhibitors of T-cell responses. Through various mechanisms, including the production of immunosuppressive cytokines and the induction of regulatory T cells, MDSCs suppress the antitumor immune response, thereby facilitating tumor progression. Understanding the molecular pathways governing MDSC activation and function is pivotal for the development of targeted immunotherapies [9–11].

Similarly, macrophages, versatile immune cells, adopt diverse phenotypes in response to cues from the TME. They can polarize into M1 macrophages with pro-inflammatory and antitumor properties or M2 macrophages, which promote an anti-inflammatory environment and support tumor growth [12–14]. The balance between these macrophage subsets can significantly impact HCC progression [9, 15]. Molecular signaling pathways and immunometabolic processes play a crucial role in determining macrophage polarization within the TME.

In this review, we embark on a comprehensive exploration of the roles of MDSCs and macrophages in the context of HCC, shedding light on their contributions to immunosuppression and tumor progression. We will delve into the intricate molecular pathways and immunometabolic processes that govern their activities within the TME. Additionally, we will discuss the implications of these findings for the development of innovative immunotherapeutic strategies in HCC, offering a glimpse of hope for improved outcomes for patients grappling with this formidable disease.

2. Myeloid-derived suppressor cells (MDSCs)

MDSCs represent a heterogeneous population of myeloid cells with potent immunosuppressive properties. They are characterized by their ability to suppress the immune response, particularly the activation and effector functions of T cells and natural killer (NK) cells [16, 17]. MDSCs play a significant role in promoting tumor immune evasion and have been extensively studied in the context of cancer immunology [18–20].

2.1 MDSC subsets

MDSCs can be broadly categorized into two main subsets: granulocytic MDSCs (G-MDSCs) and monocytic MDSCs (M-MDSCs) [21]. G-MDSCs are morphologically similar to neutrophils and are characterized by the expression of cell surface markers such as CD11b + and Ly6G+. M-MDSCs share phenotypic similarities with monocytes and are typically identified as CD11b + and Ly6C+ cells. These subsets may exhibit distinct mechanisms of immunosuppression and differentially impact tumor progression.

2.2 Origin and expansion of MDSCs in cancer

MDSCs originate from myeloid precursor cells in the bone marrow. Under pathological conditions, such as cancer, chronic inflammation, or infection, a dysregulated myelopoiesis process leads to the accumulation and expansion of MDSCs. Factors within the tumor microenvironment, including tumor-derived soluble mediators (cytokines and growth factors), can drive the recruitment and expansion of MDSCs. MDSC expansion is also influenced by the crosstalk between tumor cells and immune cells, leading to an immunosuppressive feedback loop [20, 22, 23].

2.3 Immunosuppressive mechanisms of MDSCs

MDSCs employ various mechanisms to suppress the immune response, primarily targeting T cells [19, 24, 25]: T-cell suppression: MDSCs inhibit T-cell activation and proliferation through direct cell-cell contact or the production of immunosuppressive molecules. Cytokine production: MDSCs secrete immunosuppressive cytokines such as interleukin-10 (IL-10), transforming growth facto beta (TGF-β), and interleukin-6 (IL-6), which dampen T-cell functions and promote regulatory T-cell (Treg) expansion. Induction of T-cell anergy: MDSCs induce T-cell dysfunction and exhaustion, leading to reduced cytotoxicity and cytokine production.

2.4 Molecular pathways and immunometabolic processes regulating MDSC functions

MDSC functions are tightly regulated by molecular pathways and immunometabolic processes. Key aspects include [26–28] signal transducer and activator of transcription 3 (STAT3) and nuclear factor-kappa B (NF-κB) signaling: these transcription factors are activated in MDSCs, driving the expression of immunosuppressive molecules and cytokines. Metabolic reprogramming: MDSCs exhibit metabolic

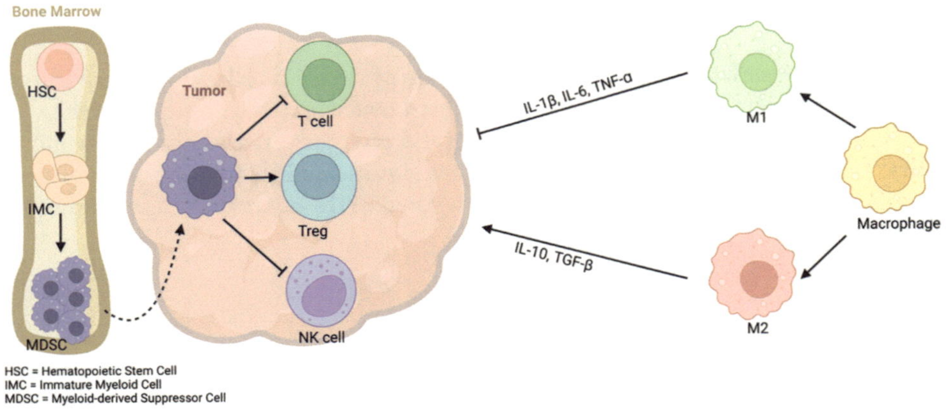

Figure 1.
MDSCs establish an immunosuppressive milieu within tumors by impeding the activity of T effector cells and NK cells while enhancing the functionality of Tregs. Macrophages polarized into M1 and M2 macrophages, producing an anti-inflammatory and pro-inflammatory microenvironment within the tumor.

changes, such as increased glycolysis and upregulated arginase-1 activity, which contribute to their immunosuppressive functions. Reactive oxygen species (ROS) production: MDSCs generate ROS, which not only suppress T-cell responses but also modulate immune cells in the TME [16, 19, 29]. Understanding these molecular and metabolic processes is critical for the development of targeted therapies aimed at disrupting MDSC-mediated immunosuppression in cancer, including hepatocellular carcinoma (**Figure 1**). Strategies to inhibit MDSC recruitment, differentiation, or function hold promise for enhancing the efficacy of immunotherapies in HCC and other cancers.

3. Macrophages

Macrophages are versatile immune cells that play a pivotal role in the tumor microenvironment (TME) [30–32]. They exhibit remarkable plasticity, allowing them to adopt different phenotypes and functions depending on local cues. In the context of cancer, macrophages can be broadly categorized into two polarized states: M1 (pro-inflammatory) and M2 (anti-inflammatory) phenotypes, each with distinct roles and functions [33–35].

3.1 Polarization of macrophages

3.1.1 M1 macrophages (pro-inflammatory)

M1 macrophages are classically activated and driven by pro-inflammatory signals, such as interferon-gamma (IFN-γ) and lipopolysaccharide (LPS). They are characterized by M1 macrophages release cytokines, such as interleukin-1 beta (IL-1β), interleukin-6 (IL-6), and tumor necrosis factor-alpha (TNF-α). These cytokines promote inflammation and activate immune responses. M1 macrophages have an increased ability to present antigens to T cells, thereby stimulating cytotoxic T-cell responses. This is crucial for combating infections and initiating adaptive immunity.

M1 macrophages play a key role in host defense by efficiently clearing pathogens and exhibiting cytotoxic activity against tumor cells [35–39].

3.1.2 M2 macrophages (anti-inflammatory)

M2 macrophages are alternatively activated and influenced by anti-inflammatory signals such as interleukin-4 (IL-4) and interleukin-13 (IL-13). They exhibit: M2 macrophages are characterized by the secretion of anti-inflammatory cytokines, including IL-10 and transforming growth factor-beta (TGF-β). These cytokines help to suppress inflammatory responses, thereby promoting tissue repair and resolution of inflammation. M2 macrophages play a crucial role in tissue repair and remodeling. They contribute to the resolution of inflammation by promoting the clearance of cellular debris and facilitating tissue regeneration. Additionally, M2 macrophages produce factors that stimulate the proliferation and differentiation of fibroblasts, aiding in the deposition of extracellular matrix components necessary for tissue healing. M2 macrophages are involved in angiogenesis, the process of forming new blood vessels. They release angiogenic factors, such as vascular endothelial growth factor (VEGF) and platelet-derived growth factor (PDGF), which promote the growth of blood vessels. Angiogenesis is essential for supplying oxygen and nutrients to tissues undergoing repair and regeneration. M2 macrophages possess immunosuppressive properties, which help to dampen immune responses and maintain tissue homeostasis. They inhibit the activity of immune cells, such as T cells and NK cells, and contribute to the establishment of an immunosuppressive microenvironment. This immunosuppression can be exploited by tumors to evade immune surveillance and promote tumor growth. M2 macrophages play a significant role in promoting tumor growth and metastasis. They create an immunosuppressive microenvironment that supports tumor cell survival and proliferation. Additionally, M2 macrophages contribute to tumor angiogenesis, extracellular matrix remodeling, and the suppression of antitumor immune responses, thereby facilitating tumor growth and metastatic spread. Understanding the functions of M2 macrophages in promoting tissue repair, angiogenesis, immunosuppression, and tumor progression is crucial for developing therapeutic strategies targeting these cells in various pathological conditions, including cancer. Modulating the activity of M2 macrophages holds promise for improving clinical outcomes and reducing the progression of diseases characterized by chronic inflammation and tissue damage.

3.2 Plasticity of macrophages and their diverse roles in cancer

Macrophages are highly plastic and can transition between M1 and M2 states in response to changing microenvironmental signals. In cancer, macrophages can exert both pro-tumorigenic and antitumorigenic effects:

3.2.1 Pro-tumorigenic roles

M2-like macrophages are often associated with tumor promotion. They can stimulate angiogenesis, suppress antitumor immunity, and support tumor invasion and metastasis. Angiogenesis promotion: M2-like macrophages can secrete pro-angiogenic factors, such as VEGF and matrix metalloproteinases (MMPs), promoting the formation of new blood vessels that support tumor growth and metastasis. M2-like macrophages produce anti-inflammatory cytokines, such as IL-10 and TGF-β, dampening antitumor immune responses and creating an immunosuppressive microenvironment that facilitates tumor evasion from immune surveillance. Tumor invasion and metastasis: M2-like macrophages contribute to tumor invasion and metastasis by promoting extracellular matrix remodeling, facilitating cancer cell migration, and enhancing the establishment of metastatic niches in distant organs [35, 40, 41].

3.2.2 Antitumorigenic roles

Conversely, M1-like macrophages have the potential to inhibit tumor growth through various mechanisms: M1-like macrophages produce pro-inflammatory cytokines, such as TNF-α and interleukin-1 beta (IL-1β), promoting inflammation within the tumor microenvironment and activating antitumor immune responses. M1-like macrophages possess enhanced phagocytic activity, allowing them to engulf and eliminate cancer cells directly, thereby inhibiting tumor growth. M1-like macrophages express increased levels of major histocompatibility complex (MHC) molecules and co-stimulatory molecules, facilitating the presentation of tumor antigens to T cells and enhancing antitumor immune responses.

3.3 Molecular pathways and immunometabolic processes shaping macrophage phenotypes

Macrophage polarization is intricately regulated by molecular pathways and immunometabolic processes:

3.3.1 Signal transduction pathways

Key signaling pathways, such as signal transducer and activator of transcription 1/signal transducer and activator of transcription 6 (STAT1/STAT6), NF-κB, and janus kinase (JAK)/STAT, play crucial roles in driving M1 or M2 polarization in response to cytokines and other signals: activation of the STAT1 pathway by interferon-gamma (IFN-γ) promotes M1 polarization, leading to the expression of pro-inflammatory genes. Conversely, activation of the STAT6 pathway by interleukin-4 (IL-4) and interleukin-13 (IL-13) induces M2 polarization, resulting in the expression of anti-inflammatory and tissue repair genes. NF-κB signaling is involved in M1 polarization in response to pro-inflammatory stimuli, such as lipopolysaccharide (LPS) and TNF-α. Activation of NF-κB leads to the expression of pro-inflammatory cytokines and antimicrobial effectors characteristic of M1 macrophages. The JAK/STAT pathway is essential for transmitting signals from cytokine receptors to the nucleus, regulating gene expression in response to extracellular stimuli. Cytokines, such as IFN-γ and IL-4, activate JAK/STAT signaling pathways, driving M1 or M2 polarization, respectively.

3.3.2 Immunometabolism

Metabolic reprogramming is crucial for macrophage polarization, with distinct metabolic profiles characterizing M1 and M2 macrophages: M1 macrophages exhibit enhanced glycolytic metabolism to meet the energy demands of their pro-inflammatory functions. Glycolysis supports the rapid production of adenosine triphosphate (ATP) and provides intermediates for the biosynthesis of pro-inflammatory cytokines and effector molecules. In contrast, M2 macrophages rely on oxidative phosphorylation and fatty acid metabolism for energy production. Oxidative phosphorylation is more efficient in generating ATP and supports the biosynthetic requirements of M2 macrophages involved in tissue repair and immunosuppression.

3.3.3 Epigenetic regulation

Epigenetic modifications, including DNA methylation and histone acetylation, play critical roles in controlling gene expression patterns that define macrophage phenotypes: DNA methylation regulates gene expression by altering chromatin structure and accessibility. Changes in DNA methylation patterns can influence macrophage polarization by modulating the expression of genes involved in inflammatory responses and metabolic pathways. Histone acetylation is associated with transcriptional activation, promoting an open chromatin conformation that facilitates gene expression. Histone acetylation patterns are dynamically regulated during macrophage polarization, influencing the expression of genes associated with M1 or M2 phenotypes. Understanding the molecular underpinnings of macrophage polarization and their immunometabolic adaptations is vital for targeting them effectively in cancer therapy. Strategies to modulate macrophage polarization, inhibit pro-tumorigenic functions, and enhance anti-tumorigenic properties are under investigation to improve cancer treatment outcomes, including those in hepatocellular carcinoma (HCC). Metabolism plays a central role in cancer biology, influencing various aspects of tumor development and progression. Altered metabolic processes in cancer cells not only support their rapid proliferation but also have profound effects on the tumor microenvironment (TME), including immune cells. Here, we delve into the key metabolic changes in cancer cells, the metabolic crosstalk within the TME, and the role of tumor metabolism in immune evasion and immunosuppression [39, 42–44].

4. Altered metabolic processes in cancer cells

Cancer cells often exhibit enhanced glycolysis, even in the presence of oxygen, a phenomenon known as the Warburg effect. This increased glucose metabolism provides a rapid source of energy and biosynthetic precursors for cell growth (**Figure 2**). Key features of glycolysis in cancer cells include Refs. [45–47].

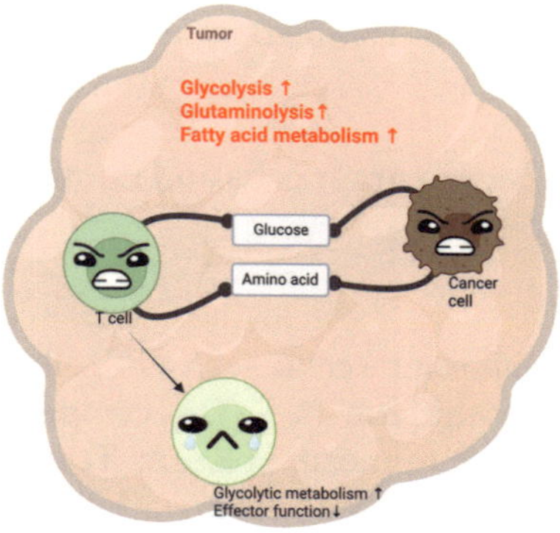

Figure 2.
T cells and cancer cells disrupt glucose and amino acids. T cell loss effector function and glycolytic metabolism are elevated in the tumor microenvironment.

4.1 Glycolysis

Cancer cells upregulate glucose transporters, such as glucose transporter type 1 (GLUT1), to enhance glucose uptake from the extracellular environment. Glycolytic enzymes are upregulated in cancer cells, leading to increased flux through the glycolytic pathway. This results in the production of ATP and metabolic intermediates necessary for cellular proliferation. Cancer cells convert a significant portion of glucose-derived pyruvate to lactate, even under aerobic conditions. Lactate production contributes to the acidic microenvironment of tumors and may promote cancer cell invasion and metastasis.

4.2 Glutaminolysis

Glutaminolysis is upregulated in cancer cells to support the synthesis of amino acids and nucleotides. Glutamine, a non-essential amino acid, is catabolized to provide carbon and nitrogen for biosynthesis. Key aspects of glutaminolysis in cancer cells include: many cancer cells exhibit dependence on glutamine for survival and proliferation. Glutamine serves as a major nitrogen donor for nucleotide biosynthesis and a carbon source for the tricarboxylic acid (TCA) cycle. Enzymes involved in glutamine metabolism, such as glutaminase and glutamate dehydrogenase, are upregulated in cancer cells to facilitate glutamine catabolism. Glutamine-derived metabolites contribute to the synthesis of amino acids, nucleotides, and other macromolecules essential for cancer cell growth and proliferation.

4.3 Fatty acid metabolism

Lipid metabolism is rewired in cancer cells, with increased fatty acid synthesis and lipid droplet formation to support membrane biogenesis and energy storage. Key features of fatty acid metabolism in cancer cells include: cancer cells upregulate enzymes involved in *de novo* fatty acid synthesis, such as fatty acid synthase (FASN), to meet the demands for membrane biogenesis and lipid signaling. Cancer cells accumulate lipid droplets, which serve as reservoirs for stored energy and essential lipids. Lipid droplets play roles in maintaining lipid homeostasis and supporting cancer cell survival under metabolic stress. Lipids and lipid-derived signaling molecules regulate various cellular processes in cancer, including proliferation, migration, and survival. Alterations in lipid metabolism contribute to the dysregulated signaling pathways observed in cancer cells.

4.4 Metabolic crosstalk between tumor cells and immune cells

4.4.1 Metabolic competition

Tumor cells compete with immune cells, such as T cells, for essential nutrients like glucose and amino acids within the TME. This competition can impair immune cell function and contribute to immunosuppression. Tumor cells can consume large amounts of glucose and amino acids, depriving nearby immune cells of these essential nutrients necessary for their activation and effector functions. Nutrient competition within the TME can impair the function of immune cells, including T cells and antigen-presenting cells (APCs), leading to reduced antitumor immune responses and immune evasion by the tumor [48–50].

4.4.2 Metabolic reprogramming of immune cells

Immune cells within the TME can undergo metabolic reprogramming. For example, T cells can shift toward glycolytic metabolism when exposed to the TME, which can limit their effector functions. Immune cells within the TME can undergo metabolic reprogramming in response to environmental cues. For example: T cells exposed to the TME often undergo metabolic reprogramming, shifting from oxidative phosphorylation to glycolytic metabolism. This metabolic shift can limit their effector functions, including cytokine production and cytotoxicity, thereby compromising antitumor immune responses. Immune cells, such as macrophages and dendritic cells, may also undergo changes in amino acid metabolism within the TME, impacting their polarization and function.

4.4.3 Metabolites as signaling molecules

Metabolites produced by cancer cells (e.g., lactate and kynurenine) can act as signaling molecules that modulate the behavior of immune cells, promoting an immunosuppressive environment. Metabolites produced by cancer cells, such as lactate and kynurenine, can act as signaling molecules that modulate the behavior of immune cells. Accumulation of lactate within the TME can suppress the function of immune cells, including T cells and NK cells, leading to immunosuppression. Lactate can also promote the polarization of immune cells toward immunosuppressive phenotypes, such as M2-like macrophages. Metabolism of tryptophan by indoleamine 2,3-dioxygenase (IDO) in cancer cells results in the production of kynurenine, which has immunosuppressive effects. Kynurenine can inhibit the proliferation and function of T cells and promote the generation of regulatory T cells (Tregs), contributing to immune evasion by the tumor.

4.4.4 Role of tumor metabolism in immune evasion and immunosuppression

Cancer cells can produce metabolites that inhibit immune responses. For example, the production of adenosine within the TME can suppress T-cell activity. Altered tumor metabolism can lead to an acidic and hypoxic TME, which impairs immune cell function and promotes immune evasion. Metabolic changes can influence the expression of immune checkpoint molecules on both cancer cells and immune cells, regulating immune responses. Targeting specific metabolic pathways in cancer cells is being explored as a strategy to improve immunotherapy responses. For example, inhibiting glycolysis or glutaminolysis may enhance the antitumor immune response [51]. Understanding the intricate relationship between tumor metabolism and immune responses is essential for developing novel therapeutic approaches. Targeting metabolic vulnerabilities in both cancer cells and immune cells may provide new avenues for cancer treatment, with the potential to overcome immune evasion and immunosuppression in hepatocellular carcinoma (HCC) and other cancers. Immunotherapy has emerged as a promising approach for the treatment of hepatocellular carcinoma (HCC), offering the potential to harness the patient's immune system to target and destroy cancer cells. Here, we provide an overview of the current state of immunotherapeutic approaches for HCC, including immune checkpoint inhibitors and adoptive cell therapies, while also addressing the associated challenges and limitations. We further discuss potential strategies to enhance the efficacy of immunotherapy in HCC by targeting myeloid-derived suppressor cells (MDSCs) and macrophages within the tumor microenvironment (TME) [52–56].

5. Immunotherapy

5.1 Current state of immunotherapeutic approaches for HCC

5.1.1 Immune checkpoint inhibitors (ICIs)

Immune checkpoint inhibitors (ICIs), such as anti-PD-1/PD-L1 and anti-CTLA-4 (cytotoxic T-lymphocyte-associated protein 4) antibodies, have shown promise in HCC. Immune checkpoint inhibitors, such as anti-PD-1/PD-L1 and anti-CTLA-4 antibodies, have shown promise in HCC treatment. ICIs work by blocking inhibitory signals that dampen T-cell activity, thereby allowing the immune system to mount a more effective antitumor response against HCC cells. Clinical trials evaluating ICIs, both as monotherapy and in combination with other agents, have demonstrated encouraging results in terms of tumor response rates and overall survival in patients with advanced HCC [57, 58].

5.1.2 Adoptive cell therapies

Adoptive cell therapies, particularly chimeric antigen receptor (CAR) T-cell therapy and tumor-infiltrating lymphocyte (TIL) therapy, are being investigated for HCC. These therapies involve the infusion of engineered or expanded immune cells with enhanced tumor-targeting capabilities. This approach involves the engineering of T cells to express chimeric antigen receptors (CARs) targeting specific antigens expressed on HCC cells. CAR T cells are then infused into patients to selectively target and kill tumor cells. Tumor-infiltrating lymphocyte (TIL) therapy involves the isolation and expansion of T cells from tumor tissue, followed by infusion back into the patient to enhance antitumor immune responses [59, 60].

5.1.3 Cytokine-based therapies

Interleukin-2 (IL-2) and interferon-alpha (IFN-α) have been used in HCC treatment to stimulate immune responses, although their efficacy can be limited by toxicity. IL-2 stimulates the proliferation and activation of T cells and NK cells, enhancing antitumor immune responses. However, its use in HCC may be limited by toxicity, including cytokine release syndrome and vascular leak syndrome. IFN-α has antiproliferative and immunomodulatory effects, including activation of immune effector cells and inhibition of angiogenesis. However, its efficacy as a monotherapy in HCC is modest, and it is often used in combination with other agents [61, 62].

5.2 Challenges and limitations of immunotherapy in HCC

5.2.1 Heterogeneity of HCC

HCC is a highly heterogeneous disease, with variations in tumor biology, genetics, and microenvironment among patients [63–65]. This heterogeneity can influence treatment response and contribute to differences in patient outcomes following immunotherapy.

5.2.2 Tumor microenvironment

The immunosuppressive tumor microenvironment (TME) in HCC poses a significant challenge to immunotherapy. MDSCs are immune cells that suppress antitumor immune responses and promote tumor growth. Their accumulation in the TME can hinder the effectiveness of immunotherapy by inhibiting the activity of T cells and other immune effector cells. M2-like macrophages, which exhibit anti-inflammatory and immunosuppressive properties, are often enriched in the HCC TME. Their presence can contribute to immune evasion and resistance to immunotherapy. Various other factors present in the HCC TME, such as regulatory T cells (Tregs), cytokines, and chemokines, contribute to immune suppression and create a hostile environment for antitumor immune responses.

5.2.3 Resistance mechanisms

Some HCC tumors develop resistance to immunotherapy through various mechanisms, including HCC tumors may upregulate alternative immune checkpoint molecules, such as T-cell immunoglobulin-3 (TIM-3), lymphocyte-activation (LAG-3), and V-domain immunoglobulin g (Ig)-containing suppressor of T-cell activation (VISTA), which can bypass inhibition by conventional immune checkpoint inhibitors (ICIs) like anti-PD-1/PD-L1 antibodies. Tumor cells may downregulate major histocompatibility complex (MHC) molecules or antigen presentation machinery, limiting the recognition of cancer cells by T cells and reducing the effectiveness of immunotherapy. Some HCC tumors may exhibit intrinsic resistance to immunotherapy due to genetic alterations, tumor cell plasticity, or other tumor-intrinsic factors.

5.3 Enhancing immunotherapy efficacy by targeting MDSCs and macrophages

5.3.1 Targeted therapies

5.3.1.1 Myeloid-derived suppressor cell targeting

Inhibitors of chemokine receptors involved in MDSC recruitment, such as CXCR2 (CXC motif chemokine receptor 2) inhibitors, can reduce the influx of MDSCs into the tumor microenvironment [18, 19, 66, 67]. Agents targeting MDSC immunosuppressive mechanisms, such as arginase-1 inhibitors or inhibitors of reactive oxygen species (ROS) production, can neutralize MDSC-mediated suppression of antitumor immune responses. Differentiation-inducing agents, such as all-trans retinoic acid (ATRA) or inhibitors of STAT3 signaling, can promote the differentiation of MDSCs into less suppressive phenotypes, such as mature dendritic cells or granulocytes.

5.3.1.2 Macrophage repolarization

Efforts to repolarize tumor-associated macrophages (TAMs) toward a pro-inflammatory M1 phenotype represent a promising strategy in cancer immunotherapy. Macrophage repolarization strategies: Targeted therapies aim to specifically modulate signaling pathways and molecules involved in macrophage polarization. Signal transducer and activator of transcription 3 (STAT3) signaling is often associated with the polarization of TAMs toward an M2 phenotype. Inhibiting STAT3 activation can shift TAMs toward an M1 phenotype. Various small molecule inhibitors of STAT3 signaling are under investigation for their potential in repolarizing TAMs. Nuclear factor-kappa B (NF-κB) signaling promotes the expression of genes associated with M2 macrophage polarization. Inhibiting NF-κB activation can promote the repolarization of TAMs toward an M1 phenotype.

5.3.2 Immunomodulatory agents

Immunomodulatory agents can stimulate the immune system and promote the repolarization of TAMs toward an M1 phenotype. Interferon-gamma (IFN-γ): IFN-γ is a cytokine known for its potent pro-inflammatory effects. It can activate macrophages and promote their polarization toward an M1 phenotype. Administration of IFN-γ or strategies to enhance IFN-γ signaling in the tumor microenvironment can repolarize TAMs and enhance antitumor immune responses. Toll-like receptor (TLR) agonists: TLR agonists are compounds that activate toll-like receptors, which play a crucial role in initiating innate immune responses. Activation of TLRs on macrophages can promote their polarization toward an M1 phenotype and enhance their antitumor activity.

5.3.2.1 Combination therapies

Combining immunotherapy with agents that target MDSCs and TAMs may synergistically enhance antitumor immune responses.

5.3.2.1.1 Targeting MDSCs and TAMs

Agents that target MDSC recruitment, function, or differentiation can reduce their immunosuppressive effects within the tumor microenvironment. This can be achieved using CXCR2 inhibitors, arginase-1 inhibitors, or differentiation-inducing agents. Strategies aimed at repolarizing TAMs toward a pro-inflammatory M1 phenotype can enhance their antitumor activity. This can involve targeted therapies directed at specific signaling pathways or immunomodulatory agents such as interferon-gamma (IFN-γ) or toll-like receptor (TLR) agonists.

5.3.2.1.2 Immunotherapy

Immune checkpoint inhibitors (ICIs) such as anti-PD-1/PD-L1 antibodies can unleash the antitumor immune responses by blocking inhibitory signals that dampen T-cell activity. They can enhance the activation and function of cytotoxic T cells within the tumor microenvironment. Adoptive cell therapies, such as chimeric antigen receptor (CAR) T-cell therapy or tumor-infiltrating lymphocyte (TIL) therapy, involve the infusion of engineered or expanded immune cells with enhanced tumor-targeting capabilities. These therapies can directly target and kill cancer cells.

5.3.2.1.3 Synergistic effects

Overcoming immunosuppression: Combining immunotherapy with agents targeting MDSCs and TAMs can alleviate immunosuppression within the tumor microenvironment. This can enhance the efficacy of immunotherapy by overcoming resistance mechanisms and promoting antitumor immune responses.

Enhancing tumor recognition: repolarization of TAMs toward an M1 phenotype can improve antigen presentation and promote the activation of cytotoxic T cells. This can enhance the recognition and elimination of tumor cells by the immune system.

Augmenting immune activation: inhibition of MDSCs and repolarization of TAMs can create a more favorable immune microenvironment, allowing for increased activation and function of immune effector cells, including T cells and NK cells. Immunotherapy holds promise as a treatment option for HCC, but challenges related to tumor heterogeneity and the immunosuppressive TME need to be addressed. Strategies to enhance immunotherapy efficacy, such as targeting MDSCs and macrophages, are actively being explored and may unlock the full potential of immunotherapy in HCC, offering hope for improved outcomes in patients with this challenging malignancy.

6. Conclusions

In this comprehensive review, we have explored the intricate interplay between myeloid-derived suppressor cells (MDSCs), macrophages, tumor metabolism, and immunotherapy in the context of hepatocellular carcinoma (HCC). The key findings and insights from this review can be summarized as follows [68–70]:

1. MDSCs and macrophages in HCC: MDSCs and macrophages are pivotal components of the tumor microenvironment in HCC, where they play multifaceted roles. MDSCs promote immunosuppression through diverse mechanisms, while macrophages exhibit plasticity, shifting between pro-inflammatory (M1) and anti-inflammatory (M2) phenotypes, influencing tumor progression.

2. Molecular pathways and immunometabolism: molecular pathways and immunometabolic processes profoundly impact the functions of MDSCs and macrophages. These immune cells undergo dynamic changes in response to the tumor microenvironment, shaping their immunosuppressive or pro-inflammatory functions. Understanding these pathways is essential for therapeutic targeting.

3. Tumor metabolism: altered metabolic processes in cancer cells, including increased glycolysis, glutaminolysis, and fatty acid metabolism, drive tumor growth and influence the immune response within the TME. Metabolic crosstalk between tumor cells and immune cells further impacts immune function.

4. Immunotherapy in HCC: immunotherapy has emerged as a promising strategy for HCC treatment, including immune checkpoint inhibitors and adoptive cell therapies. However, challenges such as tumor heterogeneity and the immunosuppressive TME must be addressed to maximize therapeutic efficacy.

5. Targeting MDSCs and macrophages: targeting MDSCs and macrophages within the TME represents a potential avenue for improving immunotherapy outcomes in HCC. Strategies to inhibit MDSC recruitment, suppress MDSC immunosuppressive functions, and repolarize macrophages toward pro-inflammatory phenotypes are actively under investigation.

7. Future directions

As we continue to explore the complexities of hepatocellular carcinoma (HCC) and its interaction with the immune system, several areas for future research and development of therapeutic strategies emerge. These directions are essential to advance our understanding of HCC immunotherapy and translate preclinical findings into clinical applications effectively.

1. Identification of novel targets: microenvironmental targets: investigate additional immune and stromal components of the TME in HCC, such as cancer-associated fibroblasts and regulatory T cells, to identify new therapeutic targets.

2. Metabolic targets: explore metabolic vulnerabilities in HCC cells and immune cells to identify novel metabolic inhibitors that can be combined with immunotherapy.

3. Epigenetic regulation: investigate the epigenetic modifications that govern MDSC and macrophage functions in the TME, with a focus on potential druggable targets.

4. Combination therapies: immunotherapy combinations: explore rational combinations of immunotherapies, such as combining immune checkpoint inhibitors with MDSC- and macrophage-targeted therapies, to overcome resistance mechanisms.

5. Metabolic modulators: evaluate the efficacy of combining metabolic inhibitors with immunotherapy to enhance antitumor immune responses while mitigating the impact of metabolic competition in the TME.

6. Patient stratification: biomarker discovery: identify reliable biomarkers that can predict response to immunotherapy in HCC, enabling patient stratification for personalized treatment approaches.

7. Genomic profiling: conduct comprehensive genomic profiling of HCC tumors to uncover genetic alterations that influence immunotherapy response.

8. Translational studies: clinical trials: design and conduct well-designed clinical trials that incorporate the insights gained from preclinical studies. Investigate the safety and efficacy of combination therapies in diverse patient populations.

9. Biomarker validation: validate promising biomarkers in clinical settings to guide treatment decisions and monitor therapeutic responses.

10. Patient-derived models: develop and utilize patient-derived models (organoids, xenografts, and patient-derived xenografts) to bridge the gap between preclinical and clinical research and assess therapeutic efficacy in a more relevant context.

11. Immunotherapy resistance mechanisms: investigate the molecular and cellular mechanisms underlying immunotherapy resistance in HCC. This includes studying the role of immune checkpoints, immune cell dysfunction, and TME alterations. Develop strategies to overcome resistance mechanisms, such as combining immunotherapy with targeted therapies or immune-potentiating agents.

In summary, the future of HCC immunotherapy research lies in the identification of novel therapeutic targets, the development of combination therapies, improved patient stratification, and a strong focus on translational studies. Bridging the gap between preclinical findings and clinical applications will be essential to bring innovative immunotherapies to HCC patients, offering them more effective and personalized treatment options in the fight against this challenging malignancy.

Acknowledgements

This study was supported by grants from the Ministry of Science and Technology (MOST), Taiwan (nos. 108-2320-B-010-045-MY3, 110-2320-B-002-080-MY3, MOST 111-2314-B-A49-072, NSTC 112-2314-B-A49-028-MY3, NSTC 113-2321-B-A49-014 , NSTC 113-2740-B-A49-003), Yen Tjing Ling Medical Foundation (nos.CI-110-22 and CI-111-24 to L.L.W), and the TYGH-NYCU Joint Research Program (no. PTH110001) and Ministry of Health and Welfare (No. 11210). We thank the Taiwan Mouse Clinic Office for their technological assistance and National Laboratory Animal Center (NLAC) (NARLabs, Taiwan) for technical assistance regarding isolators. The authors acknowledge the research collaboration and technical service supported by National Human Microbiome Core Facility, Taiwan. The authors acknowledge the use of Quillbot for language polishing of the manuscript.

Conflict of interest

The authors declare that the research was conducted in the absence of any commercial or financial relationships that could be construed as a potential conflict of interest.

Author details

Chia-Sheng Chu[1,2] and Li-Ling Wu[3,4,5*]

1 Ph.D. Program of Interdisciplinary Medicine, National Yang Ming Chiao Tung University, Taipei City, Taiwan

2 Division of Gastroenterology and Hepatology, Department of Internal Medicine, Taipei City Hospital Yang Ming Branch, Taipei City, Taiwan

3 Department and Institute of Physiology, National Yang Ming Chiao Tung University, Taipei City, Taiwan

4 Health Innovation Center, National Yang-Ming Chiao Tung University, Taipei, Taiwan

5 Microbiota Research Center, National Yang-Ming Chiao Tung University, Taipei, Taiwan

*Address all correspondence to: wuliling@nycu.edu.tw

IntechOpen

© 2024 The Author(s). Licensee IntechOpen. This chapter is distributed under the terms of the Creative Commons Attribution License (http://creativecommons.org/licenses/by/3.0), which permits unrestricted use, distribution, and reproduction in any medium, provided the original work is properly cited.

References

[1] Ferlay J, Colombet M, Soerjomataram I, Parkin DM, Piñeros M, Znaor A, et al. Cancer statistics for the year 2020: An overview. International Journal of Cancer. 2021:1-12. DOI: 10.1002/ijc.33588

[2] Sung H, Ferlay J, Siegel RL, Laversanne M, Soerjomataram I, Jemal A, et al. Global cancer statistics 2020: GLOBOCAN estimates of incidence and mortality worldwide for 36 cancers in 185 countries. CA: A Cancer Journal for Clinicians. 2021;**71**(3):209-249. DOI: 10.3322/caac.21660

[3] Singal AG, Llovet JM, Yarchoan M, Mehta N, Heimbach JK, Dawson LA, et al. AASLD practice guidance on prevention, diagnosis, and treatment of hepatocellular carcinoma. Hepatology. 2023;**78**(6):1922-1965. DOI: 10.1097/HEP.0000000000000466

[4] Llovet JM, Pinyol R, Kelley RK, El-Khoueiry A, Reeves HL, Wang XW, et al. Molecular pathogenesis and systemic therapies for hepatocellular carcinoma. Nature Cancer. 2022;**3**(4):386-401. DOI: 10.1038/s43018-022-00357-2

[5] Yang C, Zhang H, Zhang L, Zhu AX, Bernards R, Qin W, et al. Evolving therapeutic landscape of advanced hepatocellular carcinoma. Nature Reviews. Gastroenterology & Hepatology. 2023;**20**(4):203-222. DOI: 10.1038/s41575-022-00704-9

[6] Chen C, Wang Z, Ding Y, Qin Y. Tumor microenvironment-mediated immune evasion in hepatocellular carcinoma. Frontiers in Immunology. 2023;**14**:1133308. DOI: 10.3389/fimmu.2023.1133308

[7] Sas Z, Cendrowicz E, Weinhäuser I, Rygiel TP. Tumor microenvironment of hepatocellular carcinoma: Challenges and opportunities for new treatment options. International Journal of Molecular Sciences. 2022;**23**(7):778. DOI: 10.3390/ijms23073778

[8] Donne R, Lujambio A. The liver cancer immune microenvironment: Therapeutic implications for hepatocellular carcinoma. Hepatology. 2023;**77**(5):1773-1796. DOI: 10.1002/hep.32740

[9] Lu C, Rong D, Zhang B, Zheng W, Wang X, Chen Z, et al. Current perspectives on the immunosuppressive tumor microenvironment in hepatocellular carcinoma: Challenges and opportunities. Molecular Cancer. 2019;**18**(1):130. DOI: 10.1186/s12943-019-1047-6

[10] Wu Y, Yi M, Niu M, Mei Q, Wu K. Myeloid-derived suppressor cells: An emerging target for anticancer immunotherapy. Molecular Cancer. 2022;**21**(1):184. DOI: 10.1186/s12943-022-01657-y

[11] Barry ST, Gabrilovich DI, Sansom OJ, Campbell AD, Morton JP. Therapeutic targeting of tumour myeloid cells. Nature Reviews. Cancer. 2023;**23**(4):216-237. DOI: 10.1038/s41568-022-00546-2

[12] Quail DF, Joyce JA. Microenvironmental regulation of tumor progression and metastasis. Nature Medicine. 2013;**19**(11):1423-1437. DOI: 10.1038/nm.3394

[13] Wu K, Lin K, Li X, Yuan X, Xu P, Ni P, et al. Redefining tumor-associated macrophage subpopulations and functions in the

tumor microenvironment. Frontiers in Immunology. 2020;**11**:1731. DOI: 10.3389/fimmu.2020.01731

[14] Li S, Yu J, Huber A, Kryczek I, Wang Z, Jiang L, et al. Metabolism drives macrophage heterogeneity in the tumor microenvironment. Cell Reports. 2022;**39**(1):110609. DOI: 10.1016/j.celrep.2022.110609

[15] Liu Y, Xun Z, Ma K, Liang S, Li X, Zhou S, et al. Identification of a tumour immune barrier in the HCC microenvironment that determines the efficacy of immunotherapy. Journal of Hepatology. 2023;**78**(4):770-782. DOI: 10.1016/j.hep.2023.01.011

[16] Gabrilovich DI, Nagaraj S. Myeloid-derived suppressor cells as regulators of the immune system. Nature Reviews. Immunology. 2009;**9**(3):162-174. DOI: 10.1038/nri2506

[17] Gabrilovich DI. Myeloid-derived suppressor cells. Cancer Immunology Research. 2017;**5**(1):3-8. DOI: 10.1158/2326-6066.CIR-16-0297

[18] Chesney JA, Mitchell RA, Yaddanapudi K. Myeloid-derived suppressor cells-a new therapeutic target to overcome resistance to cancer immunotherapy. Journal of Leukocyte Biology. 2017;**102**(3):727-740. DOI: 10.1189/jlb.5VMR1116-458RRR

[19] Li K, Shi H, Zhang B, Ou X, Ma Q, Chen Y, et al. Myeloid-derived suppressor cells as immunosuppressive regulators and therapeutic targets in cancer. Signal Transduction and Targeted Therapy. 2021;**6**(1):362. DOI: 10.1038/s41392-021-00670-9

[20] Groth C, Hu X, Weber R, Fleming V, Altevogt P, Utikal J, et al. Immunosuppression mediated by myeloid-derived suppressor cells (MDSCs) during tumour progression. British Journal of Cancer. 2019;**120**(1):16-25. DOI: 10.1038/s41416-018-0333-1

[21] Bronte V, Brandau S, Chen SH, Colombo MP, Frey AB, Greten TF, et al. Recommendations for myeloid-derived suppressor cell nomenclature and characterization standards. Nature Communications. 2016;**7**:12150. DOI: 10.1038/ncomms12150

[22] Zhao Y, Du J, Shen X. Targeting myeloid-derived suppressor cells in tumor immunotherapy: Current, future and beyond. Frontiers in Immunology. 2023;**14**:1157537. DOI: 10.3389/fimmu.2023.1157537

[23] Umansky V, Blattner C, Gebhardt C, Utikal J. The role of myeloid-derived suppressor cells (MDSC) in cancer progression. Vaccines (Basel). 2016;**4**(4):36. DOI: 10.3390/vaccines4040036

[24] Krishnamoorthy M, Gerhardt L, Maleki VS. Immunosuppressive effects of myeloid-derived suppressor cells in cancer and immunotherapy. Cells. 2021;**10**(5):1170. DOI: 10.3390/cells10051170

[25] Yang Y, Li C, Liu T, Dai X, Bazhin AV. Myeloid-derived suppressor cells in tumors: From mechanisms to antigen specificity and microenvironmental regulation. Frontiers in Immunology. 2020;**11**:1371. DOI: 10.3389/fimmu.2020.01371

[26] Su YL, Banerjee S, White SV, Kortylewski M. STAT3 in tumor-associated myeloid cells: Multitasking to disrupt immunity. International Journal of Molecular Sciences. 2018;**19**(6):1803. DOI: 10.3390/ijms19061803

[27] Wang Y, Jia A, Bi Y, Wang Y, Liu G. Metabolic regulation of myeloid-derived

suppressor cell function in cancer. Cells. 2020;**9**(4):1011. DOI: 10.3390/cells9041011

[28] Dysthe M, Parihar R. Myeloid-derived suppressor cells in the tumor microenvironment. Advances in Experimental Medicine and Biology. 2020;**1224**:117-140. DOI: 10.1007/978-3-030-35723-8_8

[29] Huang J, Zhao Y, Zhao K, Yin K, Wang S. Function of reactive oxygen species in myeloid-derived suppressor cells. Frontiers in Immunology. 2023;**14**:1226443. DOI: 10.3389/fimmu.2023.1226443

[30] Wang H, Yung MMH, Ngan HYS, Chan KKL, Chan DW. The impact of the tumor microenvironment on macrophage polarization in cancer metastatic progression. International Journal of Molecular Sciences. 2021;**22**(12):6560. DOI: 10.3390/ijms22126560

[31] Bied M, Ho WW, Ginhoux F, Blériot C. Roles of macrophages in tumor development: A spatiotemporal perspective. Cellular & Molecular Immunology. 2023;**20**(9):983-992. DOI: 10.1038/s41423-023-01061.6

[32] Ji ZZ, Chan MK, Chan AS, Leung KT, Jiang X, To KF, et al. Tumour-associated macrophages: Versatile players in the tumour microenvironment. Frontiers in Cell and Development Biology. 2023;**11**:1261749. DOI: 10.3389/fcell.2023.1261749

[33] Atri C, Guerfali FZ, Laouini D. Role of human macrophage polarization in inflammation during infectious diseases. International Journal of Molecular Sciences. 2018;**19**(6):1801. DOI: 10.3390/ijms19061801

[34] Strizova Z, Benesova I, Bartolini R, Novysedlak R, Cecrdlova E, Foley LK, et al. M1/M2 macrophages and their overlaps - myth or reality? Clinical Science (London, England). 2023;**137**(15):1067-1093. DOI: 10.1042/CS20220531

[35] Wang N, Liang H, Zen K. Molecular mechanisms that influence the macrophage m1-m2 polarization balance. Frontiers in Immunology. 2014;**5**:614. DOI: 10.3389/fimmu.2014.00614

[36] Yao Y, Xu XH, Jin L. Macrophage polarization in physiological and pathological pregnancy. Frontiers in Immunology. 2019;**10**:792. DOI: 10.3389/fimmu.2019.00792

[37] Orecchioni M, Ghosheh Y, Pramod AB, Ley K. Macrophage polarization: Different gene signatures in M1(LPS+) vs. classically and M2(LPS-) vs. alternatively activated macrophages. Frontiers in Immunology. 2019;**10**:1084. DOI: 10.3389/fimmu.2019.01084

[38] Boutilier AJ, Elsawa SF. Macrophage polarization states in the tumor microenvironment. International Journal of Molecular Sciences. 2021;**22**(13):6995. DOI: 10.3390/ijms22136995

[39] Chen S, Saeed A, Liu Q, Jiang Q, Xu H, Xiao GG, et al. Macrophages in immunoregulation and therapeutics. Signal Transduction and Targeted Therapy. 2023;**8**(1):207. DOI: 10.1038/s41392-023-01452-1

[40] Smith TD, Tse MJ, Read EL, Liu WF. Regulation of macrophage polarization and plasticity by complex activation signals. Integrative Biology (Camb). 2016;**8**(9):946-955. DOI: 10.1039/c6ib00105j

[41] Chen Y, Song Y, Du W, Gong L, Chang H, Zou Z. Tumor-associated macrophages: An accomplice in solid tumor progression. Journal of Biomedical

Science. 2019;**26**(1):78. DOI: 10.1186/s12929-019-0568-z

[42] Kerneur C, Cano CE, Olive D. Major pathways involved in macrophage polarization in cancer. Frontiers in Immunology. 2022;**13**:1026954. DOI: 10.3389/fimmu.2022.1026954

[43] Wang S, Liu G, Li Y, Pan Y. Metabolic reprogramming induces macrophage polarization in the tumor microenvironment. Frontiers in Immunology. 2022;**13**:840029. DOI: 10.3389/fimmu.2022.840029

[44] Komal S, Han SN, Cui LG, Zhai MM, Zhou YJ, Wang P, et al. Epigenetic regulation of macrophage polarization in cardiovascular diseases. Pharmaceuticals (Basel). 2023;**16**(2):141. DOI: 10.3390/ph16020141

[45] Schiliro C, Firestein BL. Mechanisms of metabolic reprogramming in cancer cells supporting enhanced growth and proliferation. Cells. 2021;**10**(5):1056. DOI: 10.3390/cells10051056

[46] Lu J, Tan M, Cai Q. The Warburg effect in tumor progression: Mitochondrial oxidative metabolism as an anti-metastasis mechanism. Cancer Letters. 2015;**356**(2 Pt A):156-164. DOI: 10.1016/j.canlet.2014.04.001

[47] Jang M, Kim SS, Lee J. Cancer cell metabolism: Implications for therapeutic targets. Experimental & Molecular Medicine. 2013;**45**(10):e45. DOI: 10.1038/emm.2013.85

[48] Cadenas-De Miguel S, Lucianer G, Elia I. The metabolic cross-talk between cancer and T cells. Trends in Biochemical Sciences. 2023;**48**(7):597-609. DOI: 10.1016/j.tibs.2023.03.004

[49] Wei F, Wang D, Wei J, Tang N, Tang L, Xiong F, et al. Metabolic crosstalk in the tumor microenvironment regulates antitumor immunosuppression and immunotherapy resistance. Cellular and Molecular Life Sciences. 2021;**78**(1):173-193. DOI: 10.1007/s00018-020-03581-0

[50] Wang J, Li D, Cang H, Guo B. Crosstalk between cancer and immune cells: Role of tumor-associated macrophages in the tumor microenvironment. Cancer Medicine. 2019;**8**(10):4709-4721. DOI: 10.1002/cam4.2327

[51] Xiao C, Tian H, Zheng Y, Yang Z, Li S, Fan T, et al. Glycolysis in tumor microenvironment as a target to improve cancer immunotherapy. Frontiers in Cell and Development Biology. 2022;**10**:1013885. DOI: 10.3389/fcell.2022.1013885

[52] Jennings MR, Munn D, Blazeck J. Immunosuppressive metabolites in tumoral immune evasion: Redundancies, clinical efforts, and pathways forward. Journal for Immunotherapy of Cancer. 2021;**9**(10):e003013. DOI: 10.1136/jitc-2021-003013

[53] Cruz-Bermúdez A, Laza-Briviesca R, Casarrubios M, Sierra-Rodero B, Provencio M. The role of metabolism in tumor immune evasion: Novel approaches to improve immunotherapy. Biomedicine. 2021;**9**(4):361. DOI: 10.3390/biomedicines9040361

[54] Ganjoo S, Gupta P, Corbali HI, Nanez S, Riad TS, Duong LK, et al. The role of tumor metabolism in modulating T-cell activity and in optimizing immunotherapy. Frontiers in Immunology. 2023;**14**:1172931. DOI: 10.3389/fimmu.2023.1172931

[55] Arner EN, Rathmell JC. Metabolic programming and immune suppression

in the tumor microenvironment. Cancer Cell. 2023;**41**(3):421-433. DOI: 10.1016/j.ccell.2023.01.009

[56] Zhang X, Song W, Gao Y, Zhang Y, Zhao Y, Hao S, et al. The role of tumor metabolic reprogramming in tumor immunity. International Journal of Molecular Sciences. 2023;**24**(24):17422. DOI: 10.3390/ijms242417422

[57] Finn RS, Qin S, Ikeda M, Galle PR, Ducreux M, Kim TY, et al. Atezolizumab plus bevacizumab in unresectable hepatocellular carcinoma. The New England Journal of Medicine. 2020;**382**(20):1894-1905. DOI: 10.1056/NEJMoa1915745

[58] Abou-Alfa GK, Lau G, Kudo M, Chan SL, Kelley RK, Furuse J, et al. Tremelimumab plus durvalumab in unresectable hepatocellular carcinoma. NEJM Evidence. 2022;**1**(8):EVIDoa2100070. DOI: 10.1056/EVIDoa2100070

[59] Wu D, Li Y. Application of adoptive cell therapy in hepatocellular carcinoma. Immunology. 2023;**170**(4):453-469. DOI: 10.1111/imm.13677

[60] Rochigneux P, Chanez B, De Rauglaudre B, Mitry E, Chabannon C, Gilabert M. Adoptive cell therapy in hepatocellular carcinoma: Biological rationale and first results in early phase clinical trials. Cancers (Basel). 2021;**13**(2):271. DOI: 10.3390/cancers13020271

[61] Cao X, Wang J, Zhang W, Chen G, Kong X, Tani K. Treatment of human hepatocellular carcinoma by fibroblast-mediated human interferon alpha gene therapy in combination with adoptive chemoimmunotherapy. Journal of Cancer Research and Clinical Oncology. 1995;**121**(8):457-462. DOI: 10.1007/BF01218361

[62] Rico Montanari N, Anugwom CM, Boonstra A, Debes JD. The role of cytokines in the different stages of hepatocellular carcinoma. Cancers (Basel). 2021;**13**(19):4876. DOI: 10.3390/cancers13194876

[63] Zhong C, Li Y, Yang J, Jin S, Chen G, Li D, et al. Immunotherapy for hepatocellular carcinoma: Current limits and prospects. Frontiers in Oncology. 2021;**11**:589680. DOI: 10.3389/fonc.2021.589680

[64] Mandlik DS, Mandlik SK, Choudhary HB. Immunotherapy for hepatocellular carcinoma: Current status and future perspectives. World Journal of Gastroenterology. 2023;**29**(6):1054-1075. DOI: 10.3748/wjg.v29.i6.1054

[65] Hagiwara S, Nishida N, Kudo M. Advances in immunotherapy for hepatocellular carcinoma. Cancers (Basel). 2023;**15**(7):2070. DOI: 10.3390/cancers15072070

[66] Li X, Zhong J, Deng X, Guo X, Lu Y, Lin J, et al. Targeting myeloid-derived suppressor cells to enhance the antitumor efficacy of immune checkpoint blockade therapy. Frontiers in Immunology. 2021;**12**:754196. DOI: 10.3389/fimmu.2021.754196

[67] Wang Y, Jia A, Bi Y, Wang Y, Yang Q, Cao Y, et al. Targeting myeloid-derived suppressor cells in cancer immunotherapy. Cancers (Basel). 2020;**12**(9):2626. DOI: 10.3390/cancers12092626

[68] Ma C, Zhang Q, Greten TF. MDSCs in liver cancer: A critical tumor-promoting player and a potential therapeutic target. Cellular Immunology. 2021;**361**:104295. DOI: 10.1016/j.cellimm.2021.104295

[69] Tian Z, Hou X, Liu W, Han Z, Wei L. Macrophages and hepatocellular carcinoma. Cell & Bioscience. 2019;**9**:79. DOI: 10.1186/s13578-019-0342-7

[70] Cheng K, Cai N, Zhu J, Yang X, Liang H, Zhang W. Tumor-associated macrophages in liver cancer: From mechanisms to therapy. Cancer Communications (London). 2022;**42**(11):1112-1140. DOI: 10.1002/cac2.12345

Chapter 4

Perspective Chapter: Monocytes on the Interface of Metabolic Disorders and Colorectal Cancer

Elena Shmakova, Irina Larionova, Tatiana Sudarskikh and Julia Kzhyshkowska

Abstract

Colorectal cancer (CRC) is a prevalent malignancy with high incidence and mortality rates worldwide. Metabolic disorders, such as obesity, dyslipidemia, hyperglycemia, and hypertension, have been identified as significant risk factors contributing to the development and progression of CRC. These metabolic conditions often result in low-grade inflammation, which plays a crucial role in tumor initiation and progression. Monocytes, which differentiate into tumor-associated macrophages (TAMs) within the tumor microenvironment (TME), are pivotal in mediating these inflammatory responses. Monocytes in the individuals with metabolic disorders exhibit altered phenotypes and functions, enhancing their pro-inflammatory and tumor-promoting activities. Our review describes the intricate links between metabolic disorders and CRC on the level of circulating monocytes, highlighting how metabolic conditions can drive CRC initiation and aggravate tumor progression via programming of immunity. Various monocyte subsets, their phenotypic changes, and their impact on CRC are elucidated, providing insights into potential therapeutic targets for CRC prevention and treatment. Understanding the interplay between metabolic alterations and programming of monocytes-derived TAMs in the TME is essential for developing effective strategies against CRC.

Keywords: colorectal cancer, metabolic syndrome, monocytes, macrophages, obesity, inflammation

1. Introduction

Colorectal cancer (CRC) is the third most common cancer globally, with impactful incidence and mortality rates [1, 2]. The burden of CRC varies significantly by the geographic regions, with higher incidence rates in developed countries, particularly in North America, Europe, and Australia/New Zealand, compared to lower rates in many parts of Africa and Asia [3]. Alarmingly, the incidence of early-onset CRC (diagnosed in individuals under 50 years) is rising, highlighting the need for earlier screening and increased awareness [1, 2, 4]. Risk factors for CRC include genetic predisposition, Western dietary habits, lifestyle choices (such as smoking, drinking, and physical inactivity), as well as metabolic diseases like obesity and insulin resistance [1, 2, 5].

Metabolic syndrome (MetS) is a cluster of pathological alterations that include abdominal obesity, hypertension, hyperglycemia, and dyslipidemia [6]. The National Cholesterol Education Program Adult Treatment Panel III (NCEP ATP III) criteria for metabolic syndrome are among the most widely used. These criteria were published in 2001 and include the following components: (1) hyperglycemia, (2) visceral obesity, (3) dyslipidemia, and (4) hypertension. According to the NCEP ATP III definition, the presence of three or more of these criteria qualifies as a diagnosis of metabolic syndrome [7, 8]. These criteria are used widely in clinical practice and research to identify individuals at increased risk of developing cardiovascular disease and type 2 diabetes. Recent studies have shown that metabolic disorders increase incidence of colon cancer, postmenopausal breast cancer, gastric cancer, ovarian cancer, liver cancer, endometrial cancer, hepatocellular carcinoma, and melanoma [9–12]. Metabolic syndrome can drive the initiation of CRC and aggravate tumor progression [13–15]. Study conducted on a Korean population–based cohort of over 9 million individuals found that MetS correlated with an increased risk of both early-onset and late-onset CRC [13]. This large-scale cohort study demonstrated that higher body mass index (BMI) and larger waist circumference strongly correlate with the development of early-onset CRC, particularly located in the distal colon and rectal sections [13]. Another study of Taiwanese cohort (N = 364,000) established that individuals with three to four MetS components (obesity, hypertension, hyperlipidemia, and/or diabetes mellitus) had a higher risk of CRC and increased all-cause mortality rate compared to those with one or two MetS components [16].

Monocytes, which are the major precursors of tissue macrophages in adult body, play essential role in the tumor development that may occur in the sites of low-grade inflammation [6]. Metabolic disorders can directly affect the functional role of monocytes in the TME [6, 17]. In obese individuals, monocytes are accumulated in adipose tissue, triggering inflammation and leading to systemic metabolic dysfunction, including insulin resistance [18]. The pro-inflammatory activity of adipose tissue induces the imbalance in energy and glucose metabolism, as well as promotes immune dysregulation in the TME supporting tumor progression [19]. Recent study demonstrated that obesity-induced monocytes promoted the development of lung metastasis in breast cancer through the activation of neutrophils in diet-induced obesity mouse model [20]. Obesity-induced monocytes exhibited characteristics of professional antigen-presenting cells expressing high levels of *MHCII* and *CXCL2* [20]. Activation of CXCL2-CXCR2 axis in monocytes led to neutrophil activation and release of neutrophil extracellular traps, which promoted metastasis in a diet-induced obesity mouse model [20]. This signaling axis was also observed in lung metastases from obese cancer patients [20].

Dyslipidemia, characterized by abnormal lipid levels, correlates with poor outcomes in cancer patients [21, 22]. It is associated with tumor invasion, metastasis, and resistance to anti-cancer drugs [21, 22]. Dyslipidemia is implicated in the development and progression of cancer, particularly in patients with type 2 diabetes mellitus [23]. Studies demonstrated a potential link between dyslipidemia and hepatocellular carcinoma (HCC) development, underscoring the impact of lipid profiles on specific cancer types [24]. Recent study demonstrated that mild dyslipidemia, induced by a high-fat high-cholesterol diet, promotes tumor growth by increasing the pool of circulating Ly6Chi monocytes, which facilitate tumor growth and angiogenesis [9].

Under high-fat high-cholesterol diet (HFHCD) conditions, monocytes promote tumor growth via VEGF-A production in mouse model of HFHCD-induced melanoma [9]. Understanding the interplay between cancer cells and the metabolic alterations in monocytes is needed for the development of targeted therapeutic strategies [19].

2. Association between metabolic disorders and colorectal cancer

Metabolic syndrome is a complex disease that is defined by a group of interrelated metabolic disorders [7, 8, 25]. Accumulated evidence demonstrates that the presence of obesity and metabolic syndrome can increase the risk of cancer that is explained by the formation of low-grade inflammation and increased secretion of factors in the TME, which stimulate cancer cell proliferation and inhibit their apoptosis [26]. Metabolic syndrome is associated with a risk of early development of colorectal cancer (CRC). The risk of CRC initiation is increased by 9% with one metabolic disorder, by 12% with 2 metabolic disorders, and by 31% with 3 or more metabolic disorders compared to individuals without any metabolic comorbid conditions [27].

2.1 Obesity and CRC

Obesity is associated with low-grade inflammation that is one of the leading causes of insulin resistance, type 2 diabetes, and cancer [28]. Obesity-related inflammation may induce an increase in circulating fatty acids and the recruitment of immune cells with pro-inflammatory activity, as well as the production of pro-inflammatory cytokines in the adipose tissue [29, 30]. Metabolic changes in obese individuals lead to the sterile inflammation within the adipose tissue. At the same time, gut microbiota can also modify metabolism by activating low-grade inflammatory response. Using a mouse model, the influence of the intestinal microbiota of obese individuals on the occurrence of CRC was demonstrated [31]. Compared to microbiota from non-obese individuals, fecal microbiota from obese individuals transferred to mice promoted colon tumorigenesis [31].

The representative cohort studies confirming the development of CRC on the background of obesity are listed in **Table 1**. A hospital-based case-control study in Malaysia (N = 313) revealed that individuals consuming foods with high pro-inflammatory potential had a higher risk of CRC than did those consuming an anti-inflammatory diet [51]. Many studies have shown a positive association between the risk of CRC and increased body weight [32–36, 52]. A 14-year prospective cohort Korean study (N = 1,213,829) found that high, but not low body mass index (BMI) was positively associated with the risk of both rectal and colon cancers. The association between the risk of CRC and BMI was statistically significant in both men and women, but in men the statistical significance was stronger than in women [32]. A cohort study of Australian patients with CRC (N = 41,114) found that high waist circumference, weight, and fat mass were associated with an increased risk of rectal cancer [33]. A case-control study conducted in Poland (N = 800) showed that increased BMI aggravated the risk of developing CRC [34]. Controversially, a study of a cohort of patients from Iran (N = 693) showed that BMI was lower in patients with colon adenocarcinoma compared to the control group [35]. A nation-wide population-based cohort study (N = 3,858,228) demonstrated that the CRC risk has been increasing with elevating body weight. The risk of development of both rectal and colon cancers was higher in obese individuals compared to normal-weight individuals. This trend was slightly more significant for men, especially in those suffered from

Metabolic disorders	Type of cancer	Patient cohorts	Relationship between CRC and disorder	Reference
Obesity	Rectal and colon cancer	Korea, N = 1,213,829, aged 30–95 years	Positively associated	[32]
	Rectal cancer	Australia, N = 41,114, aged 27–75 years	High waist circumference, high weight, and high fat mass were associated with an increased risk of rectal cancer	[33]
	Colorectal cancer	Poland, N = 800, aged 34–85 years	Positively associated	[34]
	Colon cancer	Iran, N = 693, mean age of 49–84 years	Positively associated	[35]
	Colorectal cancer	USA, N = 85,256, only women, aged 25–42 years	Positively associated	[36]
Dyslipidemia	Rectal and colon cancer	China, N = 843, average age 59 years	HDL cholesterol level was negatively correlated with tumor size; TC/HDL level was positively correlated with tumor size	[37]
	Rectal and colon cancer	UK, N = 384,862, aged 40–70 years	TG levels are higher in cancer. Low cholesterol levels negatively correlated with cancer risk	[38]
	Colorectal cancer	Taiwan, N = 6600, aged 30–80 years	High levels of TG and cholesterol positively associated with the risk of CRC development	[39]
	Colorectal cancer	Japan, N = 123, aged 34–73 years	Positive association of serum TC levels and triglyceride levels with CRC risk	[40]
	Colorectal cancer	UK, N = 2667, aged 40–69 years	No significant differences	[41]
	Colon and rectal cancer	Italy, N = 850, average age 50 years	High plasma levels of TC and LDL were associated with a high risk of CRC. Plasma TG and HDL cholesterol were not associated with the risk of CRC.	[42]
	Colon and rectal cancer	China, N = 576, aged 35–75 years	Serum free cholesterol level was higher, whereas serum TC and LDL cholesterol levels were significantly lower in patients with CRC than in healthy controls	[43]

Metabolic disorders	Type of cancer	Patient cohorts	Relationship between CRC and disorder	Reference
Hyperglycemia and diabetes mellitus	Colorectal cancer	US, N = 54,597, aged 40–79 years	Positively associated	[44]
	Colorectal cancer	Sweden, N = 12,614,256, age range at baseline 0 to 107 years	Positively associated with the risk of early-onset CRC	[45]
	Colorectal cancer	Japan, N = 1,441,311, aged 40–54 years	Fasting glucose levels and DM increased the risk of CRC in men, while in women the risk of CRC increased only with the DM	[46]
	Colorectal cancer	Iran, N = 693, mean age 49.84	No significant differences	[35]
	Colon cancer	US, N = 1923, aged ≥18 years	No significant differences in recurrence rates	[47]
Hypertension	Colorectal cancer	US, N = 54,597, mean age 44.1 years	Positively associated in men	[48]
	Colorectal cancer	Iran, N = 499, aged 30–79 years	Consumption of foods high in blood pressure–lowering ingredients was associated with a low risk of CRC in men and women	[49]
	Colorectal cancer	US, N = 121,700 female, aged 30–55 years, N = 51,529 male aged 40–75 years	No significant differences	[50]

Notes: CRC – colorectal cancer; HDL – high-density lipoproteins; TC – total cholesterol; TG – triglycerides; LDL – low-density lipoproteins; DM – diabetes mellitus.

Table 1.
Association between metabolic disorders and colorectal cancer.

colon cancer [52]. The prospective cohort study of women from the United States (N = 85,256) established that there was an increased risk of early-onset CRC with a high BMI at 18 years of age, with a higher current BMI, and with weight gain since early adulthood [36]. The association between obesity and risk of early-onset CRC was greater in young women compared to women at age 50 years or older [36].

Although the most common criterion for overweight is assessed by BMI, it was hypothesized that the risk of CRC in men is increased with a higher BMI, and the risk of CRC in women—with higher waist-to-hip ratio (WHR) [53]. Despite a wealth of evidence showing a positive association of obesity with the higher chance of developing CRC, an analysis of data from a population-based case-control study conducted in southwest Germany (N = 11,887) showed that involuntary pre-diagnostic weight loss may be an early marker of CRC [54]. It can introduce some mistakes in statistical assessment of the relationship between obesity and CRC. Weight loss in the 2 years before diagnosis was associated with an increased risk of CRC, and weight data obtained several years before diagnosis were a predictor of CRC [54].

2.2 Dyslipidemia and CRC

Dyslipidemia is a pathological condition characterized by changes in lipid levels in the blood serum. Indicators such as the level of total cholesterol (TC), low-density lipoproteins (LDL), triglycerides (TG), and high-density lipoproteins (HDL) are used to determine dyslipidemia [37, 38, 55, 56].

A retrospective analysis of a group of patients from China (N = 843) showed that serum HDL cholesterol levels and the ratio of TC, HDL cholesterol, and LDL cholesterol levels were significantly correlated with tumor size and cancer stage in patients with CRC [37]. A prospective cohort study in the UK (N = 384,862) demonstrated that individuals who took cholesterol-lowering medications had a 15% increased risk of CRC [38]. At the same time, these patients had increased levels of TG in the blood serum. This trend was observed for both men and women, as well as in cases of both rectal and colon cancers. However, among those not taking cholesterol-lowering medications, elevated TC and LDL cholesterol were moderately associated with CRC risk [38]. A prospective cohort study in Taiwan (N = 6600) showed that high levels of TG and cholesterol were positively associated with the risk of CRC [39]. A case-control study in Japan (N = 123) showed a significant positive association of serum TC levels with CRC risk and a moderate association of triglyceride levels with CRC risk [40]. A population-based prospective study in the South Caucasus (N = 2667) did not find a statistically significant association between the occurrence of CRC and serum levels of HDL, LDL, TC, and TG after such confounding factors as BMI and waist circumference [41]. A cohort study in Italy (N = 850) revealed that high plasma levels of TC and LDL, but not TG and HDL cholesterol, were associated with a high risk of CRC. When comparing the risk of CRC in men and women who have high plasma levels of TC and LDL, it was shown that for men the chance of developing CRC is higher than for women. However, among women, the increased risk is typical for postmenopausal people. The highest risk of tumor occurrence was observed in the large intestine, but in less extent in the rectum [42]. In a Chinese cohort (N = 576), the level of free cholesterol in the blood serum was increased, but the levels of TC and LDL were significantly lower in patients with CRC, compared to the control group. The levels of TC and TG in the serum of CRC patients, as well as the levels of TC and HDL cholesterol in tumor tissue, were significantly associated with the TNM stage. The differences were also observed depending on tumor location: patients with rectal cancer had significantly higher free cholesterol and TG levels, but lower HDL cholesterol levels in the blood compared to patients with colon cancer [43]. In a cohort of Chinese patients with non-metastatic CRC (N = 266), TG level was negatively correlated with N stage and Tumor-Node-Metastasis (TNM) stage, HDL cholesterol level was positively correlated with perineural invasion, and LDL cholesterol level was negatively correlated with lymphovascular invasion [57].

2.3 Hyperglycemia and diabetes mellitus

Hyperglycemia and insulin resistance are key chronic pathological changes in type 1 and type 2 diabetes mellitus [58]. Type 2 diabetes mellitus (T2DM) and hyperglycemia contribute to cancer initiation, progression, and tumor response to chemotherapy [58, 59]. In a US cohort study that predominantly included African-Americans (N = 54,597), patients with diagnosed T2DM had an increased risk of developing CRC [44]. A nation-wide cohort study in Sweden (N = 12,614,256) showed that diabetes mellitus is associated with the risk of early development of CRC [45]. An analysis of the Japan Medical Data Center (JMDC) Claims Database in Japan (N = 1,441,311) showed that high fasting blood glucose concentration and diabetes mellitus (DM) were factors that increased the risk of CRC in men, while in women higher risk of CRC was observed only in the presence of DM [46]. In a retrospective cohort study in the US (N = 136), in patients with synchronous CRC and diabetes, hyperglycemia aggravated the general condition of patients [60]. In the Chinese study, patients with concomitant stage II or III CRC (N = 203) and diabetes were more likely to have liver metastases than patients with CRC without diabetes. In addition, the survival rate of patients with concomitant CRC and DM was significantly lower than that of patients without DM [61]. Patients with CRC having DM (US cohort, N = 534) were more likely to have a high TNM stage and lymphovascular invasion, as well as a higher depth of invasion compared to CRC patients without DM [62]. A retrospective chart review of patients with metastatic CRC in South Korea (N = 206) showed that mean glucose level and the presence of DM did not affect patient survival, but elevated glucose concentration was associated with a high risk of infection-related adverse events in patients receiving palliative chemotherapy [63]. People consuming a diet high in fiber and polyunsaturated fatty acids and with low glycemic index had low risk of CRC that was confirmed in a case-control study from Italy (N = 6107) [64].

In vitro and in vivo studies also confirmed the stimulatory effect of high glucose on tumor growth. Using human CRC cell line HCT116, it was shown that insulin stimulated the growth, proliferation, and migration of tumor cells *in vitro* [65]. In a mouse model of colon adenocarcinoma, hyperglycemia stimulated tumor growth by changing the polarization of macrophages toward the pro-tumor M2 phenotype: the expression of the *IL1b, CXCL1, CCL5, S100A9,* and *S100A8* genes was suppressed, while the expression of the *CD163* and *CD276* genes was increased [66]. In addition, *in vitro* studies using human colon cancer cell lines WiDr and HT29 demonstrated that high glucose enhanced the migration and invasion of tumor cells compared to a normal glucose condition [61].

There are also studies that did not reveal the association of hyperglycemia and diabetes with the occurrence of CRC. A study of a cohort of patients from Iran (N = 693) did not show the relation of type 1 and 2 DM to the occurrence of CRC [35]. A cohort study (N = 1923) of colon adenocarcinoma patients from US found that DM was not associated with the risk of colon cancer recurrence. The risk of a second primary cancer was not significantly higher in patients with diabetes [47].

2.4 Hypertension and CRC

Arterial hypertension, manifested in increased blood pressure (BP), may be a factor affecting the course of cancer, in particular the response of tumor to chemotherapy [67, 68]. Several studies showed a positive association of hypertension with the risk of CRC [48, 69, 70]. An analysis using a nation-wide health care claims database collected from the Japan Medical Data Center claims database (N = 2,220,112) showed that the highest incidence of CRC was in the group with stage 2 hypertension with decreasing in patients with type 1 hypertension, and the lowest incidence of CRC was observed in the group with elevated BP. Increased systolic or diastolic BP was associated with a higher risk of developing CRC in men but not in women. Among men, those who suffered from type 1 or type 2 hypertension had a higher chance of developing CRC compared to men without hypertension [48].

Opposite results were also found between CRC risk and antihypertension therapy. Thus, the risk of CRC was reduced with the use of antihypertensive drugs such as angiotensin-converting enzyme inhibitors/receptor blockers and beta blockers in Europe and Asian cohorts [71–73], but others studies found that the use of beta blockers, angiotensin-converting enzyme inhibitors/receptor blockers, and calcium channel blockers did not affect survival of patients with CRC in North American and Europe cohorts [50, 74, 75]. Use of diuretics as an antihypertensive drug was associated with decreased survival in CRC patients in North American and Asian cohorts in some studies [71, 74], but other studies found no association between diuretics use and CRC risk in Asian and Western cohorts [50, 76, 77]. Interestingly, a diet aimed at lowering blood pressure was associated with a reduced risk of developing CRC; for example, a case-control study in Iran (N = 499) showed that a consumption of food high in blood pressure-lowering ingredients was associated with a low risk of developing CRC in both men and women [49].

Numerous studies have assessed the impact of hypertension on patient survival when receiving chemotherapy or targeted therapy [78–80]. In patients with metastatic CRC (N = 289) diagnosed with hypertension, longer overall survival and progression-free survival may be observed in those ones treated with vascular endothelial growth factor (VEGF) inhibitor therapy—bevacizumab, ramucirumab, and aflibercept [78]. A retrospective population-based cohort study in Taiwan (N = 3781) found that increasing age, history of hypertension, and chronic kidney disease were associated with a higher risk of cardiotoxicity in patients with CRC treated with chemotherapy (5-FU, capecitabine) and/or targeted therapy (cetuximab, bevacizumab) [79]. In patients with metastatic CRC from Finland (N = 101) who received bevacizumab, the development of arterial hypertension was the predictor of better survival [80].

3. Monocyte phenotypes in metabolic disorders

Peripheral blood monocytes are a heterogeneous cell population that are traditionally classified into three major subpopulations based on the expression of distinct surface markers: classical ($CD14^{++}CD16^{-}$), non-classical ($CD14^{+}CD16^{++}$), and intermediate monocytes ($CD14^{++}CD16^{+}$) [81–83]. These subpopulations are distinguished by their functions in homeostasis and disease [81]. The heterogeneity of monocytes strongly depends on the surrounding microenvironment that determines the complexity of monocytes in various physiological and pathological conditions, including inflammation, immune responses, metabolic disorders, and cancer progression [17, 84].

In tumors, monocytes are the major plastic source of tumor-associated macrophages (TAMs) that are an essential component of the TME. TAMs play a crucial role in tumor progression and metastasis due to their ability to interact with cancer cells and other components of the TME [85]. TAMs are crucial regulators of angiogenesis, a pivotal process for the supply of growing tumor with nutrition and oxygen [86, 87].

TAMs can exhibit different phenotypes depending on the signals from the TME. They can adopt either a pro-inflammatory (M1) or an anti-inflammatory (M2) phenotype. M1 macrophages are usually associated with anti-tumor activities, producing pro-inflammatory cytokines and reactive oxygen species (ROS), whereas M2 macrophages facilitate tumor growth by inducing immune suppression, promoting tissue remodeling, and intensifying an angiogenesis [88]. Although in many tumors TAMs predominantly display an M2-like phenotype that promotes tumor growth and suppresses anti-tumor immune responses, several recent studies identified that TAMs are not strictly dichotomous (M1 or M2) [89, 90]. Instead, they display a range of phenotypes depending on various signals from the tumor microenvironment, including cytokines, growth factors, and cellular interactions [85, 90]. TAMs can exhibit transitional states and functional plasticity, adapting dynamically to the evolving TME [91]. This plasticity is driven by signals from tumor cells, stromal cells, and other immune cells, making TAM phenotypes highly context-dependent and heterogeneous [85]. Upon recruitment to the tumor site by chemokines such as CCL2, CCL3, and CSF-1, monocytes differentiate into macrophages and are influenced by the local microenvironment to adopt an M2-like phenotype [92, 93]. These TAMs contribute to tumor growth by secreting growth factors that stimulate cell proliferation and survival, angiogenesis, and remodeling the extracellular matrix to facilitate tumor expansion [91, 94]. Clinically, high levels of TAMs are often associated with poor prognosis, and targeting TAMs through various therapeutic strategies, such as inhibiting their recruitment, blocking their differentiation, or reprogramming their phenotype, holds potential for improving cancer treatment outcomes [94–96]. Spatial transcriptomic technologies enable identification of not only diverse phenotypes of TAMs but also the molecular spatial interactions between TAMs and other cells in TME, for example fibroblasts [97].

Interesting is the fact, that instead of numerous cancers, the total amount of TAMs in CRC tumor tissue is associated with favorable prognosis [98–103]. However, the direct mechanisms are still unknown. However, several studies indicated that intestinal microenvironment could induce the pro-inflammatory programming of macrophages [104–106]. Metabolic disorders are associated with alterations in the distribution and function of monocyte subsets. Accumulating evidence demonstrates that monocytes play essential role in the pathogenesis of obesity, dyslipidemia, hypercholesterolemia, metabolic syndrome, and diabetes [107].

3.1 Monocytes in obesity

Numerous studies confirmed that patients with obesity have a higher percentage of total monocytes as well as intermediate and classical monocyte subpopulations compared to healthy individuals (**Table 2**) [110, 120].

At the same time, the number of non-classical monocytes remains similar among obese, overweight, and normal-weight individuals [110]. Elevated levels of classical and intermediate monocytes can be explained by persisting low-grade inflammation in the adipose tissue [120–122]. A recent study demonstrated substantial role of intermediate monocyte subpopulation in obesity-mediated inflammation [120]. $CD14^{++}CD16^{+}$ monocytes were increased in patients with obesity and were associated with pro-inflammatory $CD163^{low}HLA\text{-}DR^{inter}$ intestinal macrophages [120]. Adipocytes in bone marrow can regulate myelopoiesis in individuals with obesity [123]. A short-term high-fat diet caused a shift in the metabolic reprogramming of monocytes toward glycolysis, reduced oxidative potential, and increased mitochondrial fission leading to the whitening of adipose tissue and the activation of $Ly6C^{high}$ monocytes both in vivo and *in vitro* [122]. Accumulation of $Ly6C^{high}$ monocytes in the bone marrow led to increase in pro-inflammatory adipose tissue macrophages [122]. In obese patients, $CD14^{++}CD16^{-}$ and $CD14^{+}CD16^{++}$ monocyte subpopulations showed a higher response to TLR4 and TLR8 activation as compared to normal weight individuals [124]. $CD14^{++}CD16^{-}$ monocytes produced higher level of IL-1β in response to LPS and a higher level of TNF and IL-10 upon ssRNA stimulation in obese patients compared to healthy individuals [124].

Metabolic disorders	Patient cohort/study model	Method of analysis	Monocyte phenotypes	Reference
Obesity	Blood samples (n = 73) from obese patients, Netherlands	Flow cytometry, ELISA	BMI and WC are associated with lower CD14 and higher *CD300e* expression in $CD14^{++}CD16^{+}$, $CD14^{++}CD16^{-}$, and $CD14^{+}CD16^{++}$ monocyte subpopulations. A number of total monocytes and the count of $CD14^{++}CD16^{+}$ monocytes correlated positively to circulating sCD163 levels, and $CD14^{++}CD16^{-}$ monocyte counts had a positive trend to sCD163 levels in obese patients	[108]
Obesity	Blood samples from patients with obesity (n = 105), France	Flow cytometry	The percentages of $CD14^{dim}CD16^{+}$ monocytes are associated with glycemia, independent of fat mass. $CD14^{dim}CD16^{+}$ and $CD14^{+}CD16^{+}$ monocyte subsets are increased in obese patients	[109]
Obesity	Blood samples (n = 110) from obese patients (n = 60), overweight patients (n = 23), and healthy donors (n = 27), Germany	Flow cytometry	Obese patients have higher numbers of total monocytes, $CD14^{bright}/CD16^{-}$, $CD14^{bright}/CD16^{+}$, $CD56^{+}$ monocytes, and M-MDSCs. The number of $CD14^{bright}/CD16^{-}$, $CD14^{bright}/CD16^{+}$, $CD56^{+}$ monocytes, and M-MDSCs, correlated positively with body mass index, body fat, waist circumference, triglycerides, C-reactive protein, and HbA1c, and negatively with high-density lipoprotein cholesterol. Patients with obesity and type 2 diabetes had higher numbers of $CD14^{bright}/CD16^{+}$, $CD14^{dim}/CD16^{+}$, and M-MDSCs, whereas those with obesity and impaired glucose tolerance had higher numbers of $CD56^{+}$ monocytes	[110]
Obesity	Deep subcutaneous abdominal adipose tissue from lean (n = 7) and obese (n = 5) patients, USA	scRNA-seq	$FCGR3A^{+}HES4^{+}$ monocytes, $FCER1A^{+}$ monocytes, and $CSF3R^{+}FCAR^{+}$ $SELL^{+}$ monocytes are accumulated in white adipose tissue	[111]
Dyslipidemia	Blood samples from patients (n = 32) with dyslipidemia and healthy donors (n = 22), Mexico	Flow cytometry	$CD14^{++}CD68^{+}CD80^{+}$ monocytes are increased in dyslipidemia patients compared to healthy donors. Metabolically activated monocytes $CD14^{var}CD36^{+}ABCA1^{+}PLIN2^{+}$ are elevated in dyslipidemia patients	[112]
Dyslipidemia	Donors (n = 22) with a perturbed lipid profile, Australia	Flow cytometry	$IL\text{-}1\beta^{+}TLR2^{+}CD86^{+}CD319^{+}$ monocyte production was positively associated with Chol:HDL-C level in classical, intermediate, and non-classical monocyte subpopulations.	[113]
Metabolic syndrome with diagnosed hypertriglyceridemia	Patients (n = 19) with hypertriglyceridemia and metabolic syndrome, USA	Flow cytometry	*CD36* expression was higher on $CD14^{++}CD16^{-}$ and $CD14^{+}CD16^{+}$ than on $CD14^{dim}CD16^{+}$	[114]

Metabolic disorders	Patient cohort/study model	Method of analysis	Monocyte phenotypes	Reference
Hyperglycemia	*In vitro* model of hyperglycemia	Adhesion, migration, transmigration assays, and Western blot	Increase in monocyte adhesion, migration, transmigration, and pseudopodia formation under high glucose concentrations in comparison to low glucose concentrations. High glucose concentrations increase AKT-GSK phosphorylation by activating of p101 and p110γ subunits	[115]
Hyperglycemia	*In vitro* model of hyperglycemia	Seahorse Technology, cytokine release assay	Under high glucose conditions, monocytes exhibited elevated levels of pro-inflammatory cytokines (TNFα and IL1β) and an increased uptake of oxidized LDL compared to low glucose conditions. High glucose conditions led to elevated levels of glycolysis and mitochondrial respiration in monocytes	[116]
Genetic Prader-Willi syndrome	Serum samples from healthy controls (n = 13) and PWS patients (n = 10), China	65-multiplex cytokine assay	Positive correlation was observed between the IL-1β and TNF transcription levels in monocytes as well as serum IL-1β and TNF levels	[117]
Genetic Prader-Willi syndrome	PBMCs from PWS patients (n = 6) and healthy controls (n = 12), China	scRNA-seq	Expression of inflammatory activation-associated genes (*IRF1, HES1, NFKBIA, ZFP36,* and *ATF3*), and inflammation-related chemokine genes (*CXCR4, CCL3,* and *CCL3L1*) was elevated in $CD16^+$ monocytes from patients with PWS	[117]
Diabetes	Chronic diabetic wounds from STZ-induced diabetic C57BL/6 J mice. Control group—WT mice	scRNA-seq	$Arg1^+ Pdpn^+ Ccl2^+ Cxcl1^+ Fn1^+$ and Plac8 + chil3 + Vcan + $Ly6c2^{hi}CCR2^{hi}$ monocyte subpopulations were increased in diabetic mice in comparison with WT.	[118]
Diabetic macular edema (DME) patients with type 2 diabetes	PBMCs from DME patients (n = 4). Control group—healthy individuals (n = 4), China	scRNA-seq	Monocytes demonstrated increased expression of pro-inflammatory genes (*TNF, IL1B, NFKBIA, DUSP2, NLRP3,* and *TNFAIP6*), inflammation-related chemokine genes (*CCL3, CCL3L1, CCL4L2, CXCL2,* and *CXCL8*), and transcription factors (FOS, FOSB, and JUNB) in diabetic macular edema. The upregulated inflammatory genes, such as *IL1B, TNF*, and *CCL3*, were specifically found in the pro-inflammatory $CD14^{++}$ monocytes of diabetic macular edema patients	[119]

Notes: BMI—body mass index, WC—waist circumference, PWS—Prader-Willi syndrome, DME—Diabetic macular edema.

Table 2.
Monocyte phenotype in metabolic disorders.

Other pro-inflammatory subpopulations of monocytes were detected in obese patients, and included $CD56^+$, M-$MDSC^+$, and $CD163^+$ monocytes [110]. The number of $CD14^{bright}/CD56^+$ monocytes and M-MDSC monocytes among the classical monocytes was increased in obese patients compared to normal individuals [110]. $CD56^+$ monocytes were associated with higher levels of inflammation and produced more pro-inflammatory cytokines and ROS in obese individuals than healthy individuals [110]. CD163 is a receptor that is almost exclusively expressed on monocytes and perivascular macrophages, and it may participate in the modulation of inflammatory response [125]. A number of total monocytes as well as $CD14^{++}CD16^+$ monocyte count correlated positively to circulating sCD163 levels in obese patients [108]. A recent study analyzed gene expression in CD14+ monocytes and subcutaneous adipose tissue biopsies before and after diet-induced weight loss in well-defined male individuals [126]. The body mass index (BMI) declined significantly by 12.6%, serum levels of triglycerides by 30.5%, LDL cholesterol by 11.9%, HOMA-IR by 48.7%, leptin by 62.6%, IL-6 by 4.7%, and hsCRP by 45.4% in the treatment arm during the 6-month weight loss intervention [126]. Lifestyle-induced weight loss was associated with specific changes in gene expression of circulating $CD14^+$ monocytes, which may affect ubiquitination, histone methylation, and autophagy. The study provided insights into the potential effects of lifestyle-induced weight loss on gene expression in individuals with metabolic syndrome.

In vivo the population of macrophages in the adipose tissue of obese mice differed from the macrophages of non-obese mice. At the same time, macrophages from the adipose tissue of lean mice expressed markers of anti-inflammatory M2 macrophages (*YM1*, ARGINASE *1* and *IL10*), while macrophages from the adipose tissue of obese mice expressed predominantly markers of pro-inflammatory M1 macrophages (*TNF-α* and *iNOS*). It was suggested that the anti-inflammatory cytokine IL-10, secreted by macrophages from lean mice, protected adipocytes from TNF-α-induced insulin resistance [28].

3.2 Monocytes in hyperglycemic and diabetic conditions

Pro-inflammatory shifting of monocytes was demonstrated not only in obese patients but in diabetic patients and in vivo in mouse models of diabetes [119]. In patients with diabetic macular edema (DME), monocytes exhibited increased expression of pro-inflammatory genes, including *TNF*, *IL1B*, *NFKBIA*, *DUSP2*, *NLRP3*, and *TNFAIP6*, compared to healthy individuals [119]. These genes are involved in promoting inflammation and are specifically upregulated in the pro-inflammatory $CD14^{++}$ monocytes (with high expression of canonical lineage markers [*CD14* and *CD16*] and inflammatory-related markers [*IL1B* and *TNF*]) of DME patients. Additionally, monocytes also showed increased expression of inflammation-related chemokine genes such as *CCL3*, *CCL3L1*, *CCL4L2*, *CXCL2*, and *CXCL8*, as well as transcription factors including *FOS*, *FOSB*, and *JUNB*. These findings highlight the role of monocytes in promoting inflammation in the DME [119]. Another study demonstrated that diabetic mice showed an increase in monocyte subpopulations characterized by the presence of markers associated with inflammatory response (*ARG1*, *PDPN*, *CCL2*, *CXCL1*, *FN1*, *PLAC8*, *CHIL3*, *VCAN*, *LY6C2hi*, and *CCR2hi*) in comparison to wild-type mice [118]. Similar results were obtained in patients with genetic disorder Prader-Willi syndrome (PWS) closely associated with obesity and type 2 diabetes (**Figure 1**) [117]. Monocytes from patients with PWS exhibited increased expression of genes associated with inflammatory responses (*PTGS2*, *PTGER3*, and *ICAM1*),

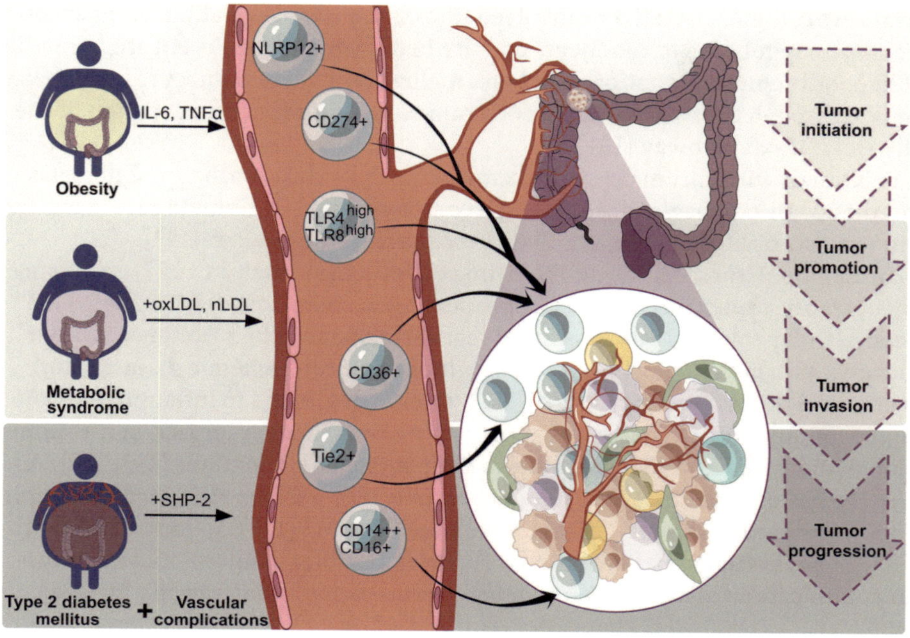

Figure 1.
The impact of metabolic disorders on programming of circulating monocytes leading to the initiation and progression of colorectal cancer. Schematic presentation of a complex network of interactions between metabolic disorders, monocyte activation, and multiple phases of cancer development. Individuals with obesity, metabolic syndrome, and type 2 diabetes mellitus characterized by elevated levels of blood inflammatory cytokines such as IL-6 and TNFα, elevate levels of oxidized LDL (oxLDL) and native LDL (nLDL), and increased levels of SHP-2 which facilitate low-grade inflammation. Low-grade inflammation is supporting by NLRP12⁺, CD274⁺, TLR4^{high}, TLR8^{high}, CD36⁺, Tie2⁺, CD14⁺⁺CD16⁺ monocytes that potentially led to tumor initiation and tumor progression.

as well as chemokine (*CCL2* and *CXCL9*) and cytokine genes (*IL-1β*, *OSM*, and *TNF*) compared to the healthy group. Furthermore, a positive correlation was observed between serum cytokine levels, IL-1β transcription levels in monocytes, and serum IL-1β levels in PWS patients [117]. A similar result was also observed for the *TNF* transcription levels in monocytes and serum TNF-α levels [117].

Monocytes exposed to high glucose conditions showed significant alteration in the metabolic programming and skewing phenotype toward pro-inflammatory one [116, 127]. Monocytes isolated from healthy individuals demonstrated a higher level of the pro-inflammatory cytokines (*TNFα* and *IL1β*) and increased oxidized LDL uptake under the high glucose conditions (16.7 mM) in comparison with low glucose conditions (5 mM) [116]. Moreover, high glucose conditions led to elevated levels of glycolysis and mitochondrial respiration in monocytes, indicating a notable change in the metabolic programming of these monocytes [116]. In patients with hyperglycemia, elevation in CD11c(+) monocytes correlated with obesity, insulin resistance, and triglyceridemia as well as with low serum levels of IL-10 [128].

Mice transplanted with bone marrow from hyperglycemic mice showed an increase in circulating levels of TNF-α after LPS treatment, in comparison to mice who received bone marrow from normoglycemic animals [129]. High glucose concentrations (10 and 20 mM) enhanced adhesion, migration, transmigration, and pseudopodia formation of THP-1 monocytes *in vitro*. Hyperglycemia enhanced monocyte activity by the activation of specific proteins, such as AKT and GSK [115]. Monocyte activation via the AKT-GSK axis involved Rho-A and Rac-1 signaling, emphasizing the complex regulation of monocyte activity in diabetes [130]. Recent study revealed that hyperglycemia in gestational diabetes mellitus enhances monocyte-endothelial adhesion through the overexpression of Connexin 43 (Cx43) and activation of the PI3K/AKT/NF-κB pathway [131].

Individuals with chronic hyperglycemia, especially those with type 2 diabetes, have compromised phagocytosis through complement or Fc-Gamma receptors, and are more susceptible to pathogens like *Mycobacterium tuberculosis* [132].

The angiopoietin receptor tunica intima endothelial kinase 2 (*Tie2*)-expressing monocytes are a specialized subset of pro-angiogenic monocytes [133, 134]. $Tie2^+$ monocytes play role in tissue repair and regeneration, and their presence is often associated with pathological conditions including cancer, ischemic diseases, and diabetes [133]. Functional activity of $Tie2^+$ monocytes linked to inflammation and immune modulation, suggesting that they may have a broader impact on the immune response and vascular remodeling due to their angiogenic functions [133, 135]. A recent study suggested that $Tie2^+$ monocytes may play a role in the vascular complications associated with type 2 diabetes mellitus (T2DM) [136]. In individuals with T2DM, there is often impaired vascular function, leading to micro- and macrovascular complications such as atherosclerosis, retinopathy, and nephropathy [136]. Patients with T2DM had higher expression of Tie2 on $CD14^{++}CD16^+$ monocytes in comparison with $CD14^{++}CD16^-$ and $CD14^+CD16^{++}$ monocytes [137]. The elevated amount of $CD14^{++}CD16^+Tie2^+$ monocytes correlated with heightened plasma concentrations of Tie2 ligands, Ang1 and Ang2, in individuals with T2DM [137]. A recent systematic review and meta-analysis demonstrated that individuals with cardiometabolic disorders like T2DM and cardiovascular disease have higher levels of intermediate and non-classical monocytes, which is attributed to an elevated release of pro-inflammatory factors [138].

3.3 Monocytes and dyslipidemia

$CD14^+CD16^+$ monocytes may play a role in detoxifying oxLDL via CD36 in familial hypercholesterolemia (FH) [107]. The expression levels of both *LRP1* and *CD36* on the surface of $CD16^-$ and $CD16^+$ FH-associated monocyte subsets were increased [107]. FH-$CD14^+CD16^+$ monocytes exhibited an increased uptake of oxLDL via CD36, whereas FH-$CD14^{++}$ $CD16^-$ monocytes preferentially engulfed native LDL (nLDL). FH-$CD14^+CD16^+$ monocytes have an increased expression of surface proteins CD68, stabilin-1, and CD11c and a higher adherence to activated endothelial cells in response to oxLDL and nLDL stimuli [107]. *CD36* expression was higher on $CD14^{++}CD16^-$ and $CD14^+CD16^+$ than on $CD14^{dim}CD16^+$ monocytes of patients with hypertriglyceridemia [114]. In patients with dyslipidemia, the counts of $CD14^{var}CD36^+ABCA1^+PLIN2^+$ monocytes were elevated compared to healthy individuals [112].

Metabolically activated monocytes, also known as MoMe cells, are a type of immune cells that undergo metabolic alteration during inflammation. Before activation, monocytes primarily use oxidative phosphorylation (OXPHOS) for energy production [139]. However, during acute inflammation, MoMe cells shift their metabolism toward increased glycogenolysis, glycolysis, and pentose phosphate pathways [140]. Additionally, MoMe facilitate low-grade inflammation in dyslipidemia patients [112]. Their presence, along with metabolically activated macrophages, contributes to the production of pro-inflammatory cytokines such as IL-6 and IL-10 in dyslipidemia patients [112]. Metabolic alteration during inflammation facilitated the adhesion and accelerated chemotaxis in monocytes in response to chemokines [141]. Dyslipidemia diet (DD) with high levels of saturated fat, cholesterol, and simple sugars led to monocyte dysfunction in non-human primates via reprogramming of the epigenetic landscape [141]. We recently demonstrated that hyperglycemia and dyslipidemia have a cooperative pro-inflammatory effect on human primary monocyte-derived macrophages. Thus, hyperglycemia elevated expression of Toll-like receptors not only in M1 but also in M2 macrophages, and sensitized M2 macrophages to dyslipidemic ligands resulting in the elevated production of L1beta and suppression of IL10 [142]. Collectively, these findings emphasize the intricate interplay between metabolic dysregulation, immune dysfunction, and the pathogenesis of various metabolic disorders, providing insights into potential therapeutic targets for intervention.

4. Monocyte phenotypes in colorectal cancer

Monocytes play a crucial role in colon cancer by contributing to tumor progression and affecting patient prognosis [143]. The characteristics of monocytes in metabolic disorders closely resemble those found in colon cancer. The incubation of PBMCs with the supernatant of the metastatic colon cancer cell line SW620 led to a moderate increase in the proportion of intermediate monocytes (37%) among $CD14^{++}$ cells after 24 hours [144]. Patients with colorectal cancer had a notable increase in levels of intermediate monocytes ($CD14^{++}CD16^{+}$) [144].

Intermediate monocytes are significantly elevated in the peripheral blood of CRC patients, particularly in stages I–III. They have been identified as a sensitive diagnostic marker for CRC with higher diagnostic potential observed in localized disease compared to metastatic CRC [144]. Single-cell profiling of immunogenic landscape of CRC patients demonstrated that monocytes were divided into four clusters according to *CD14* and *CD16* expression: Mo0 ($CD14^{++}CD16^{-}$), Mo1 ($CD14^{++}CD16^{+}$), Mo2 ($CD14^{+}CD16^{-}$), and Mo3 ($CD14^{+}CD16^{+}$) [145]. Mo0 monocytes produced cytokines and chemokines including IL6, IL1A, CXCL1, CXCL5, and CCL20, which are capable of attracting monocytes to the tumor [145]. Furthermore, Mo0 monocytes highly expressed INHBA, also known as inhibin subunit beta A, a protein that facilitates the growth of colon cancer cells [146]. Mo1 exhibited distinct gene expression patterns compared to Mo0, with increased expression of specific chemokines, including *CXCL9*, *CXCL10*, and *CXCL11* [145]. Additionally, high expression of IFN induction genes *IFIT2* and *IFIT3* as well as gene *IDO1* were observed in Mo1 monocytes [145]. The Mo2 monocytes demonstrated the elevated expression of genes of complement system (*C1QA*, *C1QB*, *C1QC*), as well as *APOE* and *APOC1*, which are related to lipid metabolism [145].

In obesity, intermediate monocytes are also significantly elevated [120]. Intermediate monocytes are known to exhibit a pro-inflammatory profile, which is further enhanced in obesity as shown by an increased migratory capacity and response upon TLR stimulation [124]. Both obesity and CRC are characterized by chronic inflammation and immune system dysregulation. Intermediate monocytes, which are elevated in both conditions, play a significant role in mediating these inflammatory responses. In obesity, the increased pro-inflammatory activity of intermediate monocytes contributes to a systemic inflammatory state that can create a favorable environment for tumor initiation and progression.

Remarkably, in T2DM, *Tie2* expression was significantly upregulated in all monocyte subpopulations [137]. However, $Tie2^{+}$ monocyte levels showed an elevation trend in patients with CRC without metastasis, despite no significant difference being observed between healthy individuals and cancer patients overall [144].

PD-L1, also known as CD274, is a protein found on cancer cells that regulates the immune system's response to cancer. Increased levels of *CD274* expression are associated with unfavorable outcomes and treatment resistance in various cancer types, including gastric and endometrial cancer [147]. Furthermore, *CD274* expression has been recognized as a predictor of how patients with CRC will respond to immunotherapy [147]. The expression of *CD274* on classical, intermediate, and non-classical monocytes was elevated in tumor samples compared to non-tumor samples in patients with liver metastasis from CRC [147]. Moreover, colorectal tumor samples with a desmoplastic growth pattern showed a notable decrease in the percentage of CD274-positive and CD206-positive cells across all monocyte populations when compared to non-desmoplastic samples [147]. IL-6, a cytokine involved in inflammation and immune responses, was shown to increase the expression of *CD274* in monocytes and macrophages in both in vivo and *in vitro* models of hepatocellular carcinoma and colorectal cancer [148, 149]. IL-6 downregulates the expression of protein tyrosine phosphatase receptor type O (PTPRO) in monocytes [149]. This downregulation led to an increase in CD274 expression in monocytes, contributing to the immunosuppressive environment that supported tumor survival and progression of HCC [149]. Although the detailed mechanism of $CD274^+$ monocytes' interaction with components of CRC microenvironment are not clear, their roles in hepatocellular carcinoma might share similarities.

Different populations of monocytes have tumor-specific programming and express markers indicating metastasis [150]. Monocytes infiltrate colon tumors and differentiate into TAMs, which further contribute to cancer progression [143]. The peripheral monocyte count has also been linked to prognosis, serving as a useful marker reflecting the TME [143]. CRC patients have elevated levels of monocytes compared to controls, and those with liver metastasis demonstrated even higher monocyte levels in comparison to patients with the primary disease [151]. Our most recent study compared transcriptome of monocytes in patients with colon and rectal cancer, and identified overexpression of PFKFB3, a critical factor that facilitates glycolysis providing energy for inflammatory macrophage reactions [152]. Spatial transcriptomic analysis identified correlation of PFKFB3 with amount and tumor-promoting properties of TAMs in colon but not in rectal cancer. PFKFB3 appeared to be a biomarker for bad prognosis and was indicative for tumor relapse specifically in patients with colon cancer [152]. It remains to be explored whether PFKFB3 facilitates hyperglycemia-mediated low-grade inflammation resulting in CRC progression.

In colon cancer, monocytes can be fused with colon cancer cells to form tumor hybrid cells (THCs) [153]. THCs are a unique population of cells that arise from the fusion of different cell types within the TME. This fusion gives rise to hybrid cells with a mixed genetic and functional profile, thereby possessing unique characteristics distinct from their parental cell types [153]. One of the prominent features of tumor hybrid cells is their enhanced migratory potential [154, 155]. Due to the fusion of different cell types, these hybrid cells can acquire the ability to migrate more effectively, potentially contributing to cancer metastasis [153]. Additionally, tumor hybrid cells may exhibit altered immunogenic properties, allowing them to evade immune surveillance and persistence within the host [154]. The fusion of colorectal cancer stem cells with monocytes results in the formation of tumor hybrid cells that possess unique characteristics [153]. These hybrid cells are reported to have increased migratory capabilities and the ability to evade the immune system, contributing to the spread and progression of CRC [153]. CD45$^+$CD14$^+$EpCAM$^+$ THCs created by co-culture of CRC stem cells with human monocytes exhibit enhanced migratory, proliferative, and immune evasion abilities [153]. The presence of CD45$^+$CD14$^+$EpCAM$^+$ THCs is considered as a poor prognosis marker in CRC patients [153].

CD36, a scavenger receptor expressed on various immune cells, including monocytes, macrophages, dendritic cells, and T cells, plays a significant role in the development and progression of CRC [156–158]. CD36 is a protein involved in fatty acid uptake and lipid metabolism in cancer cells [156]. CD36 facilitated colorectal cancer invasion *in vitro* and metastasis in vivo in mouse model of CRC [156]. Overexpression of CD36 enhanced the expression of the matrix metalloproteinase MMP28 in CRC cells [156]. Furthermore, MMP28 cleaved and reduced the expression of E-cadherin, a marker of epithelial-to-mesenchymal transition in CRC [156]. Single-cell sequencing data of PBMCs verified the highest level of *CD36* in monocytes among PBMCs in CRC patients [159]. CD36$^+$ monocytes were elevated in metabolic disorders such as dyslipidemia and hypertriglyceridemia, but the role of CD36$^+$ monocytes in colon cancer is still not clear.

Colon cancer cell lines HCT8 and HCT116 secreted EGF to activate PI3K/AKT/mTOR pathway in THP-1 cell via binding to EGFR [160]. Levels of cytokines IL-6 and IL-1β decreased by approximately 25% in THP-1 co-cultured with colon cancer cells, whereas the level of IL-10 and Arginase-1 increased by about 100% in THP-1 co-cultured with colon cancer cells compared to THP-1 group [160]. Western blot analysis exhibited significantly higher level of phosphorylated form of PI3K, AKT, and mTOR in THP-1 cells co-cultured with HCT8 or HCT116 cells relative to THP-1 cells alone [160].

Pattern recognition receptors (PRRs) play a crucial role in immune responses by recognizing specific molecular patterns on pathogens and damaged cells [161, 162]. The main types of PRRs are Toll-like receptors (TLRs), nucleotide oligomerization domain (NOD)-like receptors (NLRs), retinoic acid–inducible gene-I (RIG-I)-like receptors (RLRs), C-type lectin receptors (CLRs), and absent in melanoma-2 (AIM2)-like receptors (ALRs) [161, 163]. PRRs can shift TME toward pro-inflammatory direction to support chronic inflammation in CRC [163]. Expression of pattern recognition receptor (PRR)-related genes *TLR2*, *TLR4*, *GAL1*, and *MBL1* were significantly higher in monocytes from CRC patients compared to healthy controls [164]. NLRP12 is a member of PRRs that has a therapeutic potential for CRC treatment. NLRP12 knockout mice exhibit increased colon inflammation and CRC due to enhanced non-canonical NF-κB, ERK, and AKT pathway activation in both macrophages and tumor cells [165]. NLRP12 suppressed inflammation and helped to regulate the levels of Lachnospiraceae, a family of bacteria that produces short-chain fatty acids beneficial for metabolic health. In NLRP12-deficient mice, an imbalance in gut microbiota led to increased inflammation and susceptibility to obesity. In obesity, NLRP12 regulated the activity of monocytes, preventing excessive inflammation [166]. The RNA-seq profile of LPS-treated CD14$^+$ monocytes showed that NLRP12 expression decreased, while *IL1B, TNF,* and *IL6* expression increased in monocytes. Thus, NLRP12 allowed maintaining gut microbiota composition by modulating monocyte activity and inflammation.

5. Conclusions and perspectives

The intricate interplay between metabolic disorders and CRC has significant implications for understanding the pathogenesis of CRC as well as development of personalized therapeutic approaches. Monocytes, as key players in the innate immune system, exhibit considerable heterogeneity and plasticity in response to various signals from the TME and metabolic state of the host. Firstly, it is evident that monocytes are pivotal in shaping the TME. TAMs, derived from monocytes, can develop a range of phenotypes from pro-inflammatory (M1) to anti-inflammatory (M2), depending on the signals they receive from the TME. M2-like TAMs, which are predominant in many tumors, facilitate tumor growth and metastasis by promoting angiogenesis, remodeling the extracellular matrix, and suppressing anti-tumor immune responses [167, 168]. Such plasticity and functional diversity make TAMs attractive targets for therapeutic interventions aimed at reprogramming them to support anti-tumor immunity [167]. Monocytes also sense and modify their phenotypes and transcriptional programs in response to all types of anti-cancer therapies (surgery, radiotherapy, chemotherapy, immunotherapy), and can also predict the sensitivity of patients to therapy [169, 170]. It is of particular interest to identify how monocyte interaction with anti-cancer therapy changes in patients with metabolic conditions.

Obesity, a major component of metabolic syndrome, is particularly associated with increased CRC risk [32–36, 52]. Obesity-induced inflammation results in the accumulation of fatty acids and the recruitment of pro-inflammatory immune cells in adipose tissue [29, 30]. This pro-inflammatory environment not only enhances insulin resistance and type 2 diabetes but also creates a conducive environment for tumor cell growth and metastasis [28–30]. Studies involving human cohorts and mouse models have demonstrated that microbiota from obese individuals can promote colon tumorigenesis, underscoring the multifactorial influence of obesity on CRC development [31, 166]. Moreover, metabolic disorders such as obesity, dyslipidemia, and type 2 diabetes mellitus (T2DM) significantly influence monocyte behavior and function [120, 122, 123]. Obesity, characterized by chronic low-grade inflammation, increases the proportion of pro-inflammatory intermediate monocytes, which can enhance systemic inflammation and create a favorable environment for tumor initiation and progression [120, 122, 123]. Similarly, dyslipidemia and T2DM alter monocyte metabolism and function, leading to increased production of pro-inflammatory cytokines and altered immune responses [107, 112, 114].

Dyslipidemia, characterized by abnormal lipid levels, is another metabolic disorder that impacts CRC risk [37, 38, 55, 56]. Dyslipidemia is associated with changes in lipid metabolism that influence monocyte function and inflammation [37, 38, 55, 56, 107, 112, 114]. Elevated triglyceride levels and altered cholesterol ratios are positively correlated with increased CRC risk, as evidenced by several cohort studies across different populations [37–40, 42, 43]. Notably, dyslipidemia-induced changes in monocyte subsets, such as increased CD36 expression, further highlight the role of lipid metabolism in CRC pathogenesis [107, 112, 114].

Hyperglycemia and diabetes mellitus also play crucial roles in CRC development. High glucose levels and insulin resistance promote cancer cell proliferation and alter immune cell function, particularly macrophage polarization toward a pro-tumor M2 phenotype [58, 59, 66]. Studies demonstrated that hyperglycemia enhances the migration and invasion of tumor cells, emphasizing the direct impact of metabolic dysregulation on cancer progression [61, 65]. Hypertension, another component of metabolic syndrome, has been linked to CRC through various mechanisms. Increased blood pressure can affect tumor response to chemotherapy [78–80]. While some studies show a positive association between hypertension and CRC risk [48, 49], the usage of antihypertensive drugs presents mixed results, with certain classes of drugs potentially reducing CRC risk in specific populations [71, 72, 74, 75, 171].

Interestingly, the study of monocyte subpopulations in CRC patients has revealed potential diagnostic markers [144–146]. Intermediate monocytes ($CD14^{++}CD16^{+}$) are elevated in the early stages of CRC and show promise as sensitive diagnostic markers [144–146]. Understanding the distinct roles and dynamics of these monocyte subsets in CRC could aid in developing targeted therapies and improving diagnostic strategies.

Furthermore, the expression of specific regulators of metabolism like PFKFB3, such as CD36 and Tie2 on monocytes, provides insights into their roles in metabolic disorders and CRC. CD36, involved in lipid metabolism, is upregulated in monocytes from patients with dyslipidemia and familial hypercholesterolemia, contributing to lipid uptake and inflammation [107]. Tie2-expressing monocytes (TEMs) are associated with angiogenesis and tissue repair, and their elevated levels in T2DM highlight the link between metabolic dysregulation and vascular complications [136–138]. PFKFB3 activates glycolysis and can potentially amplify the pro-inflammatory effects of hyperglycemia [152].

Further levels of monocyte programming in cancer can be on the level of their amino acid metabolism. In monocytes of CRC patients, we found that aspartic acid and citrulline are specifically elevated in monocytes of patients with colorectal cancer compared to other cancer types [172]. Our current interpretation is that such changes contribute to the anti-tumor activity of monocyte-derived TAMs in CRC patients. How metabolic conditions can affect amino acid metabolism in monocytes of cancer patients remains to be identified.

Overall, the accumulated data justify the importance of monocytes in the intersection of metabolic disorders and CRC. The interplay between metabolic disorders and CRC is mediated through complex changes in monocyte function and phenotype. Understanding these mechanisms offers potential therapeutic targets for CRC prevention and treatment, particularly in patients with concurrent metabolic disorders. The next task for the research community is to unravel the precise molecular pathways linking metabolic alterations to monocyte-driven tumor progression, paving the way for personalized therapeutic strategies in CRC management.

Acknowledgements

This work was funded by Russian Science Foundation, grant number 24-25-00455 (EK).

Abbreviations

BMI	body mass index
CM	classical monocyte subpopulation
CRB	C-reactive protein
CRC	colorectal cancer
DM	diabetes mellitus
HDL	high-density lipoprotein
IM	intermediate monocyte subpopulation
LDL	low-density lipoproteins
NCM	non-classical monocyte subpopulation
ScRNA-seq	single-cell sequencing

TAM	tumor-associated macrophage
TC	total cholesterol
TG	triglycerides
THCs	tumor hybrid cells
TLR	toll-like receptor
WC	waist circumference

Author details

Elena Shmakova[1,2,3], Irina Larionova[1,2], Tatiana Sudarskikh[1,3] and Julia Kzhyshkowska[1,3,4,5]*

1 Laboratory of Translational Cellular and Molecular Biomedicine, National Research Tomsk State University, Tomsk, Russia

2 Laboratory of Molecular Therapy of Cancer, Cancer Research Institute, Tomsk National Research Medical Center, Russian Academy of Sciences, Tomsk, Russia

3 Institute of Fundamental Medicine, Bashkir State Medical University, Ufa, Russia

4 Medical Faculty Mannheim, Institute of Transfusion Medicine and Immunology, University of Heidelberg, Mannheim, Germany

5 German Red Cross Blood Service Baden-Württemberg – Hessen, Mannheim, Germany

*Address all correspondence to: julia.kzhyshkowska@medma.uni-heidelberg.de

IntechOpen

© 2024 The Author(s). Licensee IntechOpen. This chapter is distributed under the terms of the Creative Commons Attribution License (http://creativecommons.org/licenses/by/3.0), which permits unrestricted use, distribution, and reproduction in any medium, provided the original work is properly cited.

References

[1] Roshandel G, Ghasemi-Kebria F, Malekzadeh R. Colorectal cancer: Epidemiology, risk factors, and prevention. Cancers (Basel). 2024;**16**(8):1530. DOI: 10.3390/cancers16081530

[2] World Health Organization. Colorectal cancer [Internet]. 2023. Available from: https://www.who.int/news-room/fact-sheets/detail/colorectal-cancer [Accessed: June 01, 2024]

[3] Morgan E, Arnold M, Gini A, Lorenzoni V, Cabasag CJ, Laversanne M, et al. Global burden of colorectal cancer in 2020 and 2040: Incidence and mortality estimates from GLOBOCAN. Gut. 2023;**72**(2):338-344. DOI: 10.1136/gutjnl-2022-327736

[4] Wang Y, Huang X, Cheryala M, Aloysius M, Zheng B, Yang K, et al. Global increase of colorectal cancer in young adults over the last 30 years: An analysis of the global burden of disease study 2019. Journal of Gastroenterology and Hepatology. 2023;**38**(9):1552-1558. DOI: 10.1111/jgh.16220

[5] Rawla P, Sunkara T, Barsouk A. Epidemiology of colorectal cancer: Incidence, mortality, survival, and risk factors. Przegląd Gastroenterologiczny. 2019;**14**(2):89-103. DOI: 10.5114/pg.2018.81072

[6] Zhao H, Wu L, Yan G, Chen Y, Zhou M, Wu Y, et al. Inflammation and tumor progression: Signaling pathways and targeted intervention. Signal Transduction and Targeted Therapy. 2021;**6**(1):263. DOI: 10.1038/s41392-021-00658-5

[7] Kassi E, Pervanidou P, Kaltsas G, Chrousos G. Metabolic syndrome: Definitions and controversies. BMC Medicine. 2011;**9**:48. DOI: 10.1186/1741-7015-9-48

[8] Ambroselli D, Masciulli F, Romano E, Catanzaro G, Besharat ZM, Massari MC, et al. New advances in metabolic syndrome, from prevention to treatment: The role of diet and food. Nutrients. 2023;**15**(3):640. DOI: 10.3390/nu15030640

[9] Tran T, Lavillegrand JR, Lereverend C, Esposito B, Cartier L, Montabord M, et al. Mild dyslipidemia accelerates tumorigenesis through expansion of Ly6Chi monocytes and differentiation to pro-angiogenic myeloid cells. Nature Communications. 2022;**13**(1):5399. DOI: 10.1038/s41467-022-33034-0

[10] Bin LY, Moon H, Lee JH, Cho EJ, Yu SJ, Kim YJ, et al. Association of metabolic risk factors with risks of cancer and all-cause mortality in patients with chronic hepatitis B. Hepatology. 2021;**73**(6):2266-2277. DOI: 10.1002/hep.31612

[11] Feliciano E, Zimbalist A, Caan BJ, Mittendorf EA, Dillon D, Quesenberry CP, et al. Association of metabolic risk factors with breast cancer survival in a population-based cohort. Journal of Clinical Oncology. 2022;**40**(Suppl. 16):12089. DOI: 10.1200/JCO.2022.40.16_suppl.12089

[12] American Association for Cancer Research. Your Metabolic Health and Your Risk of Cancer [Internet]. Available from: https://www.aacr.org/patients-caregivers/progress-against-cancer/metabolic-health-and-cancer%20risk/ [Accessed: June 01, 2024]

[13] Jin EH, Han K, Lee DH, Shin CM, Lim JH, Choi YJ, et al. Association

between metabolic syndrome and the risk of colorectal cancer diagnosed before age 50 years according to tumor location. Gastroenterology. 2022;**163**(3):637-648. e2. DOI: 10.1053/j.gastro.2022.05.032

[14] Harlid S, Myte R, Van GB. The metabolic syndrome, inflammation, and colorectal cancer risk: An evaluation of large panels of plasma protein markers using repeated, prediagnostic samples. Mediators of Inflammation. 2017;**2017**:4803156. DOI: 10.1155/2017/4803156

[15] Pothiwala P, Jain SK, Yaturu S. Metabolic syndrome and cancer. Metabolic Syndrome and Related Disorders. 2009;7(4):279-288. DOI: 10.1089/met.2008.0065

[16] Chung KC, Juang SE, Chen HH, Cheng KC, Wu KL, Song LC, et al. Association between metabolic syndrome and colorectal cancer incidence and all-cause mortality: A hospital-based observational study. BMC Gastroenterology. 2022;**22**(1):453. DOI: 10.1186/s12876-022-02505-5

[17] Olingy CE, Dinh HQ, Hedrick CC. Monocyte heterogeneity and functions in cancer. Journal of Leukocyte Biology. 2019;**106**(2):309-322. DOI: 10.1002/JLB.4RI0818-311R

[18] Scheurlen KM, Billeter AT, O'Brien SJ, Galandiuk S. Metabolic dysfunction and early-onset colorectal cancer - how macrophages build the bridge. Cancer Medicine. 2020;**9**(18):6679-6693. DOI: 10.1002/cam4.3315

[19] Richards DM, Hettinger J, Feuerer M. Monocytes and macrophages in cancer: Development and functions. Cancer Microenvironment. 2013;**6**(2):179-191. DOI: 10.1007/s12307-012-0123-x

[20] McDowell SAC, Milette S, Doré S, Yu MW, Sorin M, Wilson L, et al. Obesity alters monocyte developmental trajectories to enhance metastasis. The Journal of Experimental Medicine. 2023;**220**(8):e20220509. DOI: 10.1084/jem.20220509

[21] de Jesus M, Mohammed T, Singh M, Tiu JG, Kim AS. Etiology and management of dyslipidemia in patients with cancer. Frontiers in Cardiovascular Medicine. 2022;**9**:892335. DOI: 10.3389/fcvm.2022.892335

[22] Ma Y, Lv M, Yuan P, Chen X, Liu Z. Dyslipidemia is associated with a poor prognosis of breast cancer in patients receiving neoadjuvant chemotherapy. BMC Cancer. 2023;**23**(1):208. DOI: 10.1186/s12885-023-10683-y

[23] Bielecka-Dąbrowa A, Hannam S, Rysz J, Banach M. Malignancy-associated dyslipidemia. Open Cardiovascular Medicine Journal. 2011;**5**:35-40. DOI: 10.2174/1874192401105010035

[24] Cho Y, Cho EJ, Yoo JJ, Chang Y, Chung GE, Jeong SM, et al. Association between lipid profiles and the incidence of hepatocellular carcinoma: A nationwide population-based study. Cancers (Basel). 2021;**13**(7):1599. DOI: 10.3390/cancers13071599

[25] Alberti KGMM, Zimmet P, Shaw J. IDF epidemiology task force consensus group. The metabolic syndrome—a new worldwide definition. Lancet. 2005;**366**(9491):1059-1062. DOI: 10.1016/S0140-6736(05)67402-8

[26] Mili N, Paschou SA, Goulis DG, Dimopoulos MA, Lambrinoudaki I, Psaltopoulou T. Obesity, metabolic syndrome, and cancer: Pathophysiological and therapeutic associations. Endocrine. 2021;**74**(3):478-497. DOI: 10.1007/s12020-021-02884-x

[27] Chen H, Zheng X, Zong X, Li Z, Li N, Hur J, et al. Metabolic syndrome,

metabolic comorbid conditions and risk of early-onset colorectal cancer. Gut. 2021;**70**(6):1147-1154. DOI: 10.1136/gutjnl-2020-321661

[28] Lumeng CN, Bodzin JL, Saltiel AR. Obesity induces a phenotypic switch in adipose tissue macrophage polarization. The Journal of Clinical Investigation. 2007;**117**(1):175-184. DOI: 10.1172/JCI29881

[29] Ramos-Nino ME. The role of chronic inflammation in obesity-associated cancers. ISRN Oncology. 2013;**2013**:697521. DOI: 10.1155/2013/697521

[30] Riondino S, Roselli M, Palmirotta R, Della-Morte D, Ferroni P, Guadagni F. Obesity and colorectal cancer: Role of adipokines in tumor initiation and progression. World Journal of Gastroenterology. 2014;**20**(18):5177-5190. DOI: 10.3748/wjg.v20.i18.5177

[31] Kang X, Ng SK, Liu C, Lin Y, Zhou Y, Kwong TNY, et al. Altered gut microbiota of obesity subjects promotes colorectal carcinogenesis in mice. eBioMedicine. 2023;**93**:104670. DOI: 10.1016/j.ebiom.2023.104670

[32] Jee SH, Yun JE, Park EJ, Cho ER, Park IS, Sull JW, et al. Body mass index and cancer risk in Korean men and women. International Journal of Cancer. 2008;**123**(8):1892-1896. DOI: 10.1002/ijc.23719

[33] MacInnis RJ, English DR, Haydon AM, Hopper JL, Gertig DM, Giles GG. Body size and composition and risk of rectal cancer (Australia). Cancer Causes & Control. 2006;**17**(10):1291-1297. DOI: 10.1007/s10552-006-0074-y

[34] Lewandowska A, Rudzki G, Lewandowski T, Stryjkowska-Góra A, Rudzki S. Risk factors for the diagnosis of colorectal cancer. Cancer Control. 2022;**29**:10732748211056692. DOI: 10.1177/10732748211056692

[35] Soltani G, Poursheikhani A, Yassi M, Hayatbakhsh A, Kerachian M, Kerachian MA. Obesity, diabetes and the risk of colorectal adenoma and cancer. BMC Endocrine Disorders. 2019;**19**(1):113. DOI: 10.1186/s12902-019-0444-6

[36] Liu PH, Wu K, Ng K, Zauber AG, Nguyen LH, Song M, et al. Association of obesity with risk of early-onset colorectal cancer among women. JAMA Oncology. 2019;**5**(1):37-44. DOI: 10.1001/jamaoncol.2018.4280

[37] Tao JH, Wang XT, Yuan W, Chen JN, Wang ZJ, Ma YB, et al. Reduced serum high-density lipoprotein cholesterol levels and aberrantly expressed cholesterol metabolism genes in colorectal cancer. World Journal of Clinical Cases. 2022;**10**(14):4446-4459. DOI: 10.12998/wjcc.v10.i14.4446

[38] Yuan F, Wen W, Jia G, Long J, Shu XO, Zheng W. Serum lipid profiles and cholesterol-lowering medication use in relation to subsequent risk of colorectal cancer in the UK biobank cohort. Cancer Epidemiology, Biomarkers & Prevention. 2023;**32**(4):524-530. DOI: 10.1158/1055-9965.EPI-22-1170

[39] Hsu SH, Syu DK, Chen YC, Liu CK, Sun CA, Chen M. The association between hypertriglyceridemia and colorectal cancer: A Long-term community cohort study in Taiwan. International Journal of Environmental Research and Public Health. 2022;**19**(13):7804. DOI: 10.3390/ijerph19137804

[40] Yamada K, Araki S, Tamura M, Sakai I, Takahashi Y, Kashihara H, et al.

Relation of serum total cholesterol, serum triglycerides and fasting plasma glucose to colorectal carcinoma in situ. International Journal of Epidemiology. 1998;**27**(5):794-798. DOI: 10.1093/ije/27.5.794

[41] Fang Z, He M, Song M. Serum lipid profiles and risk of colorectal cancer: A prospective cohort study in the UK biobank. British Journal of Cancer. 2021;**124**(3):663-670. DOI: 10.1038/s41416-020-01143-6

[42] Agnoli C, Grioni S, Sieri S, Sacerdote C, Vineis P, Tumino R, et al. Colorectal cancer risk and dyslipidemia: A case-cohort study nested in an Italian multicentre cohort. Cancer Epidemiology. 2014;**38**(2):144-151. DOI: 10.1016/j.canep.2014.02.002

[43] Zhang X, Zhao XW, Liu DB, Han CZ, Du LL, Jing JX, et al. Lipid levels in serum and cancerous tissues of colorectal cancer patients. World Journal of Gastroenterology. 2014;**20**(26):8646-8652. DOI: 10.3748/wjg.v20.i26.8646

[44] Lawler T, Walts ZL, Steinwandel M, Lipworth L, Murff HJ, Zheng W, et al. Type 2 diabetes and colorectal cancer risk. JAMA Network Open. 2023;**6**(11):e2343333. DOI: 10.1001/jamanetworkopen.2023.43333

[45] Khan UA, Fallah M, Sundquist K, Sundquist J, Brenner H, Kharazmi E. Risk of colorectal cancer in patients with diabetes mellitus: A Swedish nationwide cohort study. PLoS Medicine. 2020;**17**(11):e1003431. DOI: 10.1371/JOURNAL.PMED.1003431

[46] Itoh H, Kaneko H, Okada A, Yano Y, Morita K, Seki H, et al. Fasting plasma glucose and incident colorectal cancer: Analysis of a nationwide epidemiological database. The Journal of Clinical Endocrinology and Metabolism. 2021;**106**(11):e4448-e4458. DOI: 10.1210/clinem/dgab466

[47] Chubak J, Yu O, Ziebell RA, Bowles EJA, Sterrett AT, Fujii MM, et al. Risk of colon cancer recurrence in relation to diabetes. Cancer Causes & Control. 2018;**29**(11):1093-1103. DOI: 10.1007/s10552-018-1083-3

[48] Kaneko H, Yano Y, Itoh H, Morita K, Kiriyama H, Kamon T, et al. Untreated hypertension and subsequent incidence of colorectal cancer: Analysis of a nationwide epidemiological database. Journal of the American Heart Association. 2021;**10**(22):e022479. DOI: 10.1161/JAHA.121.022479

[49] Jafari Nasab S, Ghanavati M, Rafiee P, Bahrami A, Majidi N, Clark CCT, et al. A case-control study of dietary approaches to stop hypertension (DASH) diets, colorectal cancer and adenomas among Iranian population. BMC Cancer. 2021;**21**(1):1050. DOI: 10.1186/s12885-021-08786-5

[50] Zhang Y, Song M, Chan AT, Meyerhardt JA, Willett WC, Giovannucci EL. Long-term use of antihypertensive medications, hypertension and colorectal cancer risk and mortality: A prospective cohort study. British Journal of Cancer. 2022;**127**(11):1974-1982. DOI: 10.1038/s41416-022-01975-4

[51] Shafiee NH, Razalli NH, Shahril MR, Muhammad Nawawi KN, Mohd Mokhtar N, Abd Rashid AA, et al. Dietary inflammatory index, obesity, and the incidence of colorectal cancer: Findings from a hospital-based case-control study in Malaysia. Nutrients. 2023;**15**(4):982. DOI: 10.3390/nu15040982

[52] Seo JY, Jin EH, Chung GE, Kim YS, Bae JH, Yim JY, et al. The

risk of colorectal cancer according to obesity status at four-year intervals: A nationwide population-based cohort study. Scientific Reports. 2023;**13**(1):8928. DOI: 10.1038/s41598-023-36111-6

[53] Bull CJ, Bell JA, Murphy N, Sanderson E, Davey Smith G, Timpson NJ, et al. Adiposity, metabolites, and colorectal cancer risk: Mendelian randomization study. BMC Medicine. 2020;**18**(1):396. DOI: 10.1186/s12916-020-01855-9

[54] Mandic M, Safizadeh F, Niedermaier T, Hoffmeister M, Brenner H. Association of overweight, obesity, and recent weight loss with colorectal cancer risk. JAMA Network Open. 2023;**6**(4):e239556. DOI: 10.1001/jamanetworkopen.2023.9556

[55] Muc-Wierzgoń M, Nowakowska-Zajdel E, Dzięgielewska-Gęsiak S, Kokot T, Klakla K, Fatyga E, et al. Specific metabolic biomarkers as risk and prognostic factors in colorectal cancer. World Journal of Gastroenterology. 2014;**20**(29):9759-9774. DOI: 10.3748/wjg.v20.i29.9759

[56] Yao X, Tian Z. Dyslipidemia and colorectal cancer risk: A meta-analysis of prospective studies. Cancer Causes & Control. 2015;**26**(2):257-268. DOI: 10.1007/s10552-014-0507-y

[57] Hong TT, Shen D, Chen XP, Wu XH, Hua D. Preoperative serum lipid profile and outcome in nonmetastatic colorectal cancer. Chronic Diseases and Translational Medicine. 2016;**2**(4):241-249. DOI: 10.1016/j.cdtm.2016.11.015

[58] Sciacca L, Vigneri R, Tumminia A, Frasca F, Squatrito S, Frittitta L, et al. Clinical and molecular mechanisms favoring cancer initiation and progression in diabetic patients. Nutrition, Metabolism, and Cardiovascular Diseases. 2013;**23**(9):808-815. DOI: 10.1016/j.numecd.2013.05.006

[59] Cheng HC, Chang TK, Su WC, Tsai HL, Wang JY. Narrative review of the influence of diabetes mellitus and hyperglycemia on colorectal cancer risk and oncological outcomes. Translational Oncology. 2021;**14**(7):101089. DOI: 10.1016/j.tranon.2021.101089

[60] Storey S, Luo X, Ofner S, Perkins SM, Von Ah D. Hyperglycemia, symptoms, and symptom clusters in colorectal cancer survivors with type 2 diabetes. Supportive Care in Cancer. 2022;**30**(12):10149-10157. DOI: 10.1007/s00520-022-07442-3

[61] Wang B, Wang S, Wang W, Liu E, Guo S, Zhao C, et al. Hyperglycemia promotes liver metastasis of colorectal cancer via upregulation of integrin αvβ6. Medical Science Monitor. 2021;**27**:e930921. DOI: 10.12659/MSM.930921

[62] Sharma A, Ng H, Kumar A, Teli K, Randhawa J, Record J, et al. Colorectal cancer: Histopathologic differences in tumor characteristics between patients with and without diabetes. Clinical Colorectal Cancer. 2014;**13**(1):54-61. DOI: 10.1016/j.clcc.2013.10.002

[63] Hong YJ, Han HS, Jeong Y, Jeong J, Lim SN, Choi HJ, et al. Impact of hyperglycemia on survival and infection-related adverse events in patients with metastatic colorectal cancer who were receiving palliative chemotherapy. Cancer Research and Treatment. 2014;**46**(3):288-296. DOI: 10.4143/crt.2014.46.3.288

[64] Natale A, Turati F, Taborelli M, Giacosa A, Augustin LSA, Crispo A, et al. Diabetes risk reduction diet and colorectal cancer risk. Cancer

Epidemiology, Biomarkers & Prevention. 2024;**33**(5):731-738. DOI: 10.1158/1055-9965.EPI-23-1400

[65] Lu CC, Chu PY, Hsia SM, Wu CH, Tung YT, Yen GC. Insulin induction instigates cell proliferation and metastasis in human colorectal cancer cells. International Journal of Oncology. 2017;**50**(2):736-744. DOI: 10.3892/ijo.2017.3844

[66] Rodrigues Mantuano N, Stanczak MA, de Oliveira IA, Kirchhammer N, Filardy AA, Monaco G, et al. Hyperglycemia enhances cancer immune evasion by inducing alternative macrophage polarization through increased O-GlcNAcylation. Cancer Immunologic Research. 2020;**8**(10):1262-1272. DOI: 10.1158/2326-6066.CIR-19-0904

[67] Elliott WJ. Systemic hypertension. Current Problems in Cardiology. 2007;**32**(4):201-259. DOI: 10.1016/j.cpcardiol.2007.01.002

[68] Milan A, Puglisi E, Ferrari L, Bruno G, Losano I, Veglio F. Arterial hypertension and cancer. International Journal of Cancer. 2014;**134**(10):2269-2277. DOI: 10.1002/ijc.28334

[69] Xuan K, Zhao T, Sun C, Patel AS, Liu H, Chen X, et al. The association between hypertension and colorectal cancer: A meta-analysis of observational studies. European Journal of Cancer Prevention. 2021;**30**(1):84-96. DOI: 10.1097/CEJ.0000000000000578

[70] Seretis A, Cividini S, Markozannes G, Tseretopoulou X, Lopez DS, Ntzani EE, et al. Association between blood pressure and risk of cancer development: A systematic review and meta-analysis of observational studies. Scientific Reports. 2019;**9**(1):8565. DOI: 10.1038/s41598-019-45014-4

[71] Cui Y, Wen W, Zheng T, Li H, Gao YT, Cai H, et al. Use of antihypertensive medications and survival rates for breast, colorectal, lung, or stomach cancer. American Journal of Epidemiology. 2019;**188**(8):1512-1528. DOI: 10.1093/aje/kwz106

[72] Deng Y, Xie Y, Wang M, Xu P, Wei B, Li N, et al. Effects of antihypertensive drugs use on risk and prognosis of colorectal cancer: A meta-analysis of 37 observational studies. Frontiers in Pharmacology. 2021;**12**:670657. DOI: 10.3389/fphar.2021.670657

[73] Makar GA, Holmes JH, Yang YX. Angiotensin-converting enzyme inhibitor therapy and colorectal cancer risk. Journal of the National Cancer Institute. 2014;**106**(2):djt374. DOI: 10.1093/jnci/djt374

[74] Holmes S, Griffith EJ, Musto G, Minuk GY. Antihypertensive medications and survival in patients with cancer: A population-based retrospective cohort study. Cancer Epidemiology. 2013;**37**(6):881-885. DOI: 10.1016/j.canep.2013.09.001

[75] Hicks BM, Murray LJ, Powe DG, Hughes CM, Cardwell CR. β-Blocker usage and colorectal cancer mortality: A nested case-control study in the UK clinical practice research datalink cohort. Annals of Oncology. 2013;**24**(12):3100-3106. DOI: 10.1093/annonc/mdt381

[76] Boudreau DM, Koehler E, Rulyak SJ, Haneuse S, Harrison R, Mandelson MT. Cardiovascular medication use and risk for colorectal cancer. Cancer Epidemiology, Biomarkers & Prevention. 2008;**17**(11):3076-3080. DOI: 10.1158/1055-9965.EPI-08-0095

[77] Qi J, An R, Bhatti P, Spinelli JJ, Murphy RA. Anti-hypertensive medications and risk of colorectal

cancer: A systematic review and meta-analysis. Cancer Causes & Control. 2022;**33**(6):801-812. DOI: 10.1007/s10552-022-01570-1

[78] Osumi H, Shinozaki E, Ooki A, Wakatsuki T, Kamiimabeppu D, Sato T, et al. Early hypertension and neutropenia are predictors of treatment efficacy in metastatic colorectal cancer patients administered FOLFIRI and vascular endothelial growth factor inhibitors as second-line chemotherapy. Cancer Medicine. 2021;**10**(2):615-625. DOI: 10.1002/cam4.3638

[79] Ho CC, Wen PC, Yu WC, Hu YW, Yang CC. Pre-existing chronic kidney disease and hypertension increased the risk of cardiotoxicity among colorectal cancer patients treated with anticancer drugs. Journal of the Chinese Medical Association. 2021;**84**(9):877-884. DOI: 10.1097/JCMA.0000000000000590

[80] Österlund P, Soveri LM, Isoniemi H, Poussa T, Alanko T, Bono P. Hypertension and overall survival in metastatic colorectal cancer patients treated with bevacizumab-containing chemotherapy. British Journal of Cancer. 2011;**104**(4):599-604. DOI: 10.1038/bjc.2011.2

[81] Kapellos TS, Bonaguro L, Gemünd I, Reusch N, Saglam A, Hinkley ER, et al. Human monocyte subsets and phenotypes in major chronic inflammatory diseases. Frontiers in Immunology. 2019;**10**:482347. DOI: 10.3389/fimmu.2019.02035

[82] Thomas GD, Hamers AAJ, Nakao C, Marcovecchio P, Taylor AM, McSkimming C, et al. Human blood monocyte subsets: A new gating strategy defined using cell surface markers identified by mass cytometry. Arteriosclerosis, Thrombosis, and Vascular Biology. 2017;**37**(8):1548-1558. DOI: 10.1161/ATVBAHA.117.309145

[83] Ziegler-Heitbrock L, Ancuta P, Crowe S, Dalod M, Grau V, Hart D, et al. Nomenclature of monocytes and dendritic cells in blood. Blood. 2010;**116**(16):e74-80. DOI: 10.1182/BLOOD-2010-02-258558

[84] Stansfield BK, Ingram DA. Clinical significance of monocyte heterogeneity. Clinical and Translational Medicine. 2015;**4**:5. DOI: 10.1186/S40169-014-0040-3

[85] Larionova I, Tuguzbaeva G, Ponomaryova A, Stakheyeva M, Cherdyntseva N, Pavlov V, et al. Tumor-associated macrophages in human breast, colorectal, lung, ovarian and prostate cancers. Frontiers in Oncology. 2020;**10**:566511. DOI: 10.3389/fonc.2020.566511

[86] Kazakova E, Rakina M, Sudarskikh T, Iamshchikov P, Tarasova A, Tashireva L, et al. Angiogenesis regulators S100A4, SPARC and SPP1 correlate with macrophage infiltration and are prognostic biomarkers in colon and rectal cancers. Frontiers in Oncology. 2023;**13**:1058337. DOI: 10.3389/FONC.2023.1058337/FULL

[87] Larionova I, Kazakova E, Gerashchenko T, Kzhyshkowska J. New angiogenic regulators produced by TAMs: Perspective for targeting tumor angiogenesis. Cancers. 2021;**13**(13):3253

[88] Mantovani A, Sozzani S, Locati M, Allavena P, Sica A. Macrophage polarization: Tumor-associated macrophages as a paradigm for polarized M2 mononuclear phagocytes. Trends in Immunology. 2002;**23**(11):549-555. DOI: 10.1016/s1471-4906(02)02302-5

[89] Noy R, Pollard JW. Tumor-associated macrophages: From mechanisms to

therapy. Immunity. 2014;**41**(1):49-61. DOI: 10.1016/j.immuni.2014.06.010

[90] Gordon S, Martinez FO. Alternative activation of macrophages: Mechanism and functions. Immunity. 2010;**32**(5):593-604. DOI: 10.1016/j.immuni.2010.05.007

[91] Larionova I, Cherdyntseva N, Liu T, Patysheva M, Rakina M, Kzhyshkowska J. Interaction of tumor-associated macrophages and cancer chemotherapy. Oncoimmunology. 2019;**8**(7):1596004. DOI: 10.1080/2162402X.2019.1596004

[92] Caverzán MD, Beaugé L, Oliveda PM, Cesca González B, Bühler EM, Ibarra LE. Exploring monocytes-macrophages in immune microenvironment of glioblastoma for the design of novel therapeutic strategies. Brain Sciences. 2023;**13**(4):542. DOI: 10.3390/brainsci13040542

[93] Ozga AJ, Chow MT, Luster AD. Chemokines and the immune response to cancer. Immunity. 2021;**54**(5):859-874. DOI: 10.1016/j.immuni.2021.01.012

[94] Dallavalasa S, Beeraka NM, Basavaraju CG, Tulimilli SV, Sadhu SP, Rajesh K, et al. The role of tumor associated macrophages (TAMs) in cancer progression, chemoresistance, angiogenesis and metastasis - current status. Current Medicinal Chemistry. 2021;**28**(39):8203-8236. DOI: 10.2174/0929867328666210720143721

[95] Li M, He L, Zhu J, Zhang P, Liang S. Targeting tumor-associated macrophages for cancer treatment. Cell & Bioscience. 2022;**12**(1):85. DOI: 10.1186/s13578-022-00823-5

[96] Pan Y, Yu Y, Wang X, Zhang T. Tumor-associated macrophages in tumor immunity. Frontiers in Immunology. 2020;**11**:583084. DOI: 10.3389/fimmu.2020.583084

[97] Rakina M, Larionova I, Kzhyshkowska J. Macrophage diversity in human cancers: New insight provided by single-cell resolution and spatial context. Heliyon. 2024;**10**(7):e28332. DOI: 10.1016/J.HELIYON.2024.E28332

[98] Han C, Deng Y, Xu W, Liu Z, Wang T, Wang S, et al. The roles of tumor-associated macrophages in prostate cancer. Journal of Oncology. 2022;**2022**:8580043. DOI: 10.1155/2022/8580043

[99] Steitz AM, Steffes A, Finkernagel F, Unger A, Sommerfeld L, Jansen JM, et al. Tumor-associated macrophages promote ovarian cancer cell migration by secreting transforming growth factor beta induced (TGFBI) and tenascin C. Cell Death & Disease. 2020;**11**(4):249. DOI: 10.1038/s41419-020-2438-8

[100] Schweer D, McAtee A, Neupane K, Richards C, Ueland F, Kolesar J. Tumor-associated macrophages and ovarian cancer: Implications for therapy. Cancers (Basel). 2022;**14**(9):2220. DOI: 10.3390/cancers14092220

[101] Makela AV, Gaudet JM, Foster PJ. Quantifying tumor associated macrophages in breast cancer: A comparison of iron and fluorine-based MRI cell tracking. Scientific Reports. 2017;7(1):42109. DOI: 10.1038/srep42109

[102] Lin Y, Xu J, Lan H. Tumor-associated macrophages in tumor metastasis: Biological roles and clinical therapeutic applications. Journal of Hematology & Oncology. 2019;**12**(1):76. DOI: 10.1186/s13045-019-0760-3

[103] Wang C, Lin Y, Zhu H, Zhou Y, Mao F, Huang X, et al. The prognostic

and clinical value of tumor-associated macrophages in patients with breast cancer: A systematic review and meta-analysis. Frontiers in Oncology. 2022;**12**:905846. DOI: 10.3389/fonc.2022.905846

[104] Wilton J, de Mendonça FL, Pereira-Castro I, Tellier M, Nojima T, Costa AM, et al. Pro-inflammatory polarization and colorectal cancer modulate alternative and intronic polyadenylation in primary human macrophages. Frontiers in Immunology. 2023;**14**:1182525. DOI: 10.3389/fimmu.2023.1182525

[105] Wang H, Wang X, Xu L, Zhang J, Cao H. Analysis of the transcriptomic features of microsatellite instability subtype colon cancer. BMC Cancer. 2019;**19**(1):605. DOI: 10.1186/s12885-019-5802-2

[106] Ong SM, Tan YC, Beretta O, Jiang D, Yeap WH, Tai JJY, et al. Macrophages in human colorectal cancer are pro-inflammatory and prime T cells towards an anti-tumour type-1 inflammatory response. European Journal of Immunology. 2012;**42**(1):89-100. DOI: 10.1002/eji.201141825

[107] Mosig S, Rennert K, Krause S, Kzhyshkowska J, Neunübel K, Heller R, et al. Different functions of monocyte subsets in familial hypercholesterolemia: Potential function of $CD14^+$ $CD16^+$ monocytes in detoxification of oxidized LDL. The FASEB Journal. 2009;**23**(3):866-874. DOI: 10.1096/fj.08-118240

[108] van der Valk ES, Mulder DS, Kouwenhoven T, Nagtzaam NMA, van Rossum EFC, Dik WA, et al. Monocyte adaptations in patients with obesity during a 1.5 year lifestyle intervention. Frontiers in Immunology. 2022;**13**:1022361. DOI: 10.3389/fimmu.2022.1022361

[109] Poitou C, Dalmas E, Renovato M, Benhamo V, Hajduch F, Abdennour M, et al. $CD14dimCD16^+$ and $CD14^+CD16^+$ monocytes in obesity and during weight loss: Relationships with fat mass and subclinical atherosclerosis. Arteriosclerosis, Thrombosis, and Vascular Biology. 2011;**31**(10):2322-2330. DOI: 10.1161/ATVBAHA.111.230979

[110] Friedrich K, Sommer M, Strobel S, Thrum S, Blüher M, Wagner U, et al. Perturbation of the monocyte compartment in human obesity. Frontiers in Immunology. 2019;**10**:1874. DOI: 10.3389/fimmu.2019.01874

[111] Hildreth AD, Ma F, Wong YY, Sun R, Pellegrini M, O'Sullivan TE. Single-cell sequencing of human white adipose tissue identifies new cell states in health and obesity. Nature Immunology. 2021;**22**(5):639-653. DOI: 10.1038/s41590-021-00922-4

[112] Berenice Martínez-Shio E, Martín Cárdenas-Hernández Á, Jiménez-Suárez V, Sherell Marín-Jáuregui L, Castillo-Martin Del Campo C, González-Amaro R, et al. Differentiation of circulating monocytes into macrophages with metabolically activated phenotype regulates inflammation in dyslipidemia patients. Clinical and Experimental Immunology. 2022;**208**(1):83-94. DOI: 10.1093/cei/uxac013

[113] Patel VK, Williams H, Li SCH, Fletcher JP, Medbury HJ. Monocyte inflammatory profile is specific for individuals and associated with altered blood lipid levels. Atherosclerosis. 2017;**263**:15-23. DOI: 10.1016/j.atherosclerosis.2017.05.026

[114] Lian Z, Perrard XYD, Antony AK, Peng X, Xu L, Ni J, et al. Dietary effects on monocyte phenotypes in subjects with hypertriglyceridemia and

metabolic syndrome. JACC Basic to Translational Science. 2023;**8**(5):460-475. DOI: 10.1016/j.jacbts.2023.02.011

[115] Nandy D, Janardhanan R, Mukhopadhyay D, Basu A. Effect of hyperglycemia on human monocyte activation. Journal of Investigative Medicine. 2011;**59**(4):661-667. DOI: 10.2310/JIM.0b013e31820ee432

[116] Castro-Grattoni AL, Oh J, Zhang RM, Dusso A, Riek AE, Bauerle KT, et al. Hyperglycemia-induced metabolic reprogramming mediates a proatherogenic phenotype in healthy human monocytes. Journal of the Endocrine Society. 2021;**5**(Supplement. 1):A321-A321. DOI: 10.1210/jendso/bvab048.655

[117] Xu Y, Hou X, Guo H, Yao Z, Fan X, Xu C, et al. $CD16^+$ monocytes are involved in the hyper-inflammatory state of Prader-Willi syndrome by single-cell transcriptomic analysis. Frontiers in Immunology. 2023;**14**:1153730. DOI: 10.3389/fimmu.2023.1153730

[118] Ma J, Song R, Liu C, Cao G, Zhang G, Wu Z, et al. Single-cell RNA-Seq analysis of diabetic wound macrophages in STZ-induced mice. Journal of Cell Communication and Signaling. 2023;**17**(1):103-120. DOI: 10.1007/s12079-022-00707-w

[119] Ma P, Zhang P, Chen S, Shi W, Ye J, Chen S, et al. Immune cell landscape of patients with diabetic macular edema by single-cell RNA analysis. Frontiers in Pharmacology. 2021;**12**:754933. DOI: 10.3389/fphar.2021.754933

[120] Rohm TV, Fuchs R, Müller RL, Keller L, Baumann Z, Bosch AJT, et al. Obesity in humans is characterized by gut inflammation as shown by pro-inflammatory intestinal macrophage accumulation. Frontiers in Immunology. 2021;**12**:668654. DOI: 10.3389/fimmu.2021.668654

[121] Hildebrandt X, Ibrahim M, Peltzer N. Cell death and inflammation during obesity: "Know my methods, WAT(son)". Cell Death and Differentiation. 2023;**30**(2):279-292. DOI: 10.1038/s41418-022-01062-4

[122] Boroumand P, Prescott DC, Mukherjee T, Bilan PJ, Wong M, Shen J, et al. Bone marrow adipocytes drive the development of tissue invasive Ly6Chigh monocytes during obesity. eLife. 2022;**11**:e65553. DOI: 10.7554/eLife.65553

[123] Todosenko N, Khaziakhmatova O, Malashchenko V, Yurova K, Bograya M, Beletskaya M, et al. Adipocyte- and monocyte-mediated vicious circle of inflammation and obesity (review of cellular and molecular mechanisms). International Journal of Molecular Sciences. 2023;**24**(15):12259. DOI: 10.3390/ijms241512259

[124] Devêvre EF, Renovato-Martins M, Clément K, Sautès-Fridman C, Cremer I, Poitou C. Profiling of the three circulating monocyte subpopulations in human obesity. Journal of Immunology. 2015;**194**(8):3917-3923. DOI: 10.4049/jimmunol.1402655

[125] Greco R, Demartini C, Zanaboni AM, Tumelero E, Persico A, Candeloro E, et al. CD163 as a potential biomarker of monocyte activation in ischemic stroke patients. International Journal of Molecular Sciences. 2021;**22**(13):6712. DOI: 10.3390/ijms22136712

[126] Biemann R, Roomp K, Noor F, Krishnan S, Li Z, Shahzad K, et al. Gene expression profile of $CD14^+$ blood monocytes following lifestyle-induced weight loss in individuals with metabolic syndrome. Scientific Reports. 2020;**10**(1):17855. DOI: 10.1038/s41598-020-74973-2

[127] Moganti K, Li F, Schmuttermaier C, Riemann S, Klüter H, Gratchev A, et al. Hyperglycemia induces mixed M1/M2 cytokine profile in primary human monocyte-derived macrophages. Immunobiology. 2017;**222**(10):952-959. DOI: 10.1016/J.IMBIO.2016.07.006

[128] Torres-Castro I, Arroyo-Camarena ÚD, Martínez-Reyes CP, Gómez-Arauz AY, Dueñas-Andrade Y, Hernández-Ruiz J, et al. Human monocytes and macrophages undergo M1-type inflammatory polarization in response to high levels of glucose. Immunology Letters. 2016;**176**:81-89. DOI: 10.1016/J.IMLET.2016.06.001

[129] Thiem K, Keating ST, Netea MG, Riksen NP, Tack CJ, van Diepen J, et al. Hyperglycemic memory of innate immune cells promotes *in vitro* proinflammatory responses of human monocytes and murine macrophages. Journal of Immunology. 2021;**206**(4):807-813. DOI: 10.4049/jimmunol.1901348

[130] Nandy D, Asmann YW, Mukhopadhyay D, Basu A. Role of AKT-glycogen synthase kinase axis in monocyte activation in human beings with and without type 2 diabetes. Journal of Cellular and Molecular Medicine. 2010;**14**(6B):1396-1407. DOI: 10.1111/j.1582-4934.2009.00900.x

[131] Zhang Q, Wu S, Sun G, Zhang R, Li X, Zhang Y, et al. Hyperglycemia aggravates monocyte-endothelial adhesion in human umbilical vein endothelial cells from women with gestational diabetes mellitus by inducing Cx43 overexpression. Annals of Translational Medicine. 2021;**9**(3):234. DOI: 10.21037/atm-19-4738

[132] Restrepo BI, Twahirwa M, Rahbar MH, Schlesinger LS. Phagocytosis via complement or fc-gamma receptors is compromised in monocytes from type 2 diabetes patients with chronic hyperglycemia. PLoS One. 2014;**9**(3):e92977. DOI: 10.1371/journal.pone.0092977

[133] Teichert M, Milde L, Holm A, Stanicek L, Gengenbacher N, Savant S, et al. Pericyte-expressed Tie2 controls angiogenesis and vessel maturation. Nature Communications. 2017;**8**(1):16106. DOI: 10.1038/ncomms16106

[134] Felcht M, Luck R, Schering A, Seidel P, Srivastava K, Hu J, et al. Angiopoietin-2 differentially regulates angiogenesis through TIE2 and integrin signaling. The Journal of Clinical Investigation. 2012;**122**(6):1991-2005. DOI: 10.1172/JCI58832

[135] Duran CL, Borriello L, Karagiannis GS, Entenberg D, Oktay MH, Condeelis JS. Targeting Tie2 in the tumor microenvironment: From angiogenesis to dissemination. Cancers (Basel). 2021;**13**(22):5730. DOI: 10.3390/cancers13225730

[136] Kologrivova IV, Suslova TE, Koshelskaya OA, Kravchenko ES, Kharitonova OA, Romanova EA, et al. Intermediate monocytes and circulating endothelial cells: Interplay with severity of atherosclerosis in patients with coronary artery disease and type 2 diabetes mellitus. Biomedicine. 2023;**11**(11):2911. DOI: 10.3390/biomedicines11112911

[137] Reijrink M, van Ark J, Lexis CPH, Visser LM, Lodewijk ME, van der Horst ICC, et al. Increased frequency of proangiogenic tunica intima endothelial kinase 2 (Tie2) expressing monocytes in individuals with type 2 diabetes mellitus. Cardiovascular Diabetology. 2022;**21**(1):72. DOI: 10.1186/s12933-022-01497-6

[138] Oh ES, Na M, Rogers CJ. The association between monocyte subsets and cardiometabolic disorders/cardiovascular disease: A systematic review and meta-analysis. Frontiers in Cardiovascular Medicine. 2021;**8**:640124. DOI: 10.3389/fcvm.2021.640124

[139] Mayer D, Altvater M, Schenz J, Arif R, Karck M, Leuschner F, et al. Monocyte metabolism and function in patients undergoing cardiac surgery. Frontiers in Cardiovascular Medicine. 2022;**9**:853967. DOI: 10.3389/fcvm.2022.853967

[140] Zhu X, Meyers A, Long D, Ingram B, Liu T, Yoza BK, et al. Monocytes sequentially rewire metabolism and bioenergetics during an acute inflammatory response. Journal of Leukocyte Biology. 2019;**105**(2):215. DOI: 10.1002/JLB.3HI0918-373R

[141] Short JD, Tavakoli S, Nguyen HN, Carrera A, Farnen C, Cox LA, et al. Dyslipidemic diet-induced monocyte "priming" and dysfunction in non-human primates is triggered by elevated plasma cholesterol and accompanied by altered histone acetylation. Frontiers in Immunology. 2017;**8**:281193. DOI: 10.3389/fimmu.2017.00958

[142] Badillo-Garcia LE, Liu Q, Ziebner K, Balduff M, Sevastyanova T, Schmuttermaier C, et al. Hyperglycemia amplifies TLR-mediated inflammatory response of M(IL4) macrophages to dyslipidemic ligands. Journal of Leukocyte Biology. 2024;**116**(1):197-204. DOI: 10.1093/jleuko/qiae050

[143] Li Z, Xu Z, Huang Y, Zhao R, Cui Y, Zhou Y, et al. The predictive value and the correlation of peripheral absolute monocyte count, tumor-associated macrophage and microvessel density in patients with colon cancer. Medicine. 2018;**97**(21):e10759. DOI: 10.1097/MD.0000000000010759

[144] Schauer D, Starlinger P, Reiter C, Jahn N, Zajc P, Buchberger E, et al. Intermediate monocytes but not TIE2-expressing monocytes are a sensitive diagnostic indicator for colorectal cancer. PLoS One. 2012;**7**(9):e44450. DOI: 10.1371/JOURNAL.PONE.0044450

[145] Zhang Q, Liu Y, Wang X, Zhang C, Hou M, Liu Y. Integration of single-cell RNA sequencing and bulk RNA transcriptome sequencing reveals a heterogeneous immune landscape and pivotal cell subpopulations associated with colorectal cancer prognosis. Frontiers in Immunology. 2023;**14**:1184167. DOI: 10.3389/fimmu.2023.1184167

[146] Guo J, Liu Y. INHBA promotes the proliferation, migration and invasion of colon cancer cells through the upregulation of VCAN. The Journal of International Medical Research. 2021;**49**(6):3000605211014998. DOI: 10.1177/03000605211014998

[147] Sampaio-Ribeiro G, Ruivo A, Silva A, Santos AL, Oliveira RC, Gama J, et al. Innate immune cells in the tumor microenvironment of liver metastasis from colorectal cancer: Contribution to a comprehensive therapy. Cancers (Basel). 2023;**15**(12):3222. DOI: 10.3390/cancers15123222

[148] Ohno Y, Toyoshima Y, Yurino H, Monma N, Xiang H, Sumida K, et al. Lack of interleukin-6 in the tumor microenvironment augments type-1 immunity and increases the efficacy of cancer immunotherapy. Cancer Science. 2017;**108**(10):1959-1966. DOI: 10.1111/cas.13330

[149] Zhang W, Liu Y, Yan Z, Yang H, Sun W, Yao Y, et al. IL-6 promotes

PD-L1 expression in monocytes and macrophages by decreasing protein tyrosine phosphatase receptor type O expression in human hepatocellular carcinoma. Journal for Immunotherapy of Cancer. 2020;**8**(1):e000285. DOI: 10.1136/jitc-2019-000285

[150] Jakubowska K, Koda M, Grudzińska M, Kańczuga-Koda L, Famulski W. Monocyte-to-lymphocyte ratio as a prognostic factor in peripheral whole blood samples of colorectal cancer patients. World Journal of Gastroenterology. 2020;**26**(31):4639-4655. DOI: 10.3748/wjg.v26.i31.4639

[151] Grossman JG, Nywening TM, Belt B, Pittman E, Giorgi A, Michael A, et al. The role of inflammatory monocytes in human metastatic colorectal cancer. Journal of Clinical Oncology. 2015;**33**(Suppl. 3):624. DOI: 10.1200/jco.2015.33.3_suppl.624

[152] Larionova I, Patysheva M, Iamshchikov P, Kazakova E, Kazakova A, Rakina M, et al. PFKFB3 overexpression in monocytes of patients with colon but not rectal cancer programs pro-tumor macrophages and is indicative for higher risk of tumor relapse. Frontiers in Immunology. 2022;**13**:1080501. DOI: 10.3389/fimmu.2022.1080501

[153] Montalbán-Hernández K, Cantero-Cid R, Casalvilla-Dueñas JC, Avendaño-Ortiz J, Marín E, Lozano-Rodríguez R, et al. Colorectal cancer stem cells fuse with monocytes to form tumour hybrid cells with the ability to migrate and evade the immune system. Cancers (Basel). 2022;**14**(14):3445. DOI: 10.3390/cancers14143445

[154] Tretyakova MS, Subbalakshmi AR, Menyailo ME, Jolly MK, Denisov EV. Tumor hybrid cells: Nature and biological significance. Frontiers in Cell and Development Biology. 2022;**10**:814714. DOI: 10.3389/fcell.2022.814714

[155] Kaigorodova EV, Kozik AV, Zavaruev IS, Grishchenko MY. Hybrid/atypical forms of circulating tumor cells: Current state of the art. Biochemistry (Moscow). 2022;**87**(4):380-390. DOI: 10.1134/S0006297922040071

[156] Drury J, Rychahou PG, Kelson CO, Geisen ME, Wu Y, He D, et al. Upregulation of CD36, a fatty acid translocase, promotes colorectal cancer metastasis by increasing MMP28 and decreasing E-cadherin expression. Cancers (Basel). 2022;**14**(1):252. DOI: 10.3390/cancers14010252

[157] Fang Y, Shen ZY, Zhan YZ, Feng XC, Chen KL, Li YS, et al. CD36 inhibits β-catenin/c-myc-mediated glycolysis through ubiquitination of GPC4 to repress colorectal tumorigenesis. Nature Communications. 2019;**10**(1):3981. DOI: 10.1038/s41467-019-11662-3

[158] Niculae AM, Dobre M, Herlea V, Vasilescu F, Ceafalan LC, Trandafir B, et al. Lipid handling protein gene expression in colorectal cancer: CD36 and targeting miRNAs. Life. 2022;**12**(12):2127. DOI: 10.3390/life12122127

[159] Yang P, Qin H, Li Y, Xiao A, Zheng E, Zeng H, et al. CD36-mediated metabolic crosstalk between tumor cells and macrophages affects liver metastasis. Nature Communications. 2022;**13**(1):5782. DOI: 10.1038/s41467-022-33349-y

[160] Lian G, Chen S, Ouyang M, Li F, Chen L, Yang J. Colon cancer cell secretes EGF to promote M2 polarization of TAM through EGFR/PI3K/AKT/mTOR pathway. Technology in Cancer Research & Treatment. 2019;**18**:1533033819849068. DOI: 10.1177/1533033819849068

[161] Li D, Wu M. Pattern recognition receptors in health and diseases.

Signal Transduction and Targeted Therapy. 2021;**6**(1):291. DOI: 10.1038/s41392-021-00687-0

[162] Amarante-Mendes GP, Adjemian S, Branco LM, Zanetti LC, Weinlich R, Bortoluci KR. Pattern recognition receptors and the host cell death molecular machinery. Frontiers in Immunology. 2018;**9**:417707. DOI: 10.3389/fimmu.2018.02379

[163] Hennessy C, McKernan DP. Anti-viral pattern recognition receptors as therapeutic targets. Cells. 2021;**10**(9):2258. DOI: 10.3390/cells10092258

[164] Mohammadi M, Mehrzad J, Delirezh N, Abdollahi A. Chronic inflammation and its role in colorectal cancer development. Oncogen (Westerville). 2022;**5**(1):24. DOI: 10.35702/Onc.10024

[165] Allen IC, Wilson JE, Schneider M, Lich JD, Roberts RA, Arthur JC, et al. NLRP12 suppresses colon inflammation and tumorigenesis through the negative regulation of noncanonical NF-κB signaling. Immunity. 2012;**36**(5):742-754. DOI: 10.1016/j.immuni.2012.03.012

[166] Truax AD, Chen L, Tam JW, Cheng N, Guo H, Koblansky AA, et al. The inhibitory innate immune sensor NLRP12 maintains a threshold against obesity by regulating gut microbiota homeostasis. Cell Host & Microbe. 2018;**24**(3):364. DOI: 10.1016/J.CHOM.2018.08.009

[167] Wang S, Wang J, Chen Z, Luo J, Guo W, Sun L, et al. Targeting M2-like tumor-associated macrophages is a potential therapeutic approach to overcome antitumor drug resistance. npj Precision Oncology. 2024;**8**(1):31. DOI: 10.1038/s41698-024-00522-z

[168] Lee C, Jeong H, Bae Y, Shin K, Kang S, Kim H, et al. Targeting of M2-like tumor-associated macrophages with a melittin-based pro-apoptotic peptide. Journal for Immunotherapy of Cancer. 2019;**7**(1):147. DOI: 10.1186/S40425-019-0610-4

[169] Patysheva M, Frolova A, Larionova I, Afanas'ev S, Tarasova A, Cherdyntseva N, et al. Monocyte programming by cancer therapy. Frontiers in Immunology. 2022;**13**:994319. DOI: 10.3389/FIMMU.2022.994319

[170] Patysheva M, Larionova I, Stakheyeva M, Grigoryeva E, Iamshchikov P, Tarabanovskaya N, et al. Effect of early-stage human breast carcinoma on monocyte programming. Frontiers in Oncology. 2022;**11**:5906

[171] Jansen L, Hoffmeister M, Arndt V, Chang-Claude J, Brenner H. Stage-specific associations between beta blocker use and prognosis after colorectal cancer. Cancer. 2014;**120**(8):1178-1186. DOI: 10.1002/cncr.28546

[172] Chagovets V, Starodubtseva N, Tokareva A, Novoselova A, Patysheva M, Larionova I, et al. Specific changes in amino acid profiles in monocytes of patients with breast, lung, colorectal and ovarian cancers. Frontiers in Immunology. 2024;**14**:1332043. DOI: 10.3389/fimmu.2023.1332043

Section 3

Macrophages Involvement in Inflammation

Chapter 5

Lung Immunity to Fungal Infections by Macrophages: Mechanisms and Implications

Jaishree Sharma, Nitish Arun Kulkarni and Som Gowda Nanjappa

Abstract

Pulmonary pathogenic fungi cause severe to fatal disseminated infections, especially in immunocompromised patients. Alveolar macrophages form an essential early innate cellular barrier implicated in immunity to pulmonary mycoses. The complex interactions of alveolar macrophages with pathogenic fungi lead to either effective clearance or disease progression. After sensing fungi through pattern-recognizing receptors, alveolar macrophage activation enhances phagocytic and non-phagocytic killing, secretion of cytokines/chemokines, and activation of other immune cells, including adaptive immune cells and neutrophils. Such an orchestrated response involves transcriptomic and metabolic adaptations by macrophages and epigenomic imprinting. Despite their high plasticity with the inflammatory cues, recent studies have shed light on their longevity and functional stability. Nevertheless, some pathogenic fungi have evolved strategies to evade or subvert alveolar macrophage function, leading to persistent and disseminated infections. Understanding the mechanisms of the macrophage-fungal interface helps develop a new line of immune therapeutics and mitigates the challenges of limited arsenals of antifungals.

Keywords: alveolar macrophages, immune response, fungal infections, lung, immunocompromised individuals

1. Introduction

1.1 Pulmonary pathogenic fungi

Invasive pulmonary fungal infections cause severe complications in immunocompromised patients, resulting in at least 13 million infections and more than 1.5 million deaths annually [1]. However, these numbers are considered to be underestimated due to unconfirmed or misdiagnosed cases with challenges of pulmonary fungal infections mimicking other commonly occurring lung diseases, such as tuberculosis [2]. Underdiagnosed or misdiagnosed invasive fungal infections lead to treatment failures that increase hospitalizations, morbidity, and poor clinical outcomes [3]. Common pulmonary fungal pathogens that cause life-threatening conditions include *Aspergillus, Cryptococcus, and Pneumocystis*, and endemic fungi such as *Blastomyces, Histoplasma*, and *Coccidioides*. The most common route of infection is direct inhalation of fungal spores from the environment. With climate change and global warming, there is a threat of new fungal pathogens' emergence and the rapid spread of geographically restricted endemic fungal infections [4]. Thus, the development of new preventive and therapeutic measures is warranted.

The host-pathogen interface in the lung involves many cells, including various types of epithelial cells, goblet cells, myeloid cells, and lymphoid cells. Despite the independent and interdependent role of these cells in fungal immunity, the instrumental immune cell type that essentially orchestrates the fungal pathogenesis is alveolar macrophages (AMs), which constitute more than 80% of leukocytes in bronchoalveolar lavage in a healthy human or animal. This chapter will focus on the role of alveolar macrophages and their mechanisms of action, epigenetic imprinting, and plasticity in relevance to pulmonary fungal infections.

1.2 Development and homeostasis of alveolar macrophages

Although described as hematopoietic cells, AMs primarily derive from embryonic progenitor cells in the embryo's yolk sac and the fetus's liver [5]. The nuclear receptor and transcription factor, peroxisome proliferator-activated receptor-γ (PPAR-γ), determines the perinatal differentiation and identity of AMs [5, 6]. Once populated in the lung, AMs have a long lifespan (half-life in mice is ~30 days) and proliferate to replenish themselves *in situ* at a rate of 40% per year in the presence of granulocyte-macrophage colony-stimulating factor (GM-CSF), encoded by Csf2 gene [7, 8]. GM-CSF is mainly derived from alveolar type 2 cells that help develop and maintain the mature AM population [9]. However, the relative dispensability of M-CSF is noted in the survival of alveolar macrophages and interstitial macrophages [10, 11]. The signaling node—mTORC1 (mammalian/mechanistic target of rapamycin complex 1), supports AMs to respond optimally to GM-CSF, which in turn controls metabolic reprogramming, such as glycolysis and lipid biosynthesis, to fulfill the energy requirements for self-renewal [12]. GM-CSF also upregulates the expression of anti-apoptotic proteins, MCL-1 and BCL-2, leading to an increased lifespan of AMs [13, 14]. Despite the essentiality of GM-CSF for the homeostasis of AMs, fine-tuning of GM-CSF signaling is essential, regulated by Ssu72 phosphatase, and its loss leads to dysregulated development and functions of AMs [7, 15]. Unlike other tissue macrophages, besides GM-CSF, TGF-β is also necessary for the development, maturation, and maintenance of AMs, primarily secreted by themselves [16].

During the development and differentiation of AM (**Figure 1**), a transient monocytic stage occurs [5, 17, 18], and parabiosis and fate-mapping studies revealed that the transitional monocytes of AM fate may have both fetal and adult origins [19]. The increased demand for alveolar macrophages during acute inflammatory responses requires rapid recruitment of adult-origin monocyte-derived macrophages to the lung to eliminate pathogens [19]. During inflammation resolution, most macrophages originating from circulating monocytes undergo apoptosis, and some parenchymal macrophages derived from recruited $Ly6C^{lo}$ monocytes become phenotypically and functionally similar to resident AMs, suggesting an alternative mechanism of replenishment of AM population [20, 21]. However, in general homeostasis, circulating monocytes minimally contribute to the AM pool, and Ccr2 deficiency did not reduce the number of AMs [8, 18, 22].

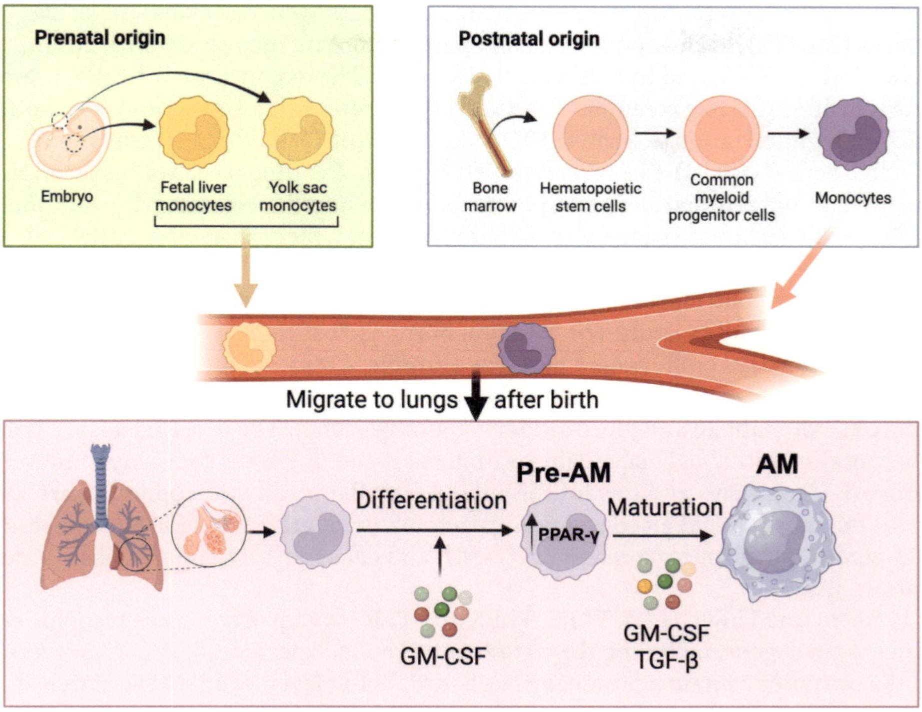

Figure 1.
Development of alveolar macrophages. Alveolar macrophages (AMs) embryonically arise from monocytes of the fetal liver or yolk sac. The postnatal origin of monocytes occurs in bone marrow from common myeloid progenitors (CMPs) derived from hematopoietic stem cells (HSCs). The monocytes migrate to the lungs to develop into pre-AMs before finally mature into AMs. AM differentiation is mediated by the presence of GM-CSF, which activates the expression of PPAR-γ to establish their identity. The maturation of pre-AMs relies on the GM-CSF and TGF-β signaling for transcriptional modifications in the signature genes of AMs. AM: alveolar macrophage; GM-CSF: granulocyte-macrophage colony-stimulating factor; PPAR-γ: peroxisome proliferator-activated receptor gamma.

2. Alveolar macrophage activation and response to fungal infections

AMs are specialized innate immune cells that maintain pulmonary homeostasis and protect against respiratory infections. The activation of AMs includes a series of steps that are essential for initiating an effective immune response. Pattern recognition receptors (PRRs) on AMs recognize antigenic/structural components of the fungal pathogens, and the recognition activates the AMs and triggers intracellular signaling cascades resulting in enhanced phagocytosis and destruction of antigens or debris larger than 0.5 μM, including inhaled pathogens and residual dead cells in the alveolar space [23]. Further, AMs release pro- and anti-inflammatory cytokines, chemokines, and ROS/RNS that aid in recruiting and activating other immune cells, killing of pathogens, and inflammation resolution [24]. These mechanisms are necessary to protect the lungs from pulmonary infections and maintain respiratory health.

2.1 Pattern-recognizing receptors

Fungal pathogens are diverse and express common and species-specific unique surface antigens involved in activating immune cells or evading host recognition. The host PRRs sense several fungal components called pathogen-associated molecular patterns (PAMPs), such as β-glucans, mannans, zymosan, mannoproteins, chitin, fungal-derived RNA, and unmethylated DNA [25]. The major classes of PRRs present in AMs include toll-like receptors (TLRs), C-type lectin receptors (CLRs), nucleotide-binding oligomerization domain (NOD)-like receptors (NLRs), and retinoic acid-inducible gene-I (RIG-I)-like receptors (RLRs) [25]. The fungal cell wall is primarily composed of polysaccharides and lipid moieties essential for cell integrity, morphology, viability, and phase transition in dimorphic fungi. More than 90% of the cell wall comprises polysaccharides arranged in layers [26], such as α-glucans, β-glucans, mannans, chitin, and chitosan, and the remaining cell wall components involve lipids, proteins, and melanin. The components of each of these vary in their amounts and types in various pathogenic fungi. For example, *Cryptococcus* species uniquely contain an immunoregulatory outer polysaccharide capsule containing primarily glucuronoxylomannan and glucuronoxylomannogalactan. The innermost layer typically contains chitin, an N-acetylglucosamine polymer, followed by highly immunoreactive β-1,3-glucans, and toward the outer cell wall, several other polysaccharides such as mannose-linked glycoproteins, galactomannan, galactosaminogalactan, and α-1,3-glucan, glucuronoxylomannan (GXM), and galactoxylomannan (GalXM) are arranged [26, 27].

TLRs such as TLR2, TLR4, TLR6, TLR7, and TLR9 are involved in the recognition of fungal pathogens, including *Aspergillus* and *Candida* species [28, 29]. *Aspergillus* conidia or spores contain a proteinaceous hydrophobin layer, whereas the active hyphal cell wall layer contains heteropolysaccharide galactosaminogalactan and galactomannan, which regulates the virulence [30, 31]. The galactosaminogalactan shields inflammatory β-glucan ligands from host detection by TLR2 [32] and Dectin-1. Upon recognition, the TLRs trigger the activation of downstream signaling adaptor protein MyD88, activating transcription factors NF-kB and MAP kinases and secreting pro-inflammatory cytokines [29]. Another TLR, TLR9, is also involved in recognizing unmethylated CpG DNA in *A. fumigatus* [33]. The data from these studies offer contrasting views on TLR's role in *A. fumigatus*-mediated immunity. TLR4 and mannose receptors on the surface of AMs bind to glycoproteins, including N- and O-linked mannans, present on the outer cell wall of *C. albicans* [34]. While the macrophage mannose receptor utilizes the FcRγ signaling chain for inducing inflammatory responses, the TLR4 signaling depends on the MyD88-dependent pathway [34]. The C. *neoformans* capsule consisting of glucuronoxylomannan and galactoxylomannan conceals chitin and β-glucan from host recognition. Glucuronoxylomannans are recognized by TLR1 and TLR2 and signal *via* the MyD88-dependent pathway [35]. In contrast, galactoxylomannan binds to CD209 (DC-SIGN) and pentraxin-3 (soluble) and activates the immune cells *via* a tyrosine-based motif, lymphocyte-specific protein 1 (LSP1).

Among C-type lectin receptors, Dectin-1 is predominantly expressed by AMs that recognize fungal cell wall component β-1,3-glucan, a highly immunogenic molecule on most pathogenic fungi such as *Aspergillus*, *Candida*, *Histoplasma*, *Coccidiosis,* and *Pneumocystis* [36, 37]. The successful recognition of β-1,3-glucans leads to downstream signaling *via* phosphorylation SYK-induced p65 at Ser276 [38], leading to NFκB-induced inflammatory cytokine production. However, some yeasts, such as *C. albicans* and *C. glabrata*, evade Dectin-1 recognition by masking β-1,3-glucan by layers of mannans [39, 40]. Similarly, the α-1,3-glucan layer in *H. capsulatum* conceals the β-1,3-glucans and prevents effective immune response following infection [41]. Other CLRs, Dectin-2 and Mincle, recognize α-mannan in the outer layer of the fungal cell wall [29] and are necessary for immunity to blastomycosis, aspergillosis, and pneumocystosis [42–44]. AMs upregulate Dectin-2 in response to α-mannan of *A. fumigatus*, *Candida*, and *C. posadasii* and the glycolipids of some *Candida spp.* bind to another CLR, Mincle (encoded by Clec4e) [34, 45]. Dectin-2 mediates an NF-kB-dependent pro-inflammatory response against fungal pathogens [28]. Glycoprotein *Blastomyces* Eng2 (Bl-Eng2) of *B. dermatitidis* binds to Dectin-2 and promotes Ag-specific Th_{17} and Th_1 cell responses, augmented activation and killing of fungi by myeloid effector cells, and protection of mice from lethal fungal challenge [46]. DC-SIGN (CD209), another CLR expressed on macrophages, binds to *Aspergillus* conidia by recognizing galactomannan [47].

NOD-like receptor (NLR) family members are being recognized as receptors for several pathogenic fungi involved in immunity. Although NLRP3's immunity against various fungal pathogens is evident by activating inflammasomes and secretion of IL-1β and IL-18 [29], the role of NOD1/2 is less clear. Intracellular NOD2 receptor in AMs recognizes *A. fumigatus* conidia and induces the production of cytokines and chemokines such as IL-12, IFN-γ, GM-CSF, CXCL2/MIP-2, CXCL1/KC, and CCL2/MIP-2 [48, 49]. Yet, the identity of fungal PAMPs for NLR recognition is not clear.

The involvement of retinoic acid-inducible gene-I (RIG-I)-like receptors (RLRs) in antifungal immunity has recently emerged. The C. *albicans* hyphae induced the expression of MDA5 (IFIHI) in macrophages, and the cells lacking MDA5 secreted lower levels of IFN-β [50]. In *Aspergillus fumigatus* infection, AMs play an important role in the induction of the MDA5/MAVS-dependent IFN responses required for host resistance [51]. The cGAS (cyclic-AMP-GMP synthase)-STING (stimulator of interferon genes) pathway is an important component of innate immunity that detects cytosolic DNA and induces IFN-stimulating genes (ISGs) and type I IFNs (α- and β-) *via* phosphorylation of transcription factor IRF3 (interferon regulatory factor 3) [52]. Recent studies show that *C. albicans* extracellular vesicles triggered the cGAS-STING pathway and induced type I IFN, ISGs, and activation of IRF3 independent of the Dectin-1-Card9 pathway and TLR9 [53]. However, the role of this mechanism in AMs is still unexplored. After recognition of PAMPs by PRRs and activation, the AMs perform effector functions such as phagocytosis and killing, secretion of cytokines and chemokines, killing by oxidative burst, and activation of other immune cells.

2.2 Phagocytic and non-phagocytic killing

AMs phagocytize and kill pathogens and secrete pro-inflammatory cytokines (**Figure 2**) that recruit other immune cells to the site of infection [54, 55]. Phagocytosis by the AMs is mediated by opsonin-dependent and independent classes (PRRs) of cell-surface receptors [23]. For opsonin-mediated phagocytosis, Fc receptors on AMs recognize the Fc portion of an immunoglobulin (IgG) bound to the fungus [56]. Cross-linking of Fc receptors is crucial for various biological and protective functions such as phagocytosis, antibody-dependent cellular cytotoxicity, and respiratory burst [57]. Opsonized particles bound with complement proteins, such as C3b and C3bi, are recognized *via* their complement receptors [58]. However, opsonization-mediated phagocytosis and killing are evaded by pathogenic fungi by antigen variation or encapsulation, resulting in increased virulence.

AM phagocytosis is influenced by FcγR expression. Sphingosine-1-phosphate enhanced the expression of FCγR and complement receptor 3 (CR3) in the AMs and promoted the opsonization and phagocytosis of *C. neoformans* spores [59–61]. The soluble receptor pentraxin-3 (PTX-3) binds to galactomannan present on *Aspergillus*

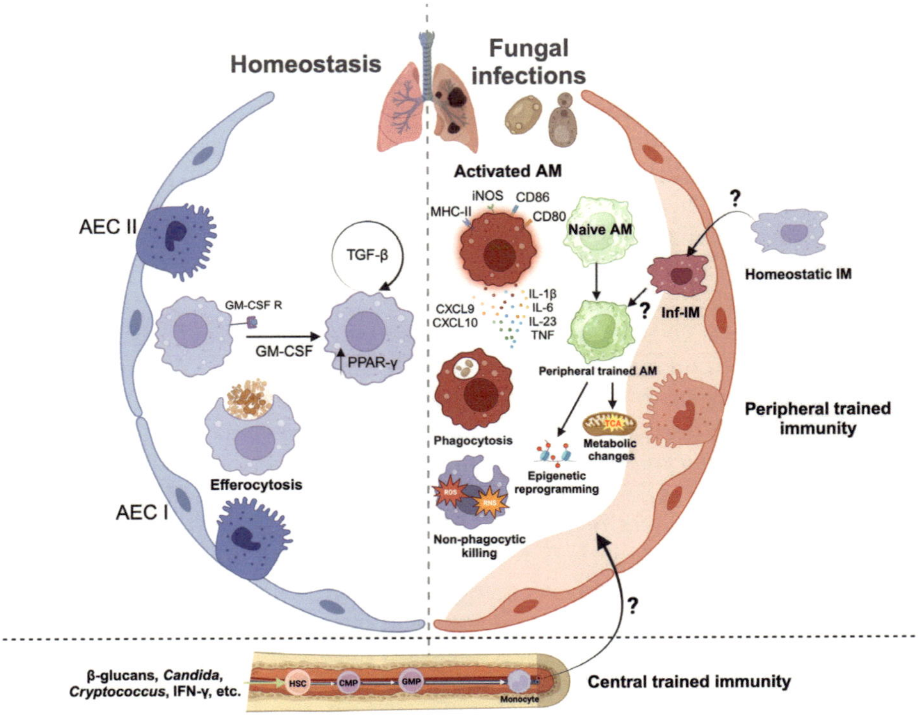

Figure 2.
Role of alveolar macrophages in homeostasis and fungal infections. Homeostasis: *Tissue-resident alveolar macrophages (AMs) undergo local proliferation utilizing GM-CSF that activates the expression of PPAR-γ and its maintenance depends on autocrine TGF-β. AMs are adept at efferocytosis of apoptotic cells and preventing pro-inflammatory responses in the alveoli.* Fungal infections: *Upon infection, the AMs are activated and express CD80, CD86, MHC-II, and iNOS (M1). Further, they secrete pro-inflammatory cytokines such as IL-1β, IL-6, IL-23, TNF, and chemokines such as CXCL9 and CXL10. AMs combat the fungi by phagocytic or ROS/RNS-mediated non-phagocytic killing. The fungal exposure may lead to the development of peripherally trained AM in the lung by epigenetic reprogramming and metabolic changes to provide trained immunological memory. Centrally trained immunity can occur to a rapid and heightened innate immune response to certain adjuvants and antigens which reprogram the HSC in the bone marrow. HSC differentiates into CMP, GMP, and then to circulating monocyte, which subsequently enter peripheral organs such as lungs to differentiate into tissue macrophages. However, this mechanism and migration of IMs into the airways is not in fungal infections. AEC I: Type I alveolar epithelial cell; AEC II: Type II alveolar epithelial cell; AM: alveolar macrophage; CMP: common myeloid progenitor; GM-CSF R: granulocyte-macrophage colony-stimulating factor receptor; GMP: granulocyte-monocyte progenitor; HSC: hematopoietic stem cell; IM: interstitial macrophage; Inf-IM: inflammatory interstitial macrophage; iNOS: inducible nitric oxide synthase; PPARγ: peroxisome proliferator-activated receptor gamma; RNS: reactive nitrogen species; ROS: reactive oxygen species; HSC: hematopoietic stem cell; CMP: common myeloid progenitors; GMP: granulocyte-macrophage progenitors.*

conidia and promotes FCγRIIA (Cd32)-dependent conidial endocytosis in an actin-dependent manner [62]. While neutrophils are the major immune cells responsible for complement-mediated opsonization, phagocytosis, and fungal killing, AMs can also kill internalized *A. fumigatus* conidia [63]. FcγR-dependent phagocytosis is enhanced by the stimulation of the PPAR-γ ligand in alveolar macrophages [64]. Similarly, leukotrienes LTB4, LTC4, and 5-hydroxyeicosatetraenoic acid (5-HETE) also stimulate AM phagocytosis [65]. During phagosome acidification, a phagosome containing conidia fuses with a lysosome to form a phagolysosome, which leads to ATPase-mediated acidification and activation of enzymes such as chitinases and proteases that lead to the degradation of the cell wall, which then exposes some of the pathogen ligands for pattern recognition receptors (PRR), TLRs, and Dectin-1 [66–68]. Syk, a protein tyrosine kinase, is essential for transporting internalized Fc receptors to lysosomes [69].

Opsonin-independent receptors, including mannose receptors, scavenger receptors, Siglecs, DC-SIGN, or Dectin-1, directly bind pathogen-associated molecular patterns, such as glycan structures with terminal mannose or sialic acid residues or fungal β-glucans [70–72] and phagocytose. Along with pathogens, opsonin-independent receptors recognize apoptotic cells and other non-opsonized materials. AM-driven efferocytosis of apoptotic cells such as neutrophils prevents immunopathology or reduces inflammation in the alveoli [73–75]. In addition, efferocytosis by AMs promotes the secretion of anti-inflammatory factors such as TGF-β, prostaglandin E2, and platelet-activating factors [76, 77].

Aging, smoking, and certain systemic diseases can significantly impair the ability of the AMs to phagocytize [78–80]. Phagocytosis is severely impaired in patients with severe asthma or COPD, increases the susceptibility to fungal infections, and reduces the uptake of apoptotic cells resulting in dysregulated anti-inflammation [81, 82]. Thus, AMs protect the hosts from fungal infections by direct phagocytosis and killing and clearing the apoptotic cells to reduce pathology and maintain host fitness.

Non-phagocytic killing by alveolar macrophages requires specific differentiation following the pathogen encounter and in cue to the inflammatory micro milieu. Type I or M1 macrophages are distinct, differentiated by inflammatory cytokines or PRR signals, have several features of pro-inflammatory type and are microbicidal. Type II or M2 macrophages differentiated by regulatory cytokines are anti-inflammatory and help in tissue repair but are implicated in fungal evasion and dissemination. One of the features of M1 macrophages is the non-phagocytic killing of fungi by secreting reactive oxygen species (ROS) and reactive nitrogen species (RNS), which include oxygen radicals ($O2^{-\cdot}$) and nitric oxide ($NO^{\cdot}$), respectively, and their derivatives [83]. These inflammatory mediators directly damage DNA, lipids, and proteins by oxidative mechanisms [84]. An enzyme, inducible nitric oxide synthase (iNOS), converts substrate L-arginine to form nitric oxide (NO) and is increased in various microbial infections and inflammatory conditions [85]. For instance, during non-tuberculosis mycobacterium (NTM), intermittently inhaled high doses of NO proved effective in reducing the bacterial burden and improving the quality of life in a cystic fibrosis patient [86]. iNOS knockout mice are more susceptible to infections, including *Mycobacterium tuberculosis* [87]. Similarly, nitric oxide production is implicated in containing fungal growth in several fungal diseases such as histoplasmosis [88], paracoccidioidomycosis [89], coccidioidomycosis [90], and cryptococcosis [91]. During aspergillosis, mitochondrial ROS enhances the fungicidal properties of AMs, although ROS is dispensable and may be compensated by other killing mechanisms [92]. ROS is produced immediately following a microbial stimulus by cytosolic and mitochondrial sources [93]; however, RNS production requires *de novo* protein synthesis since transcription of iNOS is triggered by the combined stimulation of PRRs and signaling by pro-inflammatory cytokines, such as IFNs, IL-1β, and TNF [94], activating several signaling pathways, including the p38 mitogen-activated protein kinase (MAPK), NF-κB, and Janus-activated kinase-signal transducer and activator of transcription-interferon regulatory factor 1 (JAK-STAT-IRF1) pathways [95–98]. PPAR-γ agonists reduce ROS production and decrease the expression of pro-inflammatory cytokines and iNOS [99, 100]. On the contrary, the pathogens can use various strategies to counteract or evade the effects of ROS and RNS, including but not limited to evasion, suppression, enzymatic inactivation, scavenging, iron sequestration, stress responses, and repair mechanisms [87, 101, 102]. For example, in *Blastomyces dermatitidis* and

Pneumocystis pneumonia, the nitric oxide production by AMs is inhibited, possibly by interfering with iNOS enzymatic activity and reduced dimerization of iNOS [103, 104].

2.3 Signaling and secretion of cytokines/chemokines

Another important function of AMs is the production of cytokines, chemokines, lysozyme, antimicrobial peptides, and proteases that can further enhance the immune responses to combat fungal infections in the lung [8]. AMs crosstalk with other cells of the alveolar environment by producing chemokines and cytokines, recruiting inflammatory monocytes, neutrophils, and adaptive immune cells for coordinated immune defense against pathogens.

Following the downstream activation of TLRs such as TLR2, TLR4, and TLR9, AMs secrete TNF and interleukins, IL-1β, IL-6, IL-10, and IL-12, macrophage inflammatory protein (MIP)-1α, chemokines, lysozyme, antimicrobial peptides, proteases, and other inflammatory mediators [105–109]. IL-1β produced by AMs facilitates CXC chemokine expression, such as macrophage inflammatory protein-2 (MIP-2/CXCL2) and CXCL1, to recruit neutrophils at the site of infection [110, 111]. Dectin-1-mediated recognition of β-glucans on the fungal cell surface stimulates the production of pro-inflammatory cytokines such as TNF, IL-6, and IL-18 [112, 113]. The sensing of fungi by intracellular NOD2 in AMs enhances the production of cytokines such as IFN-γ, IL-12, GM-CSF, CXCL2/MIP-2, CCL2-MCP-1, and CXCL1/KC [48, 49]. Despite most of these studies were *in vitro*, using isolated AMs or cell lines, the cytokines and chemokine expressions are noted in *in vivo*. Nevertheless, the protein expression profile of *in vivo* AMs during fungal infections needs further investigation.

The secreted inflammatory cytokines result in the polarization of macrophages into various phenotypes, mainly M1 and M2, during pulmonary fungal infections [114]. M1 macrophages are polarized due to IFN-γ secreted by T helper type 1 (Th_1) cells and natural killer (NK) [115] and secrete pro-inflammatory cytokines such as TNF, IL-12, IFN-γ, and chemokines such as CXCL9, CXCL10, and CXCL11. M1 macrophages protect against several fungi, such as *Cryptococcus neoformans, Candida albicans, Paracoccidioides brasiliensis, Histoplasma capsulatum*, and *A. fumigatus* [114].

The macrophages polarize toward the M2 phenotype due to enhanced damage to the tissue and increased production of anti-inflammatory cytokines such as IL-4 and IL-13 [116, 117]. M2a macrophages, while not efficient in fungal killing, play a significant role in the production of extracellular matrix and growth factors that aid in wound healing [115, 116, 118]. Moreover, they promote the maintenance/generation of Th2 responses and express arginase 1 (Arg1), MR (CD206), found in inflammatory zone 1 (FIZZ-1, also known as resistin-like α or Relm-α), and chitinase and chitinase-like molecules, such as YM1 (Chi3l3) and YM2 [116, 119]. M2 macrophages are be implicated in protection against *Pneumocystis spp.* but contrastingly aggravating the disease condition in *C. neoformans* [104, 120, 121]. The polarized macrophages have a special ability to change their functions depending on the cytokine microenvironment. Activated M2 macrophages increase IL-10 secretion and reduce IL-12 and IL-23 secretion, exerting anti-inflammatory effects [122]. During C. *neoformans* infection, alternative activation of AMs facilitates fungal growth and disease progression [123]. Pathogens have evolved mechanisms to interfere with macrophage polarization, exploiting the different immune functions of macrophage phenotypes [124].

Host signaling cascades activate AMs' antimicrobial responses and alter their activation state to adapt to dynamic environmental cues. Two main factors can lead to differential gene expression in AMs. First, changes in transcriptional programs may occur in response to specific stimuli, and second, metabolic reprogramming causes gene-specific transcriptional changes and alterations. Signal-regulated transcription factors activate different macrophage gene expression programs by binding to numerous cis-regulatory regions [125–127]. The major transcription factors involved in modulating macrophage functions are signal transducer and activator of transcription (STATs) [128], NF-κβ [129, 130], PPAR-γ [131, 132], IRFs [133, 134], AP-1(activator protein) [135], and cAMP-responsive element-binding protein (CREB) [136]. STAT1 and STAT2 activation in response to type-1 IFNs (α- and -β) influence macrophage polarization [137]. STAT1 signaling protects against cryptococcal infections by activating nitric-oxide-producing classical macrophages [138–140] and STAT6/IRF-4 and Dectin-1 signaling pathways trigger IL-33 production in macrophages [134] during *Histoplasma* infection. Fungal recognition by Dectin-1, Dectin-2, and Mincle leads to NF-κB signaling, promoting antifungal responses of macrophages [129]. IκBα kinase (IKK) 2-complex, which tightly controls NF-κB activity, undergoes ubiquitination-dependent proteasomal degradation, releasing NF-κB dimer to translocate into the nucleus, facilitating its target genes [141].

Alveolar macrophage differentiation regulator, PPARγ, controls the expression of Dectin-1 and enhances defense against *C. albicans* [142]. PPARγ signaling induced by IL-13 or its ligands promoted the macrophage mannose receptor (MMR) expression [132]. CREB, the IL-1β-dependent transcription factor, promotes regulatory macrophage markers [136], and *Pneumocystis* lung infection in COPD animals increased the phosphorylated CREB and exhibited elevated inflammation [143].

2.4 Activation of adaptive immune cells

Activated AMs can process and present antigens to T cells essential for the activation and proliferation of T cells against pathogens [144]. However, compared with dendritic cells, AMs are not considered good antigen presenters as they downregulate the expression of the co-stimulatory molecules, B7-1 (CD80) and B7-2 (CD86), to induce peripheral tolerance to the many continuously exposed antigens in the lung [145]. However, AMs can effectively transport the antigens to the draining lymph nodes for antigen presentation [146]. Under certain pathological states, such as sarcoidosis, AMs develop distinctive antigen-presenting characteristics of DCs [147]. Interestingly, during Influenza A virus infection, cross-presentation of viral antigens by AMs is essential for the expansion of virus-specific $CD103^{+}CD8^{+}$ tissue-resident memory (TRM) cells to inhibit virus replication in the lungs during secondary infection [148]. Thus, AMs have the potential to modulate T cell responses during fungal infections.

3. Transcriptomic and metabolic adaptations at the macrophage-fungal Interface

It is increasingly evident that innate immune cells are imparted with a memory-like phenotype during infection or inflammation that is durable called trained immunity. The trained immunity exhibits a long-lasting functional reprogramming that leads to an enhanced response to subsequent inflammatory stimuli or infections [149]. Trained immunity involves mechanisms such as epigenetic and metabolic reprogramming of innate cells that linger and help in recalling quickly and robustly following re-exposure [150]. Despite the epigenetic imprinting, the duration of trained immunity is much shorter than adaptive immune memory and is reported to be between 3 months and 1 year [149]. The induction of trained immunity can occur both at the hematopoietic region (central) and at tissues (peripheral). Central induction of trained immunity involves hematopoietic stem cells (HSCs) responding to stimuli that enhance biased, possibly, epigenetically programmed daughter cells for directed response in the periphery [150]. Whereas the peripheral induction in the cells occurs at the site of tissues responding to infection or the stimuli. In infectious disease conditions, innate immunological memory can be advantageous or detrimental, leading to disease progression or persistent immunological tolerance based on the host immune status, infectious agent, and the nature of the disease.

The epigenetic reprogramming includes chromatin remodeling, modification of histones by methylation, and acetylation [151]. Epigenetic regulation significantly impacts macrophage activity, governing the behavior of tissue-resident and activated macrophages through distinct alterations, and the changes are regulated by intricate cellular mechanisms, highlighting the importance of epigenetic modifications in the immune response [152]. The β-glucans, one of the major PAMPs in fungi, have been shown to mediate trained immunity to monocytes/macrophages by increasing the production of IL-6 and TNF in *C. albicans*, *Mycobacterium tuberculosis*, and *Pseudomonas aeruginosa* [153–155] with stable changes in histone trimethylation at H3K4 [155]. In a *Cryptococcus neoformans* infection, the transcriptome of pulmonary macrophages of immunized mice showed increased expression of genes associated with signal transducer and activator of transcription 1 (STAT1) signaling pathway [156] correlated with enhanced immunity. Further, in immunized but unchallenged pulmonary macrophages, an increased binding of STAT1 to the promoter regions of known IFN-γ-induced genes was observed, which correlates with these macrophages' ability to rapidly respond to a secondary challenge and showing memory-like responses [156]. Similarly, studies with *Cryptococcus* and *Aspergillus* infections showed epigenetic modifications of AMs that are highly plastic to produce chemoattractant CXCL2 or immunoregulatory molecules IL-10 and C1q [154, 157]. *Pneumocystis* infection in the lung elevates the concentration of chloride channel accessory 1 (hCLCA1) in the infant lung parenchyma and causes overproduction of mucin 5 AC (MUC5AC) [158]. Epigenetic regulation of innate immune cells has been comprehensively reviewed elsewhere [159].

Epigenetic stability and trained immunity durability are coupled with metabolic adaptations during polarization [160]. Classically activated macrophages (M1), necessary for antifungal immunity, utilize Warburg metabolism with lower oxygen dependency [161]. The glycolysis dependency and increased glucose-6-phosphate shuttled to the pentose phosphate pathway help the formation of NADPH, which is crucial for generating ROS in the macrophage phagosome [162]. In contrast, alternatively, activated M2 macrophages utilize oxidative phosphorylation, mainly driven by fatty acid oxidation [163, 164]. Interestingly, the trained immunity following beta-glucan exposure required the glycolysis and pharmacological inhibition of glycolysis either by 2-DG or by PFKFB3 inhibitor to prevent the formation of innate memory [165, 166]. Although there is a tremendous integration of various metabolic pathways linked to trained immunity, including glutaminolysis [167], mechanistic insights during *in vivo* infection for the development of trained immunity in different macrophage subsets are lacking during fungal infections.

4. Conclusions

Significant progress has been made in the past decade in understanding how transcriptional, epigenetic, and metabolic mechanisms affect macrophage phenotype and function. *Alveolar macrophages* are highly plastic cells that perform various functions such as pathogen defense, efferocytosis, pulmonary tolerance, and inflammation resolution. Alveolar macrophages adapt to different phenotypes in response to the inflammatory milieu and have been a target for many therapeutics. The lack of understanding of macrophage mechanisms of adaptation during pulmonary fungal infections has been a major hurdle. Further, the stability, durability, plasticity, and metabolic switches of trained immunity are not clear. Thus, identifying the AM transcriptional or metabolic pathways would significantly advance the development of AM-directed strategies to treat or develop effective fungal vaccines against pulmonary fungal diseases.

Author details

Jaishree Sharma, Nitish Arun Kulkarni and Som Gowda Nanjappa*
Department of Pathobiology, College of Veterinary Medicine, University of Illinois at Urbana-Champaign, USA

*Address all correspondence to: nanjappa@illinois.edu

IntechOpen

© 2024 The Author(s). Licensee IntechOpen. This chapter is distributed under the terms of the Creative Commons Attribution License (http://creativecommons.org/licenses/by/3.0), which permits unrestricted use, distribution, and reproduction in any medium, provided the original work is properly cited.

References

[1] Bongomin F, Gago S, Oladele RO, Denning DW. Global and multi-National Prevalence of fungal diseases-estimate precision. Journal of Fungi (Basel, Switzerland). 2017;**3**(4):57. DOI: 10.3390/jof3040057

[2] Ekeng BE, Davies AA, Osaigbovo A II, Warris ROO, Denning DW. Pulmonary and extrapulmonary manifestations of fungal infections misdiagnosed as tuberculosis: The need for prompt diagnosis and management. Journal of Fungi (Basel, Switzerland). 2022;**8**(5):460. DOI: 10.3390/jof8050460

[3] Houben R, Lalli M, Kranzer K, Menzies NA, Schumacher SG, Dowdy DW. What if they don't have tuberculosis? The consequences and trade-offs involved in false-positive diagnoses of tuberculosis. Clinical Infectious Diseases. 2019;**68**(1):150-156. DOI: 10.1093/cid/ciy544

[4] Mazi PB et al. The geographic distribution of dimorphic mycoses in the United States for the modern era. Clinical Infectious Diseases. 2023;**76**(7):1295-1301. DOI: 10.1093/cid/ciac882

[5] Guilliams M et al. Alveolar macrophages develop from fetal monocytes that differentiate into long-lived cells in the first week of life via GM-CSF. The Journal of Experimental Medicine. 2013;**210**(10):1977-1992. DOI: 10.1084/jem.20131199

[6] Schneider C, Nobs SP, Kurrer M, Rehrauer H, Thiele C, Kopf M. Induction of the nuclear receptor PPAR-gamma by the cytokine GM-CSF is critical for the differentiation of fetal monocytes into alveolar macrophages. Nature Immunology. 2014;**15**(11):1026-1037. DOI: 10.1038/ni.3005

[7] Huffman Reed JA, Rice WR, Zsengeller ZK, Wert SE, Dranoff G, Whitsett JA. GM-CSF enhances lung growth and causes alveolar type II epithelial cell hyperplasia in transgenic mice. American Journal of Physiology. Lung Cellular. 1997;**273**(4):L715-L725. DOI: 10.1152/ajplung.1997.273.4.L715

[8] Woo YD, Jeong D, Chung DH. Development and functions of alveolar macrophages. Molecules and Cells. 2021;**44**(5):292-300. DOI: 10.14348/molcells.2021.0058

[9] Gschwend J et al. Alveolar macrophages rely on GM-CSF from alveolar epithelial type 2 cells before and after birth. The Journal of Experimental Medicine. 2021;**218**(10):e20210745. DOI: 10.1084/jem.20210745

[10] Sauter KA et al. Pleiotropic effects of extended blockade of CSF1R signaling in adult mice. Journal of Leukocyte Biology. 2014;**96**(2):265-274. DOI: 10.1189/jlb.2A0114-006R

[11] Draijer C, Penke LRK, Peters-Golden M. Distinctive effects of GM-CSF and M-CSF on proliferation and polarization of two major pulmonary macrophage populations. Journal of Immunology. 2019;**202**(9):2700-2709. DOI: 10.4049/jimmunol.1801387

[12] Deng W, Yang J, Lin X, Shin J, Gao J, Zhong XP. Essential role of mTORC1 in self-renewal of murine alveolar macrophages. Journal of Immunology. 2017;**198**(1):492-504. DOI: 10.4049/jimmunol.1501845

[13] Guthridge MA et al. The phosphoserine-585-dependent pathway of the GM-CSF/IL-3/IL-5 receptors mediates hematopoietic cell survival

through activation of NF-kappaB and induction of bcl-2. Blood. 2004;**103**(3):820-827. DOI: 10.1182/blood-2003-06-1999

[14] Chao JR et al. mcl-1 is an immediate-early gene activated by the granulocyte-macrophage colony-stimulating factor (GM-CSF) signaling pathway and is one component of the GM-CSF viability response. Molecular and Cellular Biology. 1998;**18**(8):4883-4898. DOI: 10.1128/MCB.18.8.4883

[15] Woo YD et al. Ssu72 regulates alveolar macrophage development and allergic airway inflammation by fine-tuning of GM-CSF receptor signaling. The Journal of Allergy and Clinical Immunology. 2021;**147**(4):1242-1260. DOI: 10.1016/j.jaci.2020.07.038

[16] Yu X et al. The cytokine TGF-beta promotes the development and homeostasis of alveolar macrophages. Immunity. 2017;**47**(5):903-912 e4. DOI: 10.1016/j.immuni.2017.10.007

[17] Evren E, Ringqvist E, Willinger T. Origin and ontogeny of lung macrophages: From mice to humans. Immunology. 2020;**160**(2):126-138. DOI: 10.1111/imm.13154

[18] Hoeffel G et al. C-Myb(+) erythro-myeloid progenitor-derived fetal monocytes give rise to adult tissue-resident macrophages. Immunity. 2015;**42**(4):665-678. DOI: 10.1016/j.immuni.2015.03.011

[19] Misharin AV et al. Monocyte-derived alveolar macrophages drive lung fibrosis and persist in the lung over the life span. The Journal of Experimental Medicine. 2017;**214**(8):2387-2404. DOI: 10.1084/jem.20162152

[20] Landsman L, Jung S. Lung macrophages serve as obligatory intermediate between blood monocytes and alveolar macrophages. Journal of Immunology. 2007;**179**(6):3488-3494. DOI: 10.4049/jimmunol.179.6.3488

[21] Landsman L, Varol C, Jung S. Distinct differentiation potential of blood monocyte subsets in the lung. Journal of Immunology. 2007;**178**(4):2000-2007. DOI: 10.4049/jimmunol.178.4.2000

[22] Hashimoto D et al. Tissue-resident macrophages self-maintain locally throughout adult life with minimal contribution from circulating monocytes. Immunity. 2013;**38**(4):792-804. DOI: 10.1016/j.immuni.2013.04.004

[23] Groves E, Dart AE, Covarelli V, Caron E. Molecular mechanisms of phagocytic uptake in mammalian cells. Cellular and Molecular Life Sciences. 2008;**65**(13):1957-1976. DOI: 10.1007/s00018-008-7578-4

[24] Heung LJ, Wiesner DL, Wang K, Rivera A, Hohl TM. Immunity to fungi in the lung. Seminars in Immunology. 2023;**66**:101728. DOI: 10.1016/j.smim.2023.101728

[25] Hatinguais R, Willment JA, Brown GD. PAMPs of the fungal cell wall and mammalian PRRs. Current Topics in Microbiology and Immunology. 2020;**425**:187-223. DOI: 10.1007/82_2020_201

[26] Gow NA, Latge J-P, Munro CA. The fungal cell wall: Structure, biosynthesis, and function. Microbiology Spectrum. 2017;**5**(3):1-25. DOI: 10.1128/microbiolspec.funk-0035-2016

[27] Mora-Montes HM, Ponce-Noyola P, Villagómez-Castro JC, Gow NA, Flores-Carreón A, López-Romero E. Protein glycosylation in Candida. Future Microbiology. 2009;**4**(9):1167-1183

[28] Margalit A, Kavanagh K. The innate immune response to aspergillus fumigatus at the alveolar surface. FEMS Microbiology Reviews. 2015;**39**(5):670-687. DOI: 10.1093/femsre/fuv018

[29] Patin EC, Thompson A, Orr SJ. Pattern recognition receptors in fungal immunity. In: Seminars in Cell & Developmental Biology. Vol. 89. Elsevier; 2019. pp. 24-33. DOI: 10.1016/j.semcdb.2018.03.003

[30] Aimanianda V et al. Surface hydrophobin prevents immune recognition of airborne fungal spores. Nature. 2009;**460**(7259):1117-1121

[31] Lee MJ et al. The fungal exopolysaccharide galactosaminogalactan mediates virulence by enhancing resistance to neutrophil extracellular traps. PLoS Pathogens. 2015;**11**(10):e1005187. DOI: 10.1371/journal.ppat.1005187

[32] Latgé J-P, Beauvais A, Chamilos G. The cell wall of the human fungal pathogen aspergillus fumigatus: Biosynthesis, organization, immune response, and virulence. Annual Review of Microbiology. 2017;**71**:99-116

[33] Bellocchio S et al. The contribution of the toll-like/IL-1 receptor superfamily to innate and adaptive immunity to fungal pathogens in vivo. Journal of Immunology. 2004;**172**(5):3059-3069. DOI: 10.4049/jimmunol.172.5.3059

[34] Lionakis MS, Iliev ID, Hohl TM. Immunity against fungi. JCI Insight. 2017;**2**(11):1-18

[35] de Oliviera Nascimento L, Massari P, Wetzler LM. The role of TLR2 in infection and immunity. Frontiers in Immunology. 2012;**3**:20479

[36] Taylor PR et al. Dectin-1 is required for β-glucan recognition and control of fungal infection. Nature Immunology. 2007;**8**(1):31-38

[37] Drummond RA, Brown GD. The role of Dectin-1 in the host defence against fungal infections. Current Opinion in Microbiology. 2011;**14**(4):392-399. DOI: 10.1016/j.mib.2011.07.001

[38] Geijtenbeek TB, Gringhuis SI. Signalling through C-type lectin receptors: Shaping immune responses. Nature Reviews Immunology. 2009;**9**(7):465-479

[39] Navarro-Arias MJ, López MG, Gacser A, Mora-Montes HM. Members of the Candida parapsilosis complex and Candida albicans are differentially recognized by human peripheral blood mononuclear cells. Frontiers in Microbiology. 2016;**6**:174346

[40] Wheeler RT, Fink GR. A drug-sensitive genetic network masks fungi from the immune system. PLoS Pathogens. 2006;**2**(4):e35

[41] Rappleye CA, Eissenberg LG, Goldman WE. Histoplasma capsulatum α-(1, 3)-glucan blocks innate immune recognition by the β-glucan receptor. Proceedings of the National Academy of Sciences. 2007;**104**(4):1366-1370

[42] Reedy JL et al. The C-type lectin receptor Dectin-2 is a receptor for *Aspergillus fumigatus* galactomannan. Mbio. 2023;**14**(1):1-14. DOI: 10.1128/mbio.03184-22

[43] Kottom TJ et al. Dectin-2 is a C-type lectin receptor that recognizes and participates in innate immune responses. American Journal of Respiratory Cell and Molecular Biology. 2018;**58**(2):232-240. DOI: 10.1165/rcmb.2016-0335OC

[44] Wang H et al. Ligation of Dectin-2 with a novel microbial ligand promotes

adjuvant activity for vaccination. PLoS Pathogens. 2017;**13**(8):e1006568. DOI: 10.1371/journal.ppat.1006568

[45] Thompson A et al. Dependence on Mincle and Dectin-2 varies with multiple Candida species during systemic infection. Frontiers in Microbiology. 2021;**12**:633229. DOI: 10.3389/fmicb.2021.633229

[46] Beaussart A, Brandhorst T, Dufrêne YF, Klein BS. Blastomyces virulence adhesin-1 protein binding to glycosaminoglycans is enhanced by protein disulfide isomerase. MBio. 2015;**6**(5). DOI: 10.1128/mbio.01403-15

[47] Park SJ, Mehrad B. Innate immunity to *Aspergillus* species. Clinical Microbiology Reviews. 2009;**22**(4):535-551. DOI: 10.1128/CMR.00014-09

[48] Dubourdeau M et al. *Aspergillus fumigatus* induces innate immune responses in alveolar macrophages through the MAPK pathway independently of TLR2 and TLR4. Journal of Immunology. 2006;**177**(6):3994-4001. DOI: 10.4049/jimmunol.177.6.3994

[49] Zhang HJ, Qu JM, Shao CZ, Zhang J, He LX, Yuan ZH. *Aspergillus fumigatus* conidia upregulates NOD2 protein expression both in vitro and in vivo. Acta Pharmacologica Sinica. 2008;**29**(10):1202-1208. DOI: 10.1111/j.1745-7254.2008.00860.x

[50] Chen Y et al. MDA5 enhances invasive Candida albicans infection by regulating macrophage apoptosis and phagocytosis/killing functions. Inflammation. 2024;**47**(1):191-208. DOI: 10.1007/s10753-023-01903-5

[51] Wang X et al. MAVS expression in alveolar macrophages is essential for host resistance against. Journal of Immunology. 2022;**209**(2):346-353. DOI: 10.4049/jimmunol.2100759

[52] Li Q, Wu P, Du Q, Hanif U, Hu H, Li K. cGAS-STING, an important signaling pathway in diseases and their therapy. MedComm. 2020;**5**(4):e511, 2024. DOI: 10.1002/mco2.511

[53] Brown Harding H et al. Candida albicans extracellular vesicles trigger type I IFN signalling via cGAS and STING. Nature Microbiology. 2024;**9**(1):95-107. DOI: 10.1038/s41564-023-01546-0

[54] Sterkel AK, Mettelman R, Wuthrich M, Klein BS. The unappreciated intracellular lifestyle of *Blastomyces dermatitidis*. Journal of Immunology. 2015;**194**(4):1796-1805. DOI: 10.4049/jimmunol.1303089

[55] Xu-Vanpala S et al. Functional heterogeneity of alveolar macrophage population based on expression of CXCL2. Science Immunology. 2020;**5**(50):eaba7350. DOI: 10.1126/sciimmunol.aba7350

[56] Swanson JA, Hoppe AD. The coordination of signaling during FC receptor-mediated phagocytosis. Journal of Leukocyte Biology. 2004;**76**(6):1093-1103. DOI: 10.1189/jlb.0804439

[57] Laassili C et al. FC receptors act as innate immune receptors during infection? Frontiers in Immunology. 2023;**14**:1-9

[58] Mosser DM, Zhang X. Measuring opsonic phagocytosis via Fc gamma receptors and complement receptors on macrophages. Current Protocols in Immunology. Chapter 14, p. Unit 14 27. 2011;**95**. DOI: 10.1002/0471142735.im1427s95

[59] Griffin FM Jr. Roles of macrophage FC and C3b receptors in phagocytosis of

immunologically coated cryptococcus neoformans. Proceedings of the National Academy of Sciences of the United States of America. 1981;**78**(6):3853-3857. DOI: 10.1073/pnas.78.6.3853

[60] Luo Y, Tucker SC, Casadevall A. Fc- and complement-receptor activation stimulates cell cycle progression of macrophage cells from G1 to S. Journal of Immunology. 2005;**174**(11):7226-7233. DOI: 10.4049/jimmunol.174.11.7226

[61] McQuiston T, Luberto C, Del Poeta M. Role of sphingosine-1-phosphate (S1P) and S1P receptor 2 in the phagocytosis of cryptococcus neoformans by alveolar macrophages. Microbiology (Reading). 2011;**157**(Pt. 5):1416-1427. DOI: 10.1099/mic.0.045989-0

[62] Moalli F et al. Role of complement and Fc gamma receptors in the protective activity of the long pentraxin PTX3 against *Aspergillus fumigatus*. Blood. 2010;**116**(24):5170-5180. DOI: 10.1182/blood-2009-12-258376

[63] Philippe B et al. Killing of *Aspergillus fumigatus* by alveolar macrophages is mediated by reactive oxidant intermediates. Infection and Immunity. 2003;**71**(6):3034-3042. DOI: 10.1128/IAI.71.6.3034-3042.2003

[64] Aronoff DM et al. Stimulatory effects of peroxisome proliferator-activated receptor-γ on Fc γ receptor-mediated phagocytosis by alveolar macrophages. PPAR Research. 2007;**2007**:1-9

[65] Mancuso P, Standiford TJ, Marshall T, Peters-Golden M. 5-Lipoxygenase reaction products modulate alveolar macrophage phagocytosis of Klebsiella pneumoniae. Infection and Immunity. 1998;**66**(11):5140-5146. DOI: 10.1128/IAI.66.11.5140-5146.1998

[66] Ibrahim-Granet O, Philippe B, Boleti H, Boisvieux-Ulrich E, Grenet D, Stern M, et al. Phagocytosis and intracellular fate of Aspergillus fumigatus conidia in alveolar macrophages. Infection and Immunity. 2003;**71**(2):891-903. DOI: 10.1128/iai.71.2.891-903.2003

[67] Kasperkovitz PV, Cardenas ML, Vyas JM. TLR9 is actively recruited to Aspergillus fumigatus phagosomes and requires the N-terminal proteolytic cleavage domain for proper intracellular trafficking. The Journal of Immunology. 2010;**185**(12):7614-7622. DOI: 10.4049/jimmunol.1002760

[68] Faro-Trindade I, Willment JA, Kerrigan AM, Redelinghuys P, Hadebe S, Reid DM, et al. Characterisation of innate fungal recognition in the lung. PloS one. 2012;**7**(4):e35675. DOI: 10.1371/journal.pone.0035675

[69] Bonnerot C et al. Syk protein tyrosine kinase regulates Fc receptor gamma-chain-mediated transport to lysosomes. The EMBO Journal. 1998;**17**(16):4606-4616. DOI: 10.1093/emboj/17.16.4606

[70] Underhill DM, Ozinsky A. Phagocytosis of microbes: Complexity in action. Annual Review of Immunology. 2002;**20**(1):825-852. DOI: 10.1146/annurev.immunol.20.103001.114744

[71] Crocker PR, Paulson JC, Varki A. Siglecs and their roles in the immune system. Nature Reviews. Immunology. 2007;**7**(4):255-266. DOI: 10.1038/nri2056

[72] Goyal S, Castrillon-Betancur JC, Klaile E, Slevogt H. The interaction of human pathogenic fungi with C-type lectin receptors. Frontiers in Immunology. 2018;**9**:1261. DOI: 10.3389/fimmu.2018.01261

[73] Grabiec AM, Hussell T. The role of airway macrophages in apoptotic cell

clearance following acute and chronic lung inflammation. In: Seminars in Immunopathology. Vol. 38. Springer; 2016. pp. 409-423. DOI: 10.1007/s00281-016-0555-3

[74] Kim KK et al. Efferocytosis of apoptotic alveolar epithelial cells is sufficient to initiate lung fibrosis. Cell Death & Disease. 2018;**9**(11):1056. DOI: 10.1038/s41419-018-1074-z

[75] Mohning MP et al. Phagocytosis of microparticles by alveolar macrophages during acute lung injury requires MerTK. American Journal of Physiology. Lung Cellular and Molecular Physiology. 2018;**314**(1):L69-L82. DOI: 10.1152/ajplung.00058.2017

[76] Fadok VA, Bratton DL, Konowal A, Freed PW, Westcott JY, Henson PM. Macrophages that have ingested apoptotic cells in vitro inhibit proinflammatory cytokine production through autocrine/paracrine mechanisms involving TGF-beta, PGE2, and PAF. The Journal of Clinical Investigation. 1998;**101**(4):890-898. DOI: 10.1172/JCI1112

[77] Huynh ML, Fadok VA, Henson PM. Phosphatidylserine-dependent ingestion of apoptotic cells promotes TGF-beta1 secretion and the resolution of inflammation. The Journal of Clinical Investigation. 2002;**109**(1):41-50. DOI: 10.1172/JCI11638

[78] Roquilly A et al. Alveolar macrophages are epigenetically altered after inflammation, leading to long-term lung immunoparalysis. Nature Immunology. 2020;**21**(6):636-648. [Online]. Available from: https://www.nature.com/articles/s41590-020-0673-x.pdf

[79] Wong CK, Smith CA, Sakamoto K, Kaminski N, Koff JL, Goldstein DR. Aging impairs alveolar macrophage phagocytosis and increases influenza-induced mortality in mice. Journal of Immunology. 2017;**199**(3):1060-1068. DOI: 10.4049/jimmunol.1700397

[80] O'Beirne SL et al. Alveolar macrophage immunometabolism and lung function impairment in smoking and chronic obstructive pulmonary disease. American Journal of Respiratory and Critical Care Medicine. 2020;**201**(6):735-739. DOI: 10.1164/rccm.201908-1683LE

[81] Fitzpatrick AM, Holguin F, Teague WG, Brown LA. Alveolar macrophage phagocytosis is impaired in children with poorly controlled asthma. The Journal of Allergy and Clinical Immunology. 2008;**121**(6):1372-8-1378 e1-3. DOI: 10.1016/j.jaci.2008.03.008

[82] Huynh ML et al. Defective apoptotic cell phagocytosis attenuates prostaglandin E2 and 15-hydroxyeicosatetraenoic acid in severe asthma alveolar macrophages. American Journal of Respiratory and Critical Care Medicine. 2005;**172**(8):972-979. DOI: 10.1164/rccm.200501-035OC

[83] Fang FC. Antimicrobial reactive oxygen and nitrogen species: Concepts and controversies. Nature Reviews. Microbiology. 2004;**2**(10):820-832. DOI: 10.1038/nrmicro1004

[84] Li H, Zhou X, Huang Y, Liao B, Cheng L, Ren B. Reactive oxygen species in pathogen clearance: The killing mechanisms, the adaption response, and the side effects. Frontiers in Microbiology. 2021;**11**:622534. [Online]. Available from: https://www.ncbi.nlm.nih.gov/pmc/articles/PMC7889972/pdf/fmicb-11-622534.pdf

[85] MacMicking J, Xie QW, Nathan C. Nitric oxide and macrophage function.

Annual Review of Immunology. 1997;**15**(1):323-350. DOI: 10.1146/annurev.immunol.15.1.323

[86] Goldbart A, Gatt D, Golan Tripto I. Non-tuberculous mycobacteria infection treated with intermittently inhaled high-dose nitric oxide. BML Case Reports. 2021;**14**(10):e243979. DOI: 10.1136/bcr-2021-243979

[87] Nathan C, Shiloh MU. Reactive oxygen and nitrogen intermediates in the relationship between mammalian hosts and microbial pathogens. Proceedings of the National Academy of Sciences of the United States of America. 2000;**97**(16):8841-8848. DOI: 10.1073/pnas.97.16.8841

[88] Allendoerfer R, Deepe GS Jr. Blockade of endogenous TNF-alpha exacerbates primary and secondary pulmonary histoplasmosis by differential mechanisms. Journal of Immunology. 1998;**160**(12):6072-6082. [Online]. Available from: https://www.ncbi.nlm.nih.gov/pubmed/9637524

[89] Livonesi MC et al. Inducible nitric oxide synthase-deficient mice show exacerbated inflammatory process and high production of both Th1 and Th2 cytokines during paracoccidioidomycosis. Microbes and Infection. 2009;**11**(1):123-132. DOI: 10.1016/j.micinf.2008.10.015

[90] Jimenez MD, Walls L, Fierer J. High levels of interleukin-10 impair resistance to pulmonary coccidioidomycosis in mice in part through control of nitric oxide synthase 2 expression. Infection and Immunity. 2006;**74**(6):3387-3395. DOI: 10.1128/Iai.01985-05

[91] Tohyama M, Kawakami K, Futenma M, Saito A. Enhancing effect of oxygen radical scavengers on murine macrophage anticryptococcal activity through production of nitric oxide. Clinical and Experimental Immunology. 1996;**103**(3):436-441. [Online]. Available from: <Go to ISI>://WOS:A1996TZ24100014

[92] Shlezinger N, Hohl TM. Mitochondrial reactive oxygen species enhance alveolar macrophage activity against *Aspergillus fumigatus* but are dispensable for host protection. mSphere. 2021;**6**(3):e0026021. DOI: 10.1128/mSphere.00260-21

[93] Canton M et al. Reactive oxygen species in macrophages: Sources and targets. Frontiers in Immunology. 2021;**12**:734229. DOI: 10.3389/fimmu.2021.734229

[94] Stuehr DJ, Marletta MA. Mammalian nitrate biosynthesis: Mouse macrophages produce nitrite and nitrate in response to *Escherichia coli* lipopolysaccharide. Proceedings of the National Academy of Sciences of the United States of America. 1985;**82**(22):7738-7742. DOI: 10.1073/pnas.82.22.7738

[95] Xie QW, Kashiwabara Y, Nathan C. Role of transcription factor NF-kappa B/Rel in induction of nitric oxide synthase. The Journal of Biological Chemistry. 1994;**269**(7):4705-4708. [Online]. Available from: https://www.ncbi.nlm.nih.gov/pubmed/7508926

[96] Kamijo R et al. Requirement for transcription factor IRF-1 in NO synthase induction in macrophages. Science. 1994;**263**(5153):1612-1615. DOI: 10.1126/science.7510419

[97] Taylor BS, Geller DA. Molecular regulation of the human inducible nitric oxide synthase (iNOS) gene. Shock. 2000;**13**(6):413-424. DOI: 10.1097/00024382-200006000-00001

[98] Vazquez-Torres A et al. Toll-like receptor 4 dependence of innate and adaptive immunity to salmonella: Importance of the Kupffer cell network. Journal of Immunology. 2004;**172**(10):6202-6208. DOI: 10.4049/jimmunol.172.10.6202

[99] Asada K, Sasaki S, Suda T, Chida K, Nakamura H. Antiinflammatory roles of peroxisome proliferator-activated receptor gamma in human alveolar macrophages. American Journal of Respiratory and Critical Care Medicine. 2004;**169**(2):195-200. DOI: 10.1164/rccm.200207-740OC

[100] Reddy RC et al. Deactivation of murine alveolar macrophages by peroxisome proliferator-activated receptor-gamma ligands. American Journal of Physiology. Lung Cellular and Molecular Physiology. 2004;**286**(3):L613-L619. DOI: 10.1152/ajplung.00206.2003

[101] Fang FC. Nitric Oxide and Infection. Springer; 1999. Available from: https://link.springer.com/content/pdf/10.1007/b111485.pdf

[102] Miller RA, Britigan BE. Role of oxidants in microbial pathophysiology. Clinical Microbiology Reviews. 1997;**10**(1):1-18. DOI: 10.1128/CMR.10.1.1

[103] Rocco NM, Carmen JC, Klein BS. Blastomyces dermatitidis yeast cells inhibit nitric oxide production by alveolar macrophage inducible nitric oxide synthase. Infection and Immunity. 2011;**79**(6):2385-2395. DOI: 10.1128/IAI.01249-10

[104] Lasbury ME et al. Defective nitric oxide production by alveolar macrophages during pneumocystis pneumonia. American Journal of Respiratory Cell and Molecular Biology. 2011;**44**(4):540-547. DOI: 10.1165/rcmb.2009-0367OC

[105] Juarez E, Nunez C, Sada E, Ellner JJ, Schwander SK, Torres M. Differential expression of toll-like receptors on human alveolar macrophages and autologous peripheral monocytes. Respiratory Research. 2010;**11**(1):2. DOI: 10.1186/1465-9921-11-2

[106] Hoogerwerf JJ et al. Priming of alveolar macrophages upon instillation of lipopolysaccharide in the human lung. American Journal of Respiratory Cell and Molecular Biology. 2010;**42**(3):349-356. DOI: 10.1165/rcmb.2008-0362OC

[107] Bissonnette EY, Lauzon-Joset JF, Debley JS, Ziegler SF. Cross-talk between alveolar macrophages and lung epithelial cells is essential to maintain lung homeostasis. Frontiers in Immunology. 2020;**11**:583042. DOI: 10.3389/fimmu.2020.583042

[108] Alp S et al. Expression of beta-defensin 1 and 2 in nasal epithelial cells and alveolar macrophages from HIV-infected patients. European Journal of Medical Research. 2005;**10**(1):1-6. [Online]. Available from: https://www.ncbi.nlm.nih.gov/pubmed/15737946

[109] Russell RE et al. Alveolar macrophage-mediated elastolysis: Roles of matrix metalloproteinases, cysteine, and serine proteases. American Journal of Physiology. Lung Cellular and Molecular Physiology. 2002;**283**(4):L867-L873. DOI: 10.1152/ajplung.00020.2002

[110] Marriott HM et al. Interleukin-1beta regulates CXCL8 release and influences disease outcome in response to Streptococcus pneumoniae, defining intercellular cooperation between pulmonary epithelial cells and macrophages. Infection and Immunity.

2012;**80**(3):1140-1149. DOI: 10.1128/IAI.05697-11

[111] De Filippo K et al. Mast cell and macrophage chemokines CXCL1/CXCL2 control the early stage of neutrophil recruitment during tissue inflammation. Blood. 2013;**121**(24):4930-4937. DOI: 10.1182/blood-2013-02-486217

[112] Gersuk GM, Underhill DM, Zhu L, Marr KA. Dectin-1 and TLRs permit macrophages to distinguish between different *Aspergillus fumigatus* cellular states. Journal of Immunology. 2006;**176**(6):3717-3724. DOI: 10.4049/jimmunol.176.6.3717

[113] Hohl TM et al. *Aspergillus fumigatus* triggers inflammatory responses by stage-specific beta-glucan display. PLoS Pathogens. 2005;**1**(3):e30. DOI: 10.1371/journal.ppat.0010030

[114] Leopold Wager CM, Wormley FL Jr. Classical versus alternative macrophage activation: The Ying and the Yang in host defense against pulmonary fungal infections. Mucosal Immunology. 2014;7(5):1023-1035. DOI: 10.1038/mi.2014.65

[115] Mosser DM, Edwards JP. Exploring the full spectrum of macrophage activation. Nature Reviews Immunology. 2008;**8**(12):958-969. DOI: 10.1038/nri2448

[116] Stout RD, Suttles J. Functional plasticity of macrophages: Reversible adaptation to changing microenvironments. Journal of Leukocyte Biology. 2004;**76**(3):509-513. DOI: 10.1189/jlb.0504272

[117] Van Dyken SJ, Locksley RM. Interleukin-4- and interleukin-13-mediated alternatively activated macrophages: Roles in homeostasis and disease. Annual Review of Immunology. 2013;**31**:317-343. DOI: 10.1146/annurev-immunol-032712-095906

[118] Martinez FO, Helming L, Gordon S. Alternative activation of macrophages: An immunologic functional perspective. Annual Review of Immunology. 2009;**27**:451-483. DOI: 10.1146/annurev.immunol.021908.132532

[119] Murray PJ, Wynn TA. Protective and pathogenic functions of macrophage subsets. Nature Reviews Immunology. 2011;**11**(11):723-737. DOI: 10.1038/nri3073

[120] Nelson MP et al. IL-33 and M2a alveolar macrophages promote lung defense against the atypical fungal pathogen pneumocystis murina. Journal of Immunology. 2011;**186**(4):2372-2381. DOI: 10.4049/jimmunol.1002558

[121] Xiao G et al. Cryptococcus neoformans inhibits nitric oxide synthesis caused by CpG-oligodeoxynucleotide-stimulated macrophages in a fashion independent of capsular polysaccharides. Microbiology and Immunology. 2008;**52**(3):171-179. DOI: 10.1111/j.1348-0421.2008.00019.x

[122] Arora S, Dev K, Agarwal B, Das P, Syed MA. Macrophages: Their role, activation and polarization in pulmonary diseases. Immunobiology. 2018;**223**(4-5):383-396

[123] Strickland AB, Chen Y, Sun D, Shi M. Alternatively activated lung alveolar and interstitial macrophages promote fungal growth. Iscience. 2023;**26**(5):1-21

[124] Ren Y, Khan FA, Pandupuspitasari NS, Zhang S. Immune evasion strategies of pathogens in macrophages: The potential for limiting pathogen transmission. Current Issues in Molecular Biology. 2017;**21**(1):21-40

[125] Barish GD et al. Bcl-6 and NF-κB cistromes mediate opposing regulation of the innate immune response. Genes & Development. 2010;**24**(24):2760-2765

[126] Ghisletti S et al. Identification and characterization of enhancers controlling the inflammatory gene expression program in macrophages. Immunity. 2010;**32**(3):317-328

[127] Heinz S et al. Simple combinations of lineage-determining transcription factors prime cis-regulatory elements required for macrophage and B cell identities. Molecular Cell. 2010;**38**(4):576-589

[128] Lawrence T, Natoli G. Transcriptional regulation of macrophage polarization: Enabling diversity with identity. Nature Reviews Immunology. 2011;**11**(11):750-761

[129] Sun H et al. Activation of NF-κB and respiratory burst following *Aspergillus fumigatus* stimulation of macrophages. Immunobiology. 2014;**219**(1):25-36

[130] Brummer E, Choi J-H, Stevens D. Interaction between conidia, lung macrophages, immunosuppressants, proinflammatory cytokines and transcriptional regulation. Medical Mycology. 2005;**43**(Supplement. 1):S177-S179

[131] Evans RJ, Pline K, Loynes CA, Needs S, Aldrovandi M, Tiefenbach J, et al. 15-keto-prostaglandin E2 activates host peroxisome proliferator-activated receptor gamma (PPAR-γ) to promote Cryptococcus neoformans growth during infection. PLoS Pathogens. 2019;**15**(3):e1007597, 1-28. DOI: 10.1371/journal.ppat.1007597

[132] Coste A et al. PPARγ promotes mannose receptor gene expression in murine macrophages and contributes to the induction of this receptor by IL-13. Immunity. 2003;**19**(3):329-339

[133] Inglis DO, Berkes CA, Hocking Murray DR, Sil A. Conidia but not yeast cells of the fungal pathogen Histoplasma capsulatum trigger a type I interferon innate immune response in murine macrophages. Infection and Immunity. 2010;**78**(9):3871-3882

[134] Verma A, Kroetz DN, Tweedle JL, Deepe GS Jr. Type II cytokines impair host defense against an intracellular fungal pathogen by amplifying macrophage generation of IL-33. Mucosal Immunology; 2015;**8**(2):380-389. DOI: 10.1038/mi.2014.75

[135] Huang J-H et al. CR3 and dectin-1 collaborate in macrophage cytokine response through association on lipid rafts and activation of Syk-JNK-AP-1 pathway. PLoS Pathogens. 2015;**11**(7):e1004985

[136] Elcombe SE et al. Dectin-1 regulates IL-10 production via a MSK1/2 and CREB dependent pathway and promotes the induction of regulatory macrophage markers. PLoS One. 2013;**8**(3):e60086

[137] Park C, Li S, Cha E, Schindler C. Immune response in Stat2 knockout mice. Immunity. 2000;**13**(6):795-804

[138] Wager CML, Hole CR, Wozniak KL, Olszewski MA, Wormley FL Jr. STAT1 signaling is essential for protection against Cryptococcus neoformans infection in mice. Journal of Immunology (Baltimore, Md.: 1950). 2014;**193**(8):4060

[139] Hardison SE, Herrera G, Young ML, Hole CR, Wozniak KL, Wormley FL. Protective immunity against pulmonary cryptococcosis is associated with STAT1-mediated classical macrophage

activation. The Journal of Immunology. 2012;**189**(8):4060-4068

[140] Leopold Wager CM, Hole CR, Wozniak KL, Olszewski MA, Mueller M, Wormley FL Jr. STAT1 signaling within macrophages is required for antifungal activity against Cryptococcus neoformans. Infection and Immunity. 2015;**83**(12):4513-4527

[141] Kingeter LM, Lin X. C-type lectin receptor-induced NF-κB activation in innate immune and inflammatory responses. Cellular & Molecular Immunology. 2012;**9**(2):105-112

[142] Galès A et al. PPARγ controls Dectin-1 expression required for host antifungal defense against Candida albicans. PLoS Pathogens. 2010;**6**(1):e1000714

[143] Coronado K, Herrada C, Rojas DA. Role of the fungus pneumocystis in IL1β pathway activation and airways collagen deposition in elastase-induced COPD animals. International Journal of Molecular Sciences. 2024;**25**(6):3150

[144] Toews GB et al. The accessory cell function of human alveolar macrophages in specific T cell proliferation. Journal of Immunology. 1984;**132**(1):181-186. [Online]. Available from: https://www.ncbi.nlm.nih.gov/pubmed/6228577

[145] Chelen CJ, Fang Y, Freeman GJ, Secrist H, Marshall JD, Hwang PT et al. Human alveolar macrophages present antigen ineffectively due to defective expression of B7 costimulation cell surface molecules. The Journal of Clinical Investigation. 1995;**95**(3):1415-1421. DOI: 10.1172.JC1117796

[146] Kirby AC, Coles MC, Kaye PM. Alveolar macrophages transport pathogens to lung draining lymph nodes. Journal of Immunology. 2009;**183**(3):1983-1989. DOI: 10.4049/jimmunol.0901089

[147] Nicod LP, Cochand L, Dreher D. Antigen presentation in the lung: Dendritic cells and macrophages. Sarcoidosis, Vasculitis, and Diffuse Lung Diseases. 2000;**17**(3):246-255. [Online]. Available from: https://www.ncbi.nlm.nih.gov/pubmed/11033840

[148] Kawasaki T et al. Alveolar macrophages instruct CD8(+) T cell expansion by antigen cross-presentation in lung. Cell Reports. 2022;**41**(11):111828. DOI: 10.1016/j.celrep.2022.111828

[149] Netea MG et al. Defining trained immunity and its role in health and disease. Nature Reviews. Immunology. 2020;**20**(6):375-388. DOI: 10.1038/s41577-020-0285-6

[150] Dagenais A, Villalba-Guerrero C, Olivier M. Trained immunity: A "new" weapon in the fight against infectious diseases. Frontiers in Immunology. 2023;**14**:1147476. DOI: 10.3389/fimmu.2023.1147476

[151] Allis CD, Jenuwein T. The molecular hallmarks of epigenetic control. Nature Reviews Genetics. 2016;**17**(8):487-500

[152] Zhang P et al. HMGB1 mediates *Aspergillus fumigatus*-induced inflammatory response in alveolar macrophages of COPD mice via activating MyD88/NF-κB and syk/PI3K signalings. International Immunopharmacology. 2017;**53**:125-132

[153] Braian C, Karlsson L, Das J, Lerm M. Selected beta-glucans act as immune-training agents by improving anti-mycobacterial activity in human macrophages: A pilot study. Journal of Innate Immunity. 2023;**15**(1):751-764. DOI: 10.1159/000533873

[154] McBride MA et al. Bacteria- and fungus-derived PAMPs induce innate immune memory via similar functional, metabolic, and transcriptional adaptations. Journal of Leukocyte Biology. 2024;**115**(2):358-373. DOI: 10.1093/jleuko/qiad120

[155] Quintin J et al. Candida albicans infection affords protection against reinfection via functional reprogramming of monocytes. Cell Host & Microbe. 2012;**12**(2):223-232. DOI: 10.1016/j.chom.2012.06.006

[156] Leopold Wager CM et al. IFN-gamma immune priming of macrophages in vivo induces prolonged STAT1 binding and protection against cryptococcus neoformans. PLoS Pathogens. 2018;**14**(10):e1007358. DOI: 10.1371/journal.ppat.1007358

[157] Wang Y, Pawar S, Dutta O, Wang K, Rivera A, Xue C. Macrophage mediated immunomodulation during cryptococcus pulmonary infection. Frontiers in Cellular and Infection Microbiology. 2022;**12**:859049. DOI: 10.3389/fcimb.2022.859049

[158] Pérez FJ et al. Fungal colonization with pneumocystis correlates to increasing chloride channel accessory 1 (hCLCA1) suggesting a pathway for up-regulation of airway mucus responses, in infant lungs. Results in Immunology. 2014;**4**:58-61

[159] Zhang Q, Cao X. Epigenetic regulation of the innate immune response to infection. Nature Reviews Immunology. 2019;**19**(7):417-432

[160] Sprenger M, Kasper L, Hensel M, Hube B. Metabolic adaptation of intracellular bacteria and fungi to macrophages. International Journal of Medical Microbiology. 2018;**308**(1):215-227

[161] O'Neill LA, Pearce EJ. Immunometabolism governs dendritic cell and macrophage function. Journal of Experimental Medicine. 2016;**213**(1):15-23

[162] Ganeshan K, Chawla A. Metabolic regulation of immune responses. Annual Review of Immunology. 2014;**32**:609-634

[163] Galván-Peña S, O'Neill LA. Metabolic reprograming in macrophage polarization. Frontiers in Immunology. 2014;**5**:109777

[164] Wculek SK et al. Oxidative phosphorylation selectively orchestrates tissue macrophage homeostasis. Immunity. 2023;**56**(3):516-530. e9

[165] Cheng SC et al. mTOR- and HIF-1α-mediated aerobic glycolysis as metabolic basis for trained immunity. Science. 2014;**345**(6204):1579. DOI: 10.1126/science.1250684

[166] Keating ST et al. The Set7 lysine methyltransferase regulates plasticity in oxidative phosphorylation necessary for trained immunity induced by beta-Glucan. Cell Reports. 2020;**31**(3):107548. DOI: 10.1016/j.celrep.2020.107548

[167] Arts RJW et al. Immunometabolic pathways in BCG-induced trained immunity. Cell Reports. 2016;**17**(10):2562-2571. DOI: 10.1016/j.celrep.2016.11.011

Chapter 6

Macrophages in the Inner Ear: Discoveries and Innovative Techniques Illustrating Their Key Roles in Homeostasis and Inflammation

Mai Mohamed Bedeir and Yuzuru Ninoyu

Abstract

Inner ear macrophages, also known as cochlear macrophages, are immune cells that play a crucial role in maintaining the homeostasis and hearing function of the inner ear. They are responsible for responses to cochlear insults, such as noise exposure, ototoxic drugs, and surgical injuries. These cells have been shown to be present in the spiral ganglion, spiral ligament, and stria vascularis of the inner ear. As our understanding of inner ear macrophages continues to evolve, it is becoming evident that these cells are not just inert populations in the auditory system but are active participants in the complicated mechanics of inner ear homeostasis. Nevertheless, a comprehensive understanding of the roles and functions of macrophages within the auditory system is lacking. This review explores the presence, origin, and multifaceted roles of inner ear macrophages, elucidating their significance in maintaining auditory function, while also highlighting their potential inimical role in inner ear inflammation. The information collated herein has important implications for the development of therapeutic strategies aimed at preserving or restoring auditory function.

Keywords: macrophage, inner ear, hearing loss, inflammation, ototoxicity, noise exposure

1. Introduction

The inner ear is an extraordinary sensory organ responsible for two of the most vital senses: hearing and balance. Located within the labyrinth of the inner ear, sensory hair cells and neural pathways orchestrate sound perception and spatial orientation. However, the functionality of the inner ear extends beyond its sensory components; it hosts a dynamic microenvironment and is carefully regulated to ensure optimal auditory and vestibular functions [1]. Within this complex environment, immune cells, particularly macrophages, appear to maintain the proper functioning of the inner ear.

Inner ear macrophages, also known as cochlear macrophages, respond to cochlear insults such as noise exposure, ototoxic drugs, and surgical injuries. A long-held view was that the inner ear was immune-free because of the presence of the blood-labyrinth barrier, which restricts the entry of blood cells into the inner ear [2]. However, recent studies have shown that inner ear macrophages do exist and play essential roles in the inner ear [3, 4]. These cells have been shown to be present in the spiral ganglion, spiral ligament, and stria vascularis of the inner ear [3, 5–7]. The origin and distribution of these macrophages within the inner ear are linked to their functions, which are not yet entirely understood [8].

Although these macrophages are classically associated with immune defense, their roles within the inner ear are diverse. Not only are they equipped to respond to infections and inflammatory stimuli, but they also actively participate in tissue maintenance and repair and the resolution of inflammation [3, 4, 9].

The advancement of our knowledge about inner ear macrophages has made it patently apparent that these cells are not merely a passive "audience" but rather dynamic "players" in the intricate symphony of inner ear homeostasis. This chapter aims to explore in detail the current understanding of inner ear macrophages, including their origin, functions, and involvement in physiological and pathological conditions. By shedding light on their significance in maintaining cochlear homeostasis, we also unveil their potential as therapeutic targets in the management of inner ear disorders.

2. Complex origin of inner ear macrophages from embryonic development to adult maintenance

The origin of inner ear macrophages, both during embryonic development and adulthood, is a prospective field of research. The prevailing theory is that these macrophages are derived from precursors present in both the embryonic and adult stages. Resident macrophages first appear on embryonic day (E) 10 in the otic vesicle, migrating to the mesenchyme surrounding the otocyst [10, 11]. The yolk sac, which contains primitive macrophages from E7 to E9, is suggested to be the primary source, playing a vital role in early hematopoiesis and macrophage development [11, 12].

In adulthood, inner ear macrophages are thought to originate from three sources: yolk sac macrophages, fetal liver monocytes, and bone marrow-derived precursor cells [13]. The presence of distinct markers such as F4/80, Iba1, CD68, and CD11b helps categorize and track the differentiation of these macrophages during embryonic development and adulthood. Csf1 signaling plays a crucial role in the development of macrophages originating from the yolk sac, while fetal liver hematopoiesis contributes to monocyte precursors independently of Csf1 signaling (**Figure 1**) [11]. Furthermore, resident macrophages in the mature inner ear maintain a consistent presence and actively respond to stimuli. The precursors, which migrate to the cochlea, exhibit variations in gene expression depending on their origins. Studies have compared gene expression in bone marrow-derived macrophages after genotoxic irradiation [14] or after conditional macrophage depletion [15]. Thus, bone marrow precursors can differentiate into cochlear macrophages in response to injury or inflammation, as observed in the cases of noise exposure [16] or surgical stress [6].

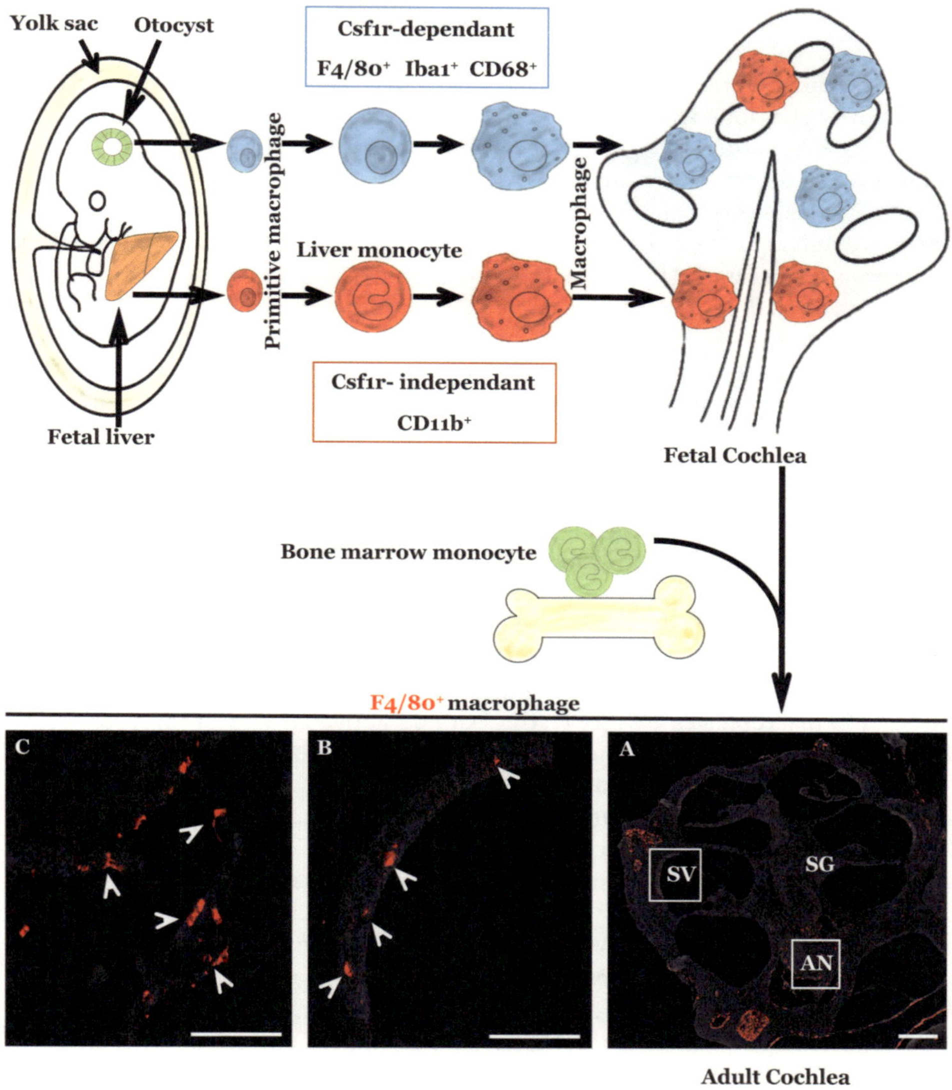

Figure 1.
A schematic view of resident macrophage origin and localization in the cochlea. This figure illustrates the developmental origins of resident macrophages in the embryonic cochlea, identifying two distinct pathways. The first subtype, originating from the yolk sac, requires Csf1r signaling for its development and is positive for F4/80, Iba1, and CD68 markers. In contrast, the second subtype arises from the fetal liver, migrating through systemic circulation, and is Csf1r signaling-independent, as indicated by CD11b positivity. Macrophages from the bone marrow continuously infiltrate the cochlea, resulting in the progressive substitution of resident macrophages with bone marrow-derived cells. In the lower panel, macrophages in the adult cochlea are stained with the F4/80 marker (red). (A) A mid-modiolar paraffin-section of the adult cochlea, highlighting macrophages located in various regions, including the stria vascularis (SV), auditory nerve (AN), and spiral ganglion (SG). Scale bar: 200 μm. (B) (C) Magnified view of the SV (B) and AN (C). Scale bar for (B) and (C): 50 μm.

Some studies have shown that inner ear macrophages can also arise from resident precursor cells in the inner ear [7, 17].

In the mature inner ear, resident macrophages, which are derived from the bone marrow, maintain a consistent presence within the spiral ligament, auditory nerve, and stria vascularis [6]. These macrophages create an active and adaptable population that is regularly renewed by monocytes in the bloodstream [7, 18]. In the stria vascularis of the mature cochlea, resident macrophages can be distinguished by the expression of markers, such as F4/80, CD68, Iba1, and CD11b [18–20], and they are primarily positioned close to blood vessels, serving as perivascular macrophages (PVMs). One hypothesis suggests that PVMs in the stria vascularis originate from cochlear melanocytes, which are neural crest derivatives that migrate to this location [21, 22]. This hypothesis has been challenged by the discrepancies observed between distinctive cell populations originating from the neural crest and CD68$^+$ cells within the embryonic cochlea [11]. Considering the different developmental pathways and phenotypes of macrophages and melanocytes, it appears unconvincing that PVMs have neural crest origins [23]. Some evidence suggests that PVMs within the stria vascularis undergo changes in their marker expression as they progress through postnatal development, ultimately being renewed by monocytes from the bloodstream in the adult inner ear [24].

3. Cochlear macrophage classification supersedes M1/M2 dichotomy, revealing diverse components

Macrophage diversity within the cochlea has emerged as a fascinating aspect of inner ear immunology, challenging traditional classification. On the basis of their activation states and functions, macrophages were initially categorized as M0, M1, and M2. M0 macrophages are the "resting" or non-activated state of macrophages. M1 macrophages or "classically activated" macrophages are activated and have pro-inflammatory functions. M2 macrophages, also known as "alternatively activated" macrophages [25, 26], are activated and have anti-inflammatory or repair functions. However, the expression of each marker alone is not sufficient to define macrophage or microglial identity, as expression levels may change depending on microglial adaptation to site-specific conditions [27, 28]. Recent advancements, particularly multi-parameter techniques, have revealed a spectrum of macrophage phenotypes beyond the established M1/M2 paradigms. In a cutting-edge study employing multiplex immunohistochemistry (mIHC) with six distinct markers, cochlear macrophages exhibited remarkable versatility in marker expression. This approach revealed a diverse array of phenotypes that contradicts the established M1/M2 dichotomy. Further, each macrophage exhibited a remarkable degree of plasticity, demonstrating its ability to express one or multiple markers. This study expanded the repertoire of macrophage phenotypes and led to the identification of a novel category termed M1/M2 mixed macrophages [3]. These findings underscore the remarkable diversity among cochlear macrophages, and the wide spectrum of responses implies that the roles of these immune cells in auditory pathology might be far more complex and multifaceted than previously envisioned. The integration of novel technologies is expected to deepen our understanding of cochlear macrophages and their contribution to the auditory immune system.

4. Advancements in techniques for studying tissue-resident macrophages bridge cellular function and spatial context

Tissue-resident macrophages, a highly diverse group of macrophages in the immune system, are influenced by factors unique to specific tissues and environmental niches. Researchers have developed and applied various pioneering techniques to understand the complex roles of these cells, particularly in immunometabolism. These methodologies aim to elucidate the functions and subtypes of these cells, with a focus on preserving their spatial context. This is crucial for the accurate localization of proteins, nucleic acids, and other elements of immunometabolism within tissue structures.

Flow cytometry, the cornerstone of immune cell profiling, can detect an array of over 20 protein markers. However, its dependence on cell suspension may modify cell properties and obscure spatial information. This limitation is particularly notable in structures such as the cochlea, where isolating cells is difficult because of tight intercellular junctions [29]. This challenge is highlighted by tissue-resident macrophages and PVMs in the lateral wall of the cochlea, which are vital for maintaining the endocochlear potential. High-throughput multi-parameter flow cytometry has been developed for cellular metabolism analyses, offering new insights into immune cell metabolism [30]. However, these approaches are time-consuming and only provide an indirect assessment of metabolic activity.

To address the limitations of flow cytometry, new iterative immunohistochemistry/immunofluorescence methods have emerged, particularly in cancer immunology. Techniques such as sequential immunoperoxidase labeling and erasing (SIMPLE) [31], chromogenic mIHC with image cytometry [3, 32, 33], and iterative bleaching extend multiplexity (IBEX) [34] have been developed. SIMPLE, introduced by Glass et al. in 2009, is a valuable tool for immune profiling of various cancers. IBEX is an ingenious method that allows for multiplexed imaging across different tissues through iterative immunolabeling and chemical bleaching. The multiple iterative labeling by antibody neodeposition (MILAN) method employs primary antibodies coupled with fluorochrome-conjugated secondary antibodies to refine staining processes [35].

Despite these advancements, challenges such as the need for highly specific antibodies, optimized staining conditions, and advanced computational tools for data analysis, persist. The integration of iterative immunohistochemistry with other omics data, such as transcriptomics and proteomics, is underway to offer a more comprehensive view of complex immune systems. Omics approaches offer unique insights into the molecular landscape of cells within tissues, enabling the measurement of gene expression and other molecular features at a single-cell resolution. By capturing the spatial context within the cellular microenvironment, spatial omics technologies provide a more comprehensive understanding of cellular heterogeneity, microenvironmental interactions, and various biological processes. Similarly, single-cell multimodal omics (scMulti-omics) techniques enable the simultaneous measurement of multiple cellular features, elucidating cellular characteristics and functional dynamics [36–38].

A particularly exciting advancement in this field is the development of subcellular imaging transcriptomics platforms, which provide high-resolution spatial mapping of gene expression [36]. Technologies such as Xenium (10x Genomics), CosMx (NanoString), Stereo-seq (BGI), and MERSCOPE (Vizen) have revolutionized our approach to biological questions, owing to their ultra-high-resolution capabilities. These tools not only enhance our understanding of tissue-resident macrophages but also pave the way for an in-depth exploration of immunometabolism and cell functions.

This underscores the importance of integrating traditional and cutting-edge techniques to unravel the complexities of these cells within the unique environment of the cochlea, thus furthering our understanding of their roles in auditory health and disease.

5. Iba1 in the cochlear microenvironment helps elucidate the dynamics of macrophages and their potential role as microglia-like cells

In the cochlear microenvironment, the presence of Iba1, a specialized calcium-binding protein associated with microglia and macrophages, signifies a crucial aspect of immune surveillance and response. Iba1$^+$ cells have been consistently observed in various regions of the cochlea, from the modiolus and spiral lamina to the spiral ganglion, spiral ligament, and organ of Corti [6, 39]. The use of Iba1 as a marker has facilitated extensive investigations into cochlear macrophages, clarifying their role in responses to stimuli or pathological conditions. Besides its conventional use in characterizing macrophages, the connection between Iba1 and microglia-like cells (MLCs) has become increasingly evident. The discovery of MLCs in the cochlea, which resemble microglia of the central nervous system, draws attention to the notable possibility that these cells contribute to neuroimmune interactions within the auditory system [40, 41].

Following exposure to oxaliplatin, a platinum-based antineoplastic agent, Iba1 expression increases notably in the nervous system [42–44]. This upregulation of Iba1 suggests increased activation of microglia and macrophages in response to oxaliplatin-induced neuropathy. An appreciable increase in Iba1$^+$ cells indicates an inflammatory response within the nervous system, wherein macrophages or MLCs, are activated and recruited. This highlights their involvement in the neuroinflammatory processes triggered by oxaliplatin.

Similarly, exposure to cisplatin, another platinum-based antineoplastic agent, causes a substantial increase in Iba1 expression in the cochlea, particularly in macrophages in the auditory nerve area. This increased expression is distinctive of neuroinflammation, as it is not significantly observed in the stria vascularis or organ of Corti [3]. The concurrent expression of markers associated with both M1 and M2 macrophages, such as Iba1, in activated macrophages adds a layer of complexity to the current understanding of cochlear immune responses. Increased Iba1 expression in response to cisplatin prompts further investigation into the precise roles of cochlear macrophages, raising notable questions about whether these cells exhibit the characteristics of true macrophages or share features with MLCs. A deeper understanding of Iba1 expression patterns after cisplatin treatment is important for resolving the questions about complicated immune processes in the cochlea.

6. Cochlear macrophages protect tissue integrity and contribute to sensory epithelium maintenance

Macrophages are being recognized as key players in cochlear dynamics, with their roles surpassing traditional immunity. Equipped with receptors that detect pathogen-derived molecules, macrophages can respond swiftly to foreign microorganisms by engulfing them and releasing harmful substances [8]. However, in the context of the ear, inflammation triggered by ototoxic drugs or excessive noise leads to a unique scenario termed sterile inflammation [45, 46]. In this setting, damage-associated molecular patterns (DAMPs) released by cochlear hair cells activate pattern recognition receptors (PRRs) [47–49]. Upon PRR activation, resident macrophages quickly become activated, leading to the release of pro-inflammatory cytokines and the generation of reactive oxygen species (ROS); this elaborate response involves the elimination of damaged cells and the initiation of wound healing by infiltrating innate immune cells [50, 51]. Infiltrating innate immune cells, including macrophages and neutrophils, respond to inflammation in early stages by eliminating damaged cells and promoting wound healing in a non-targeted manner, such as by releasing ROS and engaging in phagocytosis. In the subsequent phase, T cells from the adaptive immune system target and eliminate specific cells, releasing cytokines that regulate the activation state of innate immune cells [48, 52, 53]. Following exposure to noise or ototoxic drugs, T cells recognize self-antigens from damaged cells, whereas T regulatory cells suppress inflammation and promote wound healing. These mechanisms of the adaptive immune response aid in resolving inflammation and contribute to effective recovery [54, 55].

The multifarious functions of macrophages extend beyond immunity, with research underscoring their fundamental role in maintaining the integrity of normal tissues. By rapidly identifying and removing apoptotic cells, macrophages ensure the preservation of typical tissue structure [8, 56].

Inside the cochlea, the sensory epithelium includes inner and outer hair cells, along with various supporting cell types. Although macrophages are seldom observed within the intact cochlear sensory epithelium, they are present in adjacent tissues [57, 58]. Hair cell death initiates diverse cellular removal processes by engaging both supporting cells and macrophages. These crucial contributors to sensory epithelium maintenance likely fulfill complementary roles, implying that the suppression of the activity of one cell type prompts compensatory actions by other cell types [10].

Overall, macrophages, initially recognized for their immune functions, also play versatile roles in cochlear dynamics, including the maintenance of tissue integrity and efficient clearance of apoptotic cells. In the cochlea, the interplay between hair cells and supporting cells is integral for maintaining the sensory epithelium. Clearer insights into these mechanisms will facilitate effective therapeutic advancements for inner ear conditions and drug-induced toxicity.

7. Macrophage dynamics in ototoxicity and noise-induced hearing loss reveals neuroinflammatory responses and healing potential

In the last couple of years, there has been a growing recognition of the key role played by inflammation and immune responses in the pathophysiology of cochlear acoustic injury [5, 57]. Prolonged exposure to excessive noise is primarily associated with noise-induced hearing loss (NIHL), characterized by the damage and loss of cochlear hair cells and spiral ganglion neurons (SGNs) [59, 60]. This hair cell loss triggers the infiltration of immune cells, including macrophages and neutrophils, into the cochlea [57, 61–64]. Macrophages play a multi-pronged role in auditory pathology, particularly cochlear synaptopathy, and are important for maintaining auditory function. One significant aspect is their involvement in fractalkine signaling mediated by the ligand CX3CL1 and its receptor CX3CR1 [58, 60, 65]. This signaling pathway is pivotal for neuronal survival and communication with SGNs. Studies have demonstrated that intact fractalkine signaling promotes spontaneous recovery in response to noise-induced temporary hearing threshold shifts, even in the absence of hair cell loss. However, mice without CX3CR1 show enhanced synaptic degeneration, correlating with reduced neural responses and increased cell loss [60]. Macrophages expressing CX3CR1 migrate to damaged synaptic regions, indicating their dynamic role in the cochlear microenvironment. Macrophages also exhibit neuroprotective functions via fractalkine signaling. A disruption of this signaling pathway following hair cell death reduces macrophage recruitment to the injured cochlea, resulting in increased loss of SGNs [65]. The intricate interplay between macrophages, fractalkine signaling, and neuronal survival in injured cochlea is worth further exploration.

In the context of noise-induced synaptopathy, a recent study employed the CSF1R inhibitor PLX5622 and demonstrated the indispensable role of resident cochlear macrophages. Initial synaptic degeneration and hearing loss were not affected by macrophage elimination; however, the absence of macrophages significantly impeded the subsequent repair of damaged synapses. The ability of macrophages to facilitate synaptic repair, along with their impact on cochlear neuron survival, underscores their critical involvement in the recovery of auditory injuries [66].

Latest transcriptomic analyses have shown a remarkable upregulation of pro-inflammatory genes, including tumor necrosis factor-alpha (TNF-α), interleukin (IL)-1β, and IL-6, subsequent to noise exposure [67–69]. This increased expression has been linked to the Toll-like receptor 4 (TLR4) signaling pathway, which is recognized as a potent driver of NIHL genesis [69]. TLR4 activation triggers downstream nuclear transcription factor-kappa B (NF-κB signaling), organizing the direct targeting and amplification of pro-inflammatory genes [69]. Insights from studies using TLR4 knockout models have proven their pivotal role in inhibiting the inflammatory response and reducing cochlear damage caused by noise exposure [63, 70].

In a recent study investigating the functional consequences of extracellular high-mobility group box 1 (HMGB1)—a prototypical DAMP involved in inflammatory pathway activation—researchers explored its interaction with TLR4. Using adeno-associated virus transfection with the HMGB1-HA-tag, this study precisely examined the early cytoplasmic accumulation of HMGB1 in cochlear hair cells after noise exposure. The administration of an HMGB1-neutralizing antibody promptly after noise exposure was a potent intervention, markedly minimizing hearing loss and preventing the death of outer hair cells (OHCs). The study further identified signal transducer and activator of transcription 1 (STAT1) activation and cellular hyper-acetylation as recognized initiators of cytoplasmic accumulation of HMGB1. These findings demonstrate the detrimental effects of extracellular HMGB1 on the cochlea, identifying potential pharmacotherapeutic targets to reduce NIHL [71].

Another form of cochlear injury is ototoxicity, which refers to damage to the inner ear caused by toxic substances. More than 130 therapeutic drugs have been recognized for their ototoxic side effects. Two major classes of ototoxic drugs are aminoglycoside antibiotics and platinum-based antineoplastic agents such as cisplatin [72–75]. These medications are used extensively in medical practice and can damage hair cells, leading to hearing loss.

Extended exposure to aminoglycosides is associated with the degradation of OHCs within the organ of Corti and sensory hair cells in the vestibular organ [76]. This results in an irreversible loss of hair cells and the impairment of the hearing system, advancing from the cochlear base, which corresponds to the high-frequency sound region, to the apex, which represents the low-frequency sound area. A study investigating macrophage reactions following aminoglycoside exposure showed a direct correlation between the number of recruited macrophages and hair cell damage in mice transplanted with CX3CR1 knockout marrow but not in those transplanted with CX3CR1 wild-type or heterozygous marrow. This suggests a protective role of CX3CR1 mediated by cochlear macrophages, potentially limiting hearing impairment in aminoglycoside ototoxicity [77].

In an investigation into the response of macrophages to ototoxic injury in lateral line hair cells in larval zebrafish, macrophages rapidly migrated into neuromasts during the initial phases of ototoxic injury, where they actively engaged in both physical contact and phagocytosis of deteriorating hair cell debris. The study demonstrated that ototoxicity induces rapid externalization of phosphatidylserine to the apical surfaces of hair cells, a likely indication for their targeted removal [78].

Similarly, cisplatin targets OHCs in the basal turn of the cochlea, causing high-frequency sensorineural hearing loss [79]. This adverse effect manifests as bilateral, irreversible, and progressively worsening hearing impairment [80, 81]. Cisplatin induces a local inflammatory response in the inner ear through the generation of ROS. This activates NF-κB, which in turn regulates the expression of pro-inflammatory cytokines such as IL-1β, TNF-α, and IL-6 [82, 83]. In a previous study, we investigated the response of macrophages to acute cisplatin exposure and found a notable increase in the activated M1/M2 mixed macrophages and $Iba1^+$ macrophages, especially in the auditory nerve area, suggesting a neuroinflammatory response. It is worth noting that this activation declined starting 15 days after exposure, implying that transient macrophage activation was associated with temporary inflammation due to cisplatin. Interestingly, these activated macrophages did not strictly adhere to the conventional M1 or M2 classification. Instead, they exhibited a mixed M1/M2 phenotype, with a tendency to shift toward M2 macrophages over time. This transition toward M2 macrophages may contribute to the subsequent healing process [3].

In summary, macrophages are a major contributor to inflammatory responses following ototoxic events. A comprehensive understanding of their roles holds significant promise for uncovering potential avenues for drug discovery.

8. Re-evaluation of the role of macrophages in cochlear health identifies potential harmful impacts

Contrary to the traditional role of macrophages as protectors of the inner ear, some recent studies have proposed a divergent perspective, suggesting that macrophages may contribute to cochlear damage under certain conditions. Pertinent findings have challenged the conventional notion that depleting macrophages could potentially serve as a protective mechanism and reduce hearing loss after exposure to ototoxicity.

In a study employing kanamycin-induced hearing loss in mice, a notable increase in $Iba1^+$ activated macrophages was observed 3 days after kanamycin injection. This macrophage activation was concurrent with an increase in the number of neurons expressing activating transcription factor 3 (ATF3), a marker of early neuronal damage. Subsequent depletion of macrophages with clodronate after kanamycin administration led to reduced early neuronal damage on day 3 and overall decreased neuronal death on day 28. These findings suggest a potentially harmful role of macrophages in the case of cochlear insults [9].

Another study investigated the impact of macrophage depletion on NIHL using clodronate liposomes to target macrophages and monocytes. The results showed that mice treated with clodronate exhibited significantly lower permanent threshold shifts at specific frequencies and smaller losses of OHCs in the cochlear turn than those in controls. After noise exposure, the number of $F4/80^+$ macrophages increased, indicative of macrophage infiltration, particularly in the stria vascularis, a structure crucial for cochlear function. However, clodronate treatment suppressed this effect. Interestingly, the presence of IL-1β, which is produced by these infiltrating macrophages, was observed; however, inhibition of IL-1β did not reverse the cochlear damage induced by noise exposure [84]. These findings suggest that macrophages infiltrating the cochlea after noise exposure may play a role in NIHL.

Another study investigated the impact of macrophage migration inhibitory factor (MIF) in NIHL using MIF-deficient (MIF(−/−)) mice. Following exposure to noise, MIF(−/−) mice experienced more severe hearing loss and OHC damage compared to wild-type mice, indicating prolonged hearing impairment in the absence of MIF. These findings suggest that MIF plays a critical role in recovery from acoustic trauma. Therefore, targeting MIF might serve as an effective therapeutic strategy for the management of NIHL [85].

This emerging perspective challenges the traditional understanding of macrophages as purely protective entities in the inner ear. The notion that macrophage depletion might be a protective strategy against cochlear damage, particularly in ototoxicity and NIHL, prompts novel directions for therapeutic exploration. Meanwhile, studies on the potentially harmful role of macrophages will inspire state-of-the-art interventions and modified clinical strategies to address the challenges associated with inner ear conditions and drug-induced ototoxicity.

9. Conclusion

In-depth investigations on cochlear macrophages have revealed a complex milieu within the auditory system. The detection of MLCs in the cochlea, identified using the marker Iba1, suggests a role for MLCs in cochlear maturation and remodeling during postnatal development.

Particularly in the context of cochlear injuries, e.g., ototoxicity induced by drugs such as cisplatin, the consistent increase in Iba1 expression underscores the active involvement of macrophages. However, the exact nature of cochlear macrophages—whether they are true macrophages or share traits with MLCs—warrants further investigation. Similarly, future research must clarify their precise roles in the inner ear.

Considering the participation of macrophages in inflammation, particularly in response to cytotoxicity, their crucial role in auditory health must be highlighted. Potential therapeutic interventions aimed at preserving or restoring auditory function will hinge on a clearer understanding of the diverse phenotypes, origins, and responses of cochlear. Continued research on the complex interactions of macrophages in the cochlear microenvironment is expected to advance the fields of auditory health and pathology.

Acknowledgements

This study was supported by the Japanese Society for the Promotion of Science (JSPS) KAKENHI (JP20K18321 to Y.N.) and the Society for Promotion of International Oto-Rhino-Laryngology (SPIO) (SR21002 to M.B.). M.B. was supported by the Otsuka Toshimi Scholarship Foundation (OTSF). We thank Editage for editing and reviewing the manuscript for the English language.

Conflict of interest

The authors declare no conflict of interest.

Author details

Mai Mohamed Bedeir and Yuzuru Ninoyu*
Department of Otolaryngology, Head and Neck Surgery, Kyoto Prefectural University of Medicine, Kyoto, Japan

*Address all correspondence to: ninoyu@koto.kpu-m.ac.jp

IntechOpen

© 2024 The Author(s). Licensee IntechOpen. This chapter is distributed under the terms of the Creative Commons Attribution License (http://creativecommons.org/licenses/by/3.0), which permits unrestricted use, distribution, and reproduction in any medium, provided the original work is properly cited.

References

[1] Perin P, Marino F, Varela-Nieto I, Szczepek AJ. Editorial: Neuroimmunology of the inner ear. Frontiers in Neurology. 2021;**12**:635359. DOI: 10.3389/fneur.2021.635359

[2] Harris JP. Immunology of the inner ear: Response of the inner ear to antigen challenge. Otolaryngology Head and Neck Surgery. 1983;**91**:18-23. DOI: 10.1177/019459988309100105

[3] Bedeir MM, Ninoyu Y, Nakamura T, Tsujikawa T, Hirano S. Multiplex immunohistochemistry reveals cochlear macrophage heterogeneity and local auditory nerve inflammation in cisplatin-induced hearing loss. Frontiers in Neurology. 2022;**13**:1015014. DOI: 10.3389/FNEUR.2022.1015014

[4] Miwa T, Okano T. Role of inner ear macrophages and autoimmune/autoinflammatory mechanisms in the pathophysiology of inner ear disease. Frontiers in Neurology. 2022;**13**:861992. DOI: 10.3389/FNEUR.2022.861992

[5] Yang W, Vethanayagam RR, Dong Y, Cai Q, Hu BH. Activation of the antigen presentation function of mononuclear phagocyte populations associated with the basilar membrane of the cochlea after acoustic overstimulation. Neuroscience. 2015;**303**:1-15. DOI: 10.1016/J.NEUROSCIENCE.2015.05.081

[6] Okano T, Nakagawa T, Kita T, Kada S, Yoshimoto M, Nakahata T, et al. Bone marrow-derived cells expressing Iba1 are constitutively present as resident tissue macrophages in the mouse cochlea. Journal of Neuroscience Research. 2008;**86**:1758-1767. DOI: 10.1002/jnr.21625

[7] Miwa T, Rengasamy G, Liu Z, Ginhoux F, Okano T. Contribution of circulating monocytes in maintaining homeostasis of resident macrophages in postnatal and young adult mouse cochlea. Scientific Reports. 2024;**14**:62. DOI: 10.1038/s41598-023-50634-y

[8] Warchol ME. Interactions between macrophages and the sensory cells of the inner ear. Cold Spring Harbor Perspectives in Medicine. 2019;**9**:a033555. DOI: 10.1101/cshperspect.a033555

[9] Shimada MD, Noda M, Koshu R, Takaso Y, Sugimoto H, Ito M, et al. Macrophage depletion attenuates degeneration of spiral ganglion neurons in kanamycin-induced unilateral hearing loss model. Scientific Reports. 2023;**13**(1):16741. DOI: 10.1038/s41598-023-43927-9

[10] Hirose K, Rutherford MA, Warchol ME. Two cell populations participate in clearance of damaged hair cells from the sensory epithelia of the inner ear. Hearing Research. 2017;**352**:70-81. DOI: 10.1016/j.heares.2017.04.006

[11] Kishimoto I, Okano T, Nishimura K, Motohashi T, Omori K. Early development of resident macrophages in the mouse cochlea depends on yolk sac hematopoiesis. Frontiers in Neurology. 2019;**10**:1115. DOI: 10.3389/FNEUR.2019.01115/BIBTEX

[12] Ginhoux F, Greter M, Leboeuf M, Nandi S, See P, Gokhan S, et al. Fate mapping analysis reveals that adult microglia derive from primitive macrophages. Science (80-). 2010;**330**:841-845. DOI: 10.1126/science.1194637

[13] Ginhoux F, Guilliams M. Tissue-resident macrophage ontogeny and

homeostasis. Immunity. 2016;**44**:439-449. DOI: 10.1016/j.immuni.2016.02.024

[14] Lavin Y, Winter D, Blecher-Gonen R, David E, Keren-Shaul H, Merad M, et al. Tissue-resident macrophage enhancer landscapes are shaped by the local microenvironment. Cell. 2014;**159**:1312-1326. DOI: 10.1016/j.cell.2014.11.018

[15] Bruttger J, Karram K, Wörtge S, Regen T, Marini F, Hoppmann N, et al. Genetic cell ablation reveals clusters of local self-renewing microglia in the mammalian central nervous system. Immunity. 2015;**43**:92-106. DOI: 10.1016/J.IMMUNI.2015.06.012

[16] Sato E, Shick HE, Ransohoff RM, Hirose K. Repopulation of cochlear macrophages in murine hematopoietic progenitor cell chimeras: The role of CX3CR1. The Journal of Comparative Neurology. 2008;**506**:930-942. DOI: 10.1002/cne.21583

[17] Dong Y, Zhang C, Frye M, Yang W, Ding D, Sharma A, et al. Differential fates of tissue macrophages in the cochlea during postnatal development HHS Public Access. Hearing Research. 2018;**365**:110-126. DOI: 10.1016/j.heares.2018.05.010

[18] Shi X. Resident macrophages in the cochlear blood-labyrinth barrier and their renewal via migration of bone-marrow-derived cells. Cell and Tissue Research. 2010;**342**:21-30. DOI: 10.1007/s00441-010-1040-2

[19] Jabba SV, Oelke A, Singh R, Maganti RJ, Fleming S, Wall SM, et al. Macrophage invasion contributes to degeneration of stria vascularis in Pendred syndrome mouse model. BMC Medicine. 2006;**4**:37. DOI: 10.1186/1741-7015-4-37

[20] Steinacher C, Chacko LJ, Liu W, Rask-Andersen H, Bader W, Dudas J, et al. Visualization of macrophage subsets in the development of the fetal human inner ear. Frontiers in Immunology. 2022;**13**:965196. DOI: 10.3389/FIMMU.2022.965196

[21] Zhang W, Dai M, Fridberger A, Hassan A, DeGagne J, Neng L, et al. Perivascular-resident macrophage-like melanocytes in the inner ear are essential for the integrity of the intrastrial fluid-blood barrier. Proceedings of the National Academy of Sciences of the United States of America. 2012;**109**:10388-10393. DOI: 10.1073/PNAS.1205210109

[22] Neng L, Zhang F, Kachelmeier A, Shi X. Endothelial cell, pericyte, and perivascular resident macrophage-type melanocyte interactions regulate cochlear intrastrial fluid-blood barrier permeability. JARO - Journal of the Association for Research in Otolaryngology. 2013;**14**:175-185. DOI: 10.1007/s10162-012-0365-9

[23] Hirose K, Li SZ. The role of monocytes and macrophages in the dynamic permeability of the blood-perilymph barrier. Hearing Research. 2019;**374**:49-57. DOI: 10.1016/J.HEARES.2019.01.006

[24] Szczepek AJ, Ghosh S, Liu W, Ito T, Kurata N, Fukunaga Y. Tissue-resident macrophages in the stria vascularis. Frontiers in Neurology. 2022;**13**:818395. DOI: 10.3389/fneur.2022.818395

[25] Wynn TA, Chawla A, Pollard JW. Macrophage biology in development, homeostasis and disease. Nature. 2013;**496**:445-455. DOI: 10.1038/nature12034

[26] Van Der Vlist M, Raoof R, Willemen HLDM, Khoury-Hanold W, Meyaard L, Correspondence NE. Macrophages transfer mitochondria to

sensory neurons to resolve inflammatory pain. Neuron. 2022;**110**(4):613-626.e9. DOI: 10.1016/j.neuron.2021.11.020

[27] Ginhoux F, Schultze JL, Murray PJ, Ochando J, Biswas SK. New insights into the multidimensional concept of macrophage ontogeny, activation and function. Nature Immunology. 2015;**17**:34-40. DOI: 10.1038/ni.3324

[28] Paolicelli RC, Sierra A, Stevens B, Tremblay ME, Aguzzi A, Ajami B, et al. Microglia states and nomenclature: A field at its crossroads. Neuron. 2022;**110**:3458-3483. DOI: 10.1016/J.NEURON.2022.10.020

[29] Rai V, Wood MB, Feng H, Schabla NM, Tu S, Zuo J. The immune response after noise damage in the cochlea is characterized by a heterogeneous mix of adaptive and innate immune cells. Scientific Reports. 2020;**10**(1):15167. DOI: 10.1038/s41598-020-72181-6

[30] Fan Y, Naglich JG, Koenitzer JD, Ribeiro H, Lippy J, Blum J, et al. Miniaturized high-throughput multiparameter flow cytometry assays measuring in vitro human dendritic cell maturation and T-cell activation in mixed lymphocyte reactions. SLAS Discovery: Advancing Life Sciences R&D. 2018;**23**:742-750. DOI: 10.1177/2472555218775409

[31] Glass G, Papin JA, Mandell JW. SIMPLE: A sequential immunoperoxidase labeling and erasing method. The Journal of Histochemistry and Cytochemistry. 2009;**57**:899-905. DOI: 10.1369/JHC.2009.953612

[32] Tsujikawa T, Kumar S, Borkar RN, Azimi V, Thibault G, Chang YH, et al. Quantitative multiplex immunohistochemistry reveals myeloid-inflamed tumor-immune complexity associated with poor prognosis. Cell Reports. 2017;**19**:203-217. DOI: 10.1016/J.CELREP.2017.03.037

[33] Banik G, Betts CB, Liudahl SM, Sivagnanam S, Kawashima R, Cotechini T, et al. High-dimensional multiplexed immunohistochemical characterization of immune contexture in human cancers. Methods in Enzymology. 2020;**635**:1-20. DOI: 10.1016/BS.MIE.2019.05.039

[34] Radtke AJ, Kandov E, Lowekamp B, Speranza E, Chu CJ, Gola A, et al. IBEX: A versatile multiplex optical imaging approach for deep phenotyping and spatial analysis of cells in complex tissues. Proceedings of the National Academy of Sciences of the United States of America. 2020;**117**:33455-33465. DOI: 10.1073/PNAS.2018488117/SUPPL_FILE/PNAS.2018488117.SM09.MP4

[35] Cattoretti G, Marcelis L, Bolognesi MM. Multiple Iterative Labeling by Antibody Neodeposition (MILAN). Protocol Exchange. 2019. DOI: 10.21203/rs.2.1646/v5

[36] Lewis SM, Asselin-Labat ML, Nguyen Q, Berthelet J, Tan X, Wimmer VC, et al. Spatial omics and multiplexed imaging to explore cancer biology. Nature Methods. 2021;**18**:997-1012. DOI: 10.1038/s41592-021-01203-6

[37] Bressan D, Battistoni G, Hannon GJ. The dawn of spatial omics. Science (80-). 2023;**381**:eabq4964. DOI: 10.1126/science.abq4964

[38] Ma A, McDermaid A, Xu J, Chang Y, Ma Q. Integrative methods and practical challenges for single-cell multi-omics. Trends in Biotechnology. 2020;**38**:1007-1022. DOI: 10.1016/J.TIBTECH.2020.02.013

[39] O'Malley JT, Nadol JB, McKenna MJ. Anti CD163+, Iba1+, and CD68+ cells

in the adult human inner ear: Normal distribution of an unappreciated class of macrophages/microglia and implications for inflammatory otopathology in humans. Otology & Neurotology. 2016;**37**:99-108. DOI: 10.1097/MAO.0000000000000879

[40] Chen P, Chai Y, Liu H, Li G, Wang L, Yang T, et al. Postnatal development of microglia-like cells in mouse cochlea. Neural Plasticity. 2018;**2018**:1970150. DOI: 10.1155/2018/1970150

[41] Paciello F, Pisani A, Rolesi R, Montuoro R, Mohamed-Hizam V, Boni G, et al. Oxidative stress and inflammation cause auditory system damage via glial cell activation and dysregulated expression of gap junction proteins in an experimental model of styrene-induced oto/neurotoxicity. Journal of Neuroinflammation. 2024;**21**:4. DOI: 10.1186/S12974-023-02996-3

[42] Kim C, Lee JH, Kim W, Li D, Kim Y, Lee K, et al. The suppressive effects of cinnamomi cortex and its phytocompound coumarin on oxaliplatin-induced neuropathic cold allodynia in rats. Molecules. 2016;**21**:1253. DOI: 10.3390/MOLECULES21091253

[43] Makker PGS, Duffy SS, Lees JG, Perera CJ, Tonkin RS, Butovsky O, et al. Characterisation of immune and neuroinflammatory changes associated with chemotherapy-induced peripheral neuropathy. PLoS ONE. 2017;**12**:e0170814. DOI: 10.1371/JOURNAL.PONE.0170814

[44] Jung Y, Lee JH, Kim W, Yoon SH, Kim SK. Anti-allodynic effect of Buja in a rat model of oxaliplatin-induced peripheral neuropathy via spinal astrocytes and pro-inflammatory cytokines suppression. BMC Complementary and Alternative Medicine. 2017;**17**:1-8. DOI: 10.1186/S12906-017-1556-Z/FIGURES/3

[45] Rock KL, Latz E, Ontiveros F, Kono H. The sterile inflammatory response. Annual Review of Immunology. 2010;**28**:321-342. DOI: 10.1146/ANNUREV-IMMUNOL-030409-101311

[46] Zhang Y, Li Y, Fu X, Wang P, Wang Q, Meng W, et al. The detrimental and beneficial functions of macrophages after cochlear injury. Frontiers in Cell and Development Biology. 2021;**9**:631904. DOI: 10.3389/fcell.2021.631904

[47] Tang D, Kang R, Coyne CB, Zeh HJ, Lotze MT. PAMPs and DAMPs: Signal 0s that spur autophagy and immunity. Immunological Reviews. 2012;**249**:158-175. DOI: 10.1111/J.1600-065X.2012.01146.X

[48] Marshall JS, Warrington R, Watson W, Kim HL. An introduction to immunology and immunopathology. Allergy, Asthma & Clinical Immunology. 2018;**14**:1-10. DOI: 10.1186/S13223-018-0278-1/TABLES/4

[49] Frye MD, Ryan AF, Kurabi A. Inflammation associated with noise-induced hearing loss special collection: Noise-induced hearing loss: Translating risk from animal models to real-world environments inflammation associated with noise-induced hearing loss. The Journal of the Acoustical Society of America. 2019;**146**:4020-4032. DOI: 10.1121/1.5132545

[50] Park HS, Jung HY, Park EY, Kim J, Lee WJ, Bae YS. Cutting edge: Direct interaction of TLR4 with NAD(P)H oxidase 4 isozyme is essential for lipopolysaccharide-induced production of reactive oxygen species and activation of NF-kappa B. Journal of Immunology.

2004;**173**:3589-3593. DOI: 10.4049/JIMMUNOL.173.6.3589

[51] Tsung A, Klune JR, Zhang X, Jeyabalan G, Cao Z, Peng X, et al. HMGB1 release induced by liver ischemia involves toll-like receptor 4 dependent reactive oxygen species production and calcium-mediated signaling. The Journal of Experimental Medicine. 2007;**204**:2913-2923. DOI: 10.1084/JEM.20070247

[52] Stein M, Keshav S, Harris N, Gordon S. Interleukin 4 potently enhances murine macrophage mannose receptor activity: A marker of alternative immunologic macrophage activation. The Journal of Experimental Medicine. 1992;**176**:287-292. DOI: 10.1084/JEM.176.1.287

[53] Chaplin DD. Overview of the immune response. The Journal of Allergy and Clinical Immunology. 2010;**125**:S3. DOI: 10.1016/J.JACI.2009.12.980

[54] Fontenot JD, Gavin MA, Rudensky AY. Foxp3 programs the development and function of CD4+CD25+ regulatory T cells. Nature Immunology. 2003;**4**:986-992. DOI: 10.1038/NI904

[55] Brodeur TY, Robidoux TE, Weinstein JS, Craft J, Swain SL, Marshak-Rothstein A. IL-21 promotes pulmonary fibrosis through the induction of profibrotic CD8+ T cells. Journal of Immunology. 2015;**195**:5251-5260. DOI: 10.4049/JIMMUNOL.1500777

[56] Gregory CD, Devitt A. The macrophage and the apoptotic cell: An innate immune interaction viewed simplistically? Immunology. 2004;**113**:1. DOI: 10.1111/J.1365-2567.2004.01959.X

[57] Hirose K, Discolo CM, Keasler JR, Ransohoff R. Mononuclear phagocytes migrate into the murine cochlea after acoustic trauma. The Journal of Comparative Neurology. 2005;**489**:180-194. DOI: 10.1002/cne.20619

[58] Kaur T, Ohlemiller KK, Warchol ME. Genetic disruption of fractalkine signaling leads to enhanced loss of cochlear afferents following ototoxic or acoustic injury. The Journal of Comparative Neurology. 2018;**526**:824. DOI: 10.1002/CNE.24369

[59] He W, Yu J, Sun Y, Kong W. Macrophages in noise-exposed cochlea: Changes, regulation and the potential role. Aging and Disease. 2019;**11**:191-199. DOI: 10.14336/AD.2019.0723

[60] Kaur T, Clayman AC, Nash AJ, Schrader AD, Warchol ME, Ohlemiller KK. Lack of fractalkine receptor on macrophages impairs spontaneous recovery of ribbon synapses after moderate noise trauma in c57bl/6 mice. Frontiers in Neuroscience. 2019;**13**:620. DOI: 10.3389/FNINS.2019.00620/BIBTEX

[61] Dai M, Yang Y, Omelchenko I, Nuttall AL, Kachelmeier A, Xiu R, et al. Bone marrow cell recruitment mediated by inducible nitric oxide synthase/stromal cell-derived factor-1α signaling repairs the acoustically damaged cochlear blood-labyrinth barrier. The American Journal of Pathology. 2010;**177**:3089-3099. DOI: 10.2353/ajpath.2010.100340

[62] Fredelius L, Rask-Andersen H. The role of macrophages in the disposal of degeneration products within the organ of corti after acoustic overstimulation. Acta Oto-Laryngologica. 1990;**109**:76-82. DOI: 10.3109/00016489009107417

[63] Vethanayagam RR, Yang W, Dong Y, Hu BH. Toll-like receptor 4 modulates the cochlear immune response to acoustic injury. Cell Death & Disease.

2016;7(6):e2245. DOI: 10.1038/cddis.2016.156

[64] Shin SH, Yoo JE, Jung J, Choi JY, Bae SH. Inflammatory monocytes infiltrate the spiral ligament and migrate to the basilar membrane after noise exposure. Clinical and Experimental Otorhinolaryngology. 2022;**15**:153-159. DOI: 10.21053/CEO.2021.00857

[65] Kaur T, Zamani D, Tong L, Rube EW, Ohlemiller KK, Hirose K, et al. Fractalkine signaling regulates macrophage recruitment into the cochlea and promotes the survival of spiral ganglion neurons after selective hair cell lesion. The Journal of Neuroscience. 2015;**35**:15050-15061. DOI: 10.1523/JNEUROSCI.2325-15.2015

[66] Manickam V, Gawande DY, Stothert AR, Clayman AC, Batalkina L, Warchol ME, et al. Macrophages promote repair of inner hair cell ribbon synapses following noise-induced cochlear synaptopathy. The Journal of Neuroscience. 2023;**43**:2075-2089. DOI: 10.1523/JNEUROSCI.1273-22.2023

[67] Wang Q, Shen Y, Hu H, Fan C, Zhang A, Ding R, et al. Systematic transcriptome analysis of noise-induced hearing loss pathogenesis suggests inflammatory activities and multiple susceptible molecules and pathways. Frontiers in Genetics. 2020;**11**:968. DOI: 10.3389/fgene.2020.00968

[68] Fuentes-Santamaría V, Alvarado JC, Melgar-Rojas P, Gabaldón-Ull MC, Miller JM, Juiz JM. The role of glia in the peripheral and central auditory system following noise overexposure: Contribution of TNF-α and IL-1β to the pathogenesis of hearing loss. Frontiers in Neuroanatomy. 2017;**11**:9. DOI: 10.3389/fnana.2017.00009

[69] Zhang G, Zheng H, Pyykko I, Zou J. The TLR-4/NF-κB signaling pathway activation in cochlear inflammation of rats with noise-induced hearing loss. Hearing Research. 2019;**379**:59-68. DOI: 10.1016/J.HEARES.2019.04.012

[70] Yang S, Cai Q, Vethanayagam RR, Wang J, Yang W, Hu BH. Immune defense is the primary function associated with the differentially expressed genes in the cochlea following acoustic trauma. Hearing Research. 2016;**333**:283-294. DOI: 10.1016/J.HEARES.2015.10.010

[71] Xiao L, Zhang Z, Liu J, Zheng Z, Xiong Y, Li C, et al. HMGB1 accumulation in cytoplasm mediates noise-induced cochlear damage. Cell and Tissue Research. 2023;**391**:43-54. DOI: 10.1007/s00441-022-03696-9

[72] Francis SP, Cunningham LL. Non-autonomous cellular responses to ototoxic drug-induced stress and death. Frontiers in Cellular Neuroscience. 2017;**11**:252. DOI: 10.3389/FNCEL.2017.00252/BIBTEX

[73] Hinojosa R, Nelson EG, Lerner SA, Redleaf MI, Schramm DR. Aminoglycoside ototoxicity: A human temporal bone study. Laryngoscope. 2001;**111**:1797-1805. DOI: 10.1097/00005537-200110000-00025

[74] Wu W-J, Sha S-H, McLaren JD, Kawamoto K, Raphael Y, Schacht J. Aminoglycoside ototoxicity in adult CBA, C57BL and BALB mice and the Sprague–Dawley rat. Hearing Research. 2001;**158**:165-178. DOI: 10.1016/S0378-5955(01)00303-3

[75] Gersten BK, Fitzgerald TS, FernandezKA, CunninghamLL. Ototoxicity and platinum uptake following cyclic administration of platinum-based chemotherapeutic agents. JARO - Journal of the Association for Research

in Otolaryngology. 2020;**21**:303-321. DOI: 10.1007/s10162-020-00759-y

[76] Jiang H, Sha S-H, Forge A, Schacht J. Caspase-independent pathways of hair cell death induced by kanamycin in vivo. Cell Death and Differentiation. 2006;**13**:20-30. DOI: 10.1038/sj.cdd.4401706

[77] Sato E, Shick HE, Ransohoff RM, Hirose K. Expression of fractalkine receptor CX3CR1 on cochlear macrophages influences survival of hair cells following ototoxic injury. JARO - Journal of the Association for Research in Otolaryngology. 2010;**11**:223-234. DOI: 10.1007/s10162-009-0198-3

[78] Warchol ME, Schrader A, Sheets L. Macrophages respond rapidly to ototoxic injury of lateral line hair cells but are not required for hair cell regeneration. Frontiers in Cellular Neuroscience. 2021;**14**:613246. DOI: 10.3389/FNCEL.2020.613246/BIBTEX

[79] Jamesdaniel S, Coling D, Hinduja S, Ding D, Li J, Cassidy L, et al. Cisplatin-induced ototoxicity is mediated by nitroxidative modification of cochlear proteins characterized by nitration of Lmo4. The Journal of Biological Chemistry. 2012;**287**:18674-18686. DOI: 10.1074/JBC.M111.297960

[80] Rybak LP, Ramkumar V. Ototoxicity. Kidney International. 2007;**72**(8):931-935. DOI: 10.1038/sj.ki.5002434

[81] Callejo A, Sedó-Cabezón L, Domè Nech Juan I, Llorens J, Cavaletti G, Carozzi V. Cisplatin-induced ototoxicity: Effects, mechanisms and protection strategies. Toxics. 2015;**3**:268-293. DOI: 10.3390/toxics3030268

[82] Waissbluth S, Salehi P, He X, Daniel SJ. Systemic dexamethasone for the prevention of cisplatin-induced ototoxicity. European Archives of Oto-Rhino-Laryngology. 2013;**270**:1597-1605. DOI: 10.1007/s00405-012-2150-0

[83] Zhang N, Cai J, Xu L, Wang H, Liu W. Cisplatin-induced Stria Vascularis damage is associated with inflammation and fibrosis. Neural Plasticity. 2020;**2020**:8851525. DOI: 10.1155/2020/8851525

[84] Mizushima Y, Fujimoto C, Kashio A, Kondo K, Yamasoba T. Macrophage recruitment, but not interleukin 1 beta activation, enhances noise-induced hearing damage. Biochemical and Biophysical Research Communications. 2017;**493**:894-900. DOI: 10.1016/J.BBRC.2017.09.124

[85] Kariya S, Okano M, Maeda Y, Hirai H, Higaki T, Noyama Y, et al. Macrophage migration inhibitory factor deficiency causes prolonged hearing loss after acoustic overstimulation. Otology & Neurotology. 2015;**36**:1103-1108. DOI: 10.1097/MAO.0000000000000755

Chapter 7

Role of Macrophages in Promoting Inflammation and Fibrosis in Systemic Sclerosis

Sandra Lopez Garces, Liyang Pan and Richard Stratton

Abstract

Systemic sclerosis (SSc) is a severe autoimmune disease characterized by chronic inflammation, vascular damage and fibrosis. The hallmark clinical manifestation is fibrotic skin thickening; however, the clinical outcome is determined by the extent of internal organ fibrosis. Macrophages, integral to the innate immune system, play a crucial role in phagocytosing invading pathogens and efferocytosis of apoptotic cells, while also contributing significantly to tissue homeostasis and repair. These highly adaptable cells, particularly in the M2-like polarization state, have been associated with a pro-fibrotic environment, implicated in various fibrotic disorders as well as cancer invasion. In SSc, these cells may be dysfunctional, having the potential to produce inflammatory and pro-fibrotic cytokines, recruit other inflammatory cells and stimulate fibroblast differentiation into myofibroblast, thus promoting extracellular matrix (ECM) deposition and fibrosis. Accordingly, we hypothesize that abnormally activated macrophages have a central role in SSc, promoting inflammation and fibrosis, and driving the disease process.

Keywords: systemic sclerosis, macrophages, fibrosis, autoimmune disease, inflammation

1. Introduction

Systemic sclerosis (SSc) is a severe condition of uncertain etiology, in which dysregulated immune responses are somehow linked to vascular damage, inflammation, autoantibody production, and persisting fibroblast activation, leading to skin and organ-based fibrosis [1]. In SSc, the characteristic clinical manifestation is fibrotic thickening of the skin, which starts at the extremities and then spreads proximally to varying extents and is linked in severity to outcome and survival [2]. Moreover, the clinical outcome is strongly associated with the pattern of internal organ involvement, particularly the development of lung fibrosis (interstitial lung disease, ILD), now the leading cause of excess mortality in SSc [1].

SSc is classified into three main clinical subsets: limited cutaneous SSc (lcSSc), diffuse cutaneous SSc (dcSSc) and SSc sine scleroderma (ssSSc). This classification system is based on the pattern of fibrotic skin involvement. In lcSSc, skin thickening is confined to the extremities and face; this pattern accounting for 50–60% of cases. In contrast, in dcSSc, the thickening of the skin spreads more proximally to involve the upper arms, the torso and potentially affects skin throughout the body. This pattern of disease accounts for 30–40% of cases and is the more severe form, showing early development of visceral organ complications and rapid disease progression [3]. Finally, ssSSc is characterized by the absence of cutaneous manifestations and is identified by typical SSc vascular or organ involvement with positive SSc-associated autoantibody testing [4].

1.1 Epidemiology

The prevalence and incidence of SSc have been reported to vary widely across the globe, showing a pooled prevalence of 176 per million, with a high prevalence in North America (259 per million) and the lowest in Asia (68 per million). Incidence and prevalence are higher in women, with a 5 to 1 female-to-male ratio [5]. The incidence pooled was 14 per million person-years. A study in the United Kingdom showed a prevalence of 307 per million, age being a contributing factor and an annual incidence of 19 per million person-years, 9.7 higher in women. The reported mortality rate was 43.6 per thousand person-years, with risk factors for higher mortality being male sex and age [6].

The standardized mortality ratio for patients suffering from SSc has been reported to be 2.72–5.73. The cumulative survival rates at 5 and 10 years from diagnosis were 85.9 and 71.7% respectively. For the lcSSc subtype, the cumulative survival rates at 5 and 10 years from disease onset are estimated to be 90.9 and 78.2%, respectively. Cumulative survival is significantly lower for dcSSc, with a survival rate of 69.6 and 55.6% at 5 and 10 years [7]. Taken as a whole, these data indicate SSc as a significant healthcare burden which affects more than 2 million individuals worldwide and is linked to significant mortality and disability [6].

1.2 Current therapies

Treatment for SSc is not curative but instead focuses on managing active organ-specific complications. When treating vascular manifestations such as SSc-related pulmonary arterial hypertension (PAH), the objective is to reduce pulmonary arterial vascular resistance through the use of medications like prostacyclin analogues [8], endothelin receptor antagonists [9], and phosphodiesterase-5 inhibitors [10]; treatments which combine vasodilator activity with anti-proliferative effects against vascular smooth muscle cells [11]. Raynaud's phenomenon (RP) and the associated digital ulcers are addressed with vasodilators such as calcium channel blockers, prostacyclin infusions and topical nitroglycerin. Gastrointestinal issues are managed with proton-pump inhibitors, H2 blockers, and prokinetic agents to ameliorate acid reflux and ulcers [12]. Renal disease is commonly treated with angiotensin-converting enzyme inhibitors to control blood pressure and improve renal plasma flow [13]. Cardiac complications, which may be associated with immune cell infiltration, fibrosis and vasculopathy, are managed using strong immunosuppressive treatments such as cyclophosphamide or rituximab, combined with supportive cardiac care such as anti-arrhythmics and diuretics [14]. Individual treatment plans may vary based on the specific manifestations and severity of the disease.

Aside from organ-specific treatments, immunosuppression has been attempted and demonstrates some effectiveness in reducing skin involvement as measured by the modified Rodnan skin score (mRSS) [15] and lung fibrosis in SSc patients [16]. Commonly used immunosuppressive therapies as a first line of defense include cytotoxic drugs like mycophenolate mofetil, and cyclophosphamide. Recently, biologic agents targeting specific cells or pathways have shown promise in improving skin scores and managing organ complications. Biologics such as rituximab [17] (anti-CD20), tocilizumab [18] (anti-IL-6 receptor), and abatacept [19] (T-cell co-stimulatory modulator) fall into this category. For severe SSc cases with poor prognosis and non-responsive to traditional immunosuppression and other treatments, autologous hematopoietic stem cell transplantation (AHSCT) has been employed [20]. AHSCT has shown significant improvement in skin fibrosis and quality of life. However, it comes with a higher treatment-related mortality rate of 5–10% and an association with early and late malignancies. Therefore, careful consideration and evaluation of risks and benefits are necessary when considering AHSCT as a treatment option for severe SSc cases [21].

2. Macrophages in SSc

Macrophage infiltration in SSc was first observed by Ishikawa and Ishikawa in 1992 [22]. They observed phagocytic cells located between collagen bundles and around the skin adnexa and vessels. Later in 2009, Higashi-Kuwata et al. found an elevated number of CD68, CD163, and CD204 positive cells in SSc skin biopsies [23]. The same group found that the population of CD14+, a marker for monocytes, was significantly increased in PBMC from SSc patients compared to healthy controls [24]. These monocytes co-expressed CD204+ and CD163+, markers also used for macrophage identification, indicating a possible monocyte to macrophage differentiation. Furthermore, CD16+ monocytes were found to be increased in SSc and correlated with the severity of skin fibrosis and pulmonary function [25]. Classical monocytes, expressing CD14+CD16–, derived from hematopoietic stem and progenitor cells, appear to actively migrate into the lung tissue, and differentiate into alveolar macrophages [26], whereas non classical, CD14loCD16+, monocytes are confined to the lung vasculature and preferentially differentiate into intravascular macrophages [27, 28].

In summary, the evidence supports the notion of monocyte differentiation into macrophages in SSc, proposing that monocyte-derived macrophages might play a pivotal role in the pathogenesis of SSc. This highlights a dysregulation in monocyte-macrophage differentiation, potentially contributing to an aberrant macrophage polarization and a possible increase in migration to the fibrotic tissue in SSc. Macrophages are the bridge between innate and adaptive response, these are highly heterogeneous, and have been shown to potentially contribute to all facets of SSc pathogenesis. These cells can be of embryonic origin as well as monocyte-derived [29]. Therefore, in the context of the disease it is thought that monocytes are activated producing an initial inflammatory response, which develops to fibrosis, contributing to the disease. In the following sections we will discuss the involvement of macrophages and monocytes in promoting inflammation and fibrosis in SSc as well as crosstalk to the microenvironment.

2.1 Autoimmunity

SSc patients exhibit a wide range of autoantibodies, with antinuclear antibodies being reported in 85–99% of cases. These antibodies encompass anti-topoisomerase

I (ATA), anti-RNA polymerase (ARA), anti-centromere antibodies (ACA), anti-fibrillarin (anti-U3RNP), and anti-ribonucleoprotein (anti-Th/To). The frequency of antinuclear antibodies differs among subsets of SSc and is linked to different clinical manifestations, as seen in **Table 1**. Other autoantibodies, targeting non-nuclear autoantigens, have been less studied in the context of the disease with poor clinical characterization; these includes anti-endothelial cell antibodies (AECAs) [30], anti-fibroblast, anti-platelet-derived growth factor receptor (PDGFR), anti-fibroblast antibodies, anti-fibrillin-1 antibodies, antibodies against matrix metalloproteinases (MMPs) antibodies, and anti-epithelium antibodies (AEpCA) [31] each of which may contribute to disease pathogenesis. Their mechanisms of action involve inflammation induction, fibroblast activation, collagen accumulation induction, and endothelial cell activation [32].

It is unclear how autoantibodies contribute to pathogens and their role with macrophages. However, the initial insult to the vascular system might be related to the antigen presenting capabilities in SSc. In other rheumatic diseases such as Systemic Lupus Erythromatosis (SLE), the capabilities of antigen presenting cells including macrophages and dendritic cells have been shown to play a role in the production of autoantibodies [33]. Efferocytosis is involved in the uptake of apoptotic bodies from the environment. In macrophages efferocytosis has been shown to trigger the change from pro-inflammatory macrophages to a wound healing repair subset [34]. Failure of efferocytosis could then lead to apoptotic bodies in the extracellular space and may lead to the release of DNA and DNA associated proteins into the environment, which induce inflammation and also provide a substrate for autoantibody development [35]. In SSc, monocyte-derived macrophages have proven to be defective at clearing T cells, which might lead to the survival of autoreactive T cells [36]. This might be due to failure to trigger adequate response to apoptotic cells, as expression of mer tyrosine kinase (MERTK), a receptor that binds to apoptotic cells, has been shown to be upregulated in SSc compared to controls [37]. Failure to remove apoptotic cells could

Autoantibodies	Frequency (%)	Disease subset	Clinical association
Anti-topoisomerase I (Topo I, ATA, SCl-70)	15–24	dcSSc	Interstitial lung diseases Cardiomyopathy Renal crisis Digital ulcers
Anti-RNA polymerase (anti-RNP)	4–20	dcSSc	Esophageal involvement Renal crisis Calcinosis cutis Malignancy Myositis
Anti-centromere antibodies (ACA)	20–57.8	lcSSc	Long-standing Raynaud's phenomenon Pulmonary arterial hypertension
Anti-fibrillarin (anti-U3NP)	4–10	dcSSc	Multiple skeletal manifestations Renal crisis and cardiac involvement
Anti-Th/To ribonucleoprotein	1–13	lcSSc	Pulmonary fibrosis

Table 1.
Autoantibodies linked to Systemic Sclerosis and clinical association.

also take place in germinal zones where macrophages might fail to clear autoreactive B cells. Furthermore, polymorphisms in MHC class genes have been reported widely in SSc [38]. It is possible that certain MHC class II variants lead to an increased affinity for self-antigens, which together with macrophage activation due to vascular damage leads to exposure of self-antigens, activating the adaptive immune system [39].

Another possible explanation is that vascular damage initiates macrophage recruitment and activation. Macrophages secrete ROS and other pro-inflammatory cytokines that could trigger oxidations of autoantigens, making them more susceptible to binding to MHC class II or creating neoepitopes and triggering activation of self-reactive T-cells and B-cells [40]. In addition, SSc plasma has elevated IL-6 and other inflammatory mediators [41, 42] and SSc monocytes have been shown to secrete elevated levels of B activator factor [43], which might combine to induce B and T cell activation, altogether suggesting a role of macrophages in contributing towards autoimmunity through T cell activation and promoting autoantibody formation in SSc.

2.2 Vasculopathy

The most frequent clinical manifestation of vascular damage in systemic sclerosis is Raynaud's phenomenon, which is one of the major criteria for the diagnosis of the disease, alongside renal crisis and other vascular disease. It is thought that an initial insult such as viral infection or exposure to toxins, triggers endothelial cell activation, initiating the disease in genetically susceptible individuals. This, coupled to autoantibody driven endothelial cell dysfunction, leads to a vascular profile characteristic of limited systemic sclerosis or in some patients triggering an early inflammatory profile which can progress towards diffuse cutaneous system sclerosis [44]. Endothelial cell apoptosis and altered expression of adhesion molecules and cytokines might lead to the release of reactive oxygen species (ROS), resulting in continuous microvessel damage [45]. Serum levels of vascular dysfunction markers have been shown to correlate with the early stages of SSc [46]. ROS production and microvasculature damage promote inflammation, leading to the recruitment of immune cells.

One possible explanation for monocyte activation mediated by autoantibodies could be the release of topoisomerase I from apoptotic endothelial cells. This release might be triggered by the initial vascular damage and inflammation characteristic of the disease. Once released, topoisomerase I binds to heparin sulphate proteoglycans and CCR7 receptors expressed on the surface of fibroblasts. This binding event recruits ATA, forming immunocomplexes (IC) that subsequently trigger monocyte adhesion and activation [47]. Accumulation of apoptotic bodies, and ICs feeds inflammation which in turn polarizes macrophages towards a pro-inflammatory phenotype. In SSc, FCGR3A positive monocytes and macrophages have been shown to be expanded [48, 49]. These cells were reported to express higher inflammatory markers (ERE, S100A8, and S100A9), and to be enriched for interferon signature genes. In an SSc-related ILD study, a higher percentage of mixed M1/M2 macrophage subset was found; specifically two populations expressing CD163+, D206+, TLR4+, CD80+, CD86+ and either CD204+ or CD14+ were found in ATA positive SSc patients [50]. Further experiments need to be performed to assess whether the single cell populations and those previously reported using flow cytometry are the same, however, it suggest a link between activated macrophages and organ fibrosis in the disease.

Monocytes patrol the blood vessels and transvasate to the tissue of injury where they differentiate to monocyte-derived macrophages [51]. In SSc, CD52, an anti-adhesion molecule, has been found to be decreased in monocytes. Decreased CD52 expression was linked to enhancement of β2 integrin CD11b and CD18 complex which was observed to be upregulated in SSc. Furthermore, an increased level of VEGF165b, a VEGF isoform generated by alternative splicing in VEGF mRNA, has been shown to be elevated in SSc skin [52]. In macrophages, binding of VEGF165b to VEGFR-2 induces an antiangiogenic M1-like phenotype that directly impairs angiogenesis [53]. It is possible that vascular damage and pro-inflammatory macrophage activation occurs in a positive feedback loop failing to repair vasculature, leading vascular leakage and ultimately to vascular remodeling. M1 macrophages thus feed inflammation, and vascular damage. In an attempt to resolve inflammation, M2 macrophages secrete remodeling factors, including transforming growth factor beta (TGF-β), CCL2, IL-10 and clear debris. In SSc, genes for M1 and M2 macrophages have been shown to be enriched, including CD68, COL6A1, CXCL1, CXCL2, HLA–DRB4, IL6ST, PLAU, S100A8, SERPINE2, SERPINH1, and WDFY4 [54]. This dual macrophage signature, could be due to the presence of both M1 and M2 populations, failing in homeostasis, or a mixed M1/M2 signature where macrophages fail to polarize towards a resolving phenotype. The mixture of macrophage factors will eventually lead to activation of fibroblasts and fibrosis.

2.3 Fibrosis

Organ fibrosis, reviewed in [55], is the distinguishing hallmark of SSc. Successful wound repair that leads to localized scarring, is a transient, non-chronic process that terminates via a resolution phase, leading to the rapid restoration of local tissue integrity. However, continuing insult or inflammation results in persistently high levels of cytokines, growth factors and locally destructive enzymes such as collagenases. This process leads to persistent fibrosis and the replacement of normal tissue architecture with compact, mechanically stressed, and rigid connective tissue. Fibrogenesis is characterized by excessive ECM deposition, defective crosslinking, and poor ECM degradation. Fibroblasts and myofibroblasts produce ECM components: collagen, fibronectin, elastin, and matrix glycoproteins. These molecules interlink with each other, giving the ECM its chemical and mechanical properties. In SSc, genetic and epigenetic variations affecting fibroblast function and ECM protein expression, altering normal connective tissue structure [56]. This is exacerbated by fibroblast to myofibroblast differentiation introduced through ischaemia and local cytokine tissue environments. Additionally, the new pathogenic ECM in SSc is characterized by increased stiffness, which triggers fibroblasts to myofibroblast differentiation in a positive feedback loop via mechano-transduction [57].

As described previously, macrophages play a key role in promoting fibrosis; they feed inflammation, leading to vascular leakage and promoting immune cell recruitment, secrete pro-fibrotic mediators, activating fibroblasts, and respond to tissue stiffness in a positive feedback loop. TGFβ is a pleiotropic cytokine known to activate fibroblasts, induce endothelial-to-mesenchymal transition and enhance stem cell recruitment. Wound-healing macrophages secrete growth factors such as TGFβ, platelet derived growth factor (PDGF), fibroblast growth factor (FGF), vascular endothelial growth factor (VEGF) and insulin-like growth factor 1 (IGF-1), promoting cellular proliferation, fibroblast differentiation to myofibroblast and angiogenesis [58]. Nintedanib, a treatment licensed for interstitial lung disease in SSc, targets tyrosine kinases inhibiting PDGF, FGF, VEGF andCSF1R, which in macrophages has been shown to decrease pro-inflammatory markers including CD204, CD206, CD163 and MERTK and to reduce TGFβ secretion. Overall these data are indicating a potential role for macrophage-fibroblast activation through the secretion of TGFβ, thus promoting fibrosis [37].

Macrophages regulate wound healing by producing MMPs and tissue inhibitor of metalloproteinases (TIMPs) controlling ECM turnover; they engulf and digest dead cells, debris, and various ECM components. Activation by TGFβ leads to the heterodimerization of TGFβRII with TGFβRI, which is also known as activin receptor-like kinase 5 (ALK5). This interaction enables downstream canonical TGFβ signaling. The process involves the phosphorylation of SMAD2/3 and the translocation of phosphorylated SMAD2/3 to the nucleus, where it activates gene transcription. Research has shown that the deletion of Alk5 in monocytes inhibits proinflammatory markers while promoting anti-inflammatory macrophage markers.

Furthermore, macrophages engage in crosstalk with T and B cells to modulate immune responses. Adaptive immune cells are linked to autoimmunity in SSc, T cells and B cells interact with macrophages to exacerbate fibrosis. In mice, B cell depletion using Rituximab, has been shown to decrease M2 polarization and fibrosis and to be linked to decreased IL-6 production by B cells. T cells from SSc have been shown to secrete elevated IL-4, which polarizes macrophages towards an M2 pro-fibrotic phenotype. Similarly, T cell derived IL-4 has been shown to increase GM-CSF secretion from B cells [59]. Furthermore, Th2 cytokines including IL-4 and IL-13 have been shown to have increased levels in the serum of SSc patients compared to controls [59]. These cytokines bind to the IL4Rα and IL13Rα1 heterodimer Type II receptor. Receptor activation leads to downstream phosphorylation of STAT6 and subsequent transcription to the nucleus. Both STAT6 and SMAD2/3 signaling lead to M2 macrophage polarization and subsequent fibroblast activation. Although further research is needed to elucidate crosstalk with the adaptive immune system, there is evidence implicating this crosstalk in the pathogenesis of the disease.

Under normal wound healing conditions, macrophages orchestrate clearance of apoptotic cells and the regulation of fibroblast activation. In fact, a 3D co-culture experiment using primary human macrophages and myofibroblast has shown a decrease in myofibroblast activity dependent on the number of co-cultured macrophages [60], highlighting the essential role of healthy macrophages in modulating fibrosis. In SSc, fibroblast differentiation into myofibroblast and the consequent production of ECM products leads to tissue loss of function and tissue stiffness [1]. Macrophage activation in SSc contributes to fibrosis through the secretion of profibrotic mediators such as TGFβ and matrix remodeling proteins [61]. Additionally, CXCL10, CCL19 and CCL7 (MCP3) chemokines have been observed to be upregulated in SSc, with CCL19 being expressed adjacent to CD163 macrophages [39]. In addition, SSc macrophages have been shown to have an increased level of CCL2, TGF-β, and IL-6 [54]. This increase is further exacerbated by autologous plasma stimulation, indicating a possible systemic macrophage activation that might lead to continuing macrophage induction. Furthermore, a higher proportion of CD163 and CD204 positive macrophages have been reported in blood and skin biopsies from SSc patients. This provides evidence for the recruitment of macrophages and monocytes to the tissue in SSc. The phenotype of these macrophages seems to be disrupted; this disruption is probably the end result of genetic and epigenetic modifications which lead to silencing or overexpression of proteins mediating fibrosis. FLI1, a member of the Ets family of transcription factors, is expressed in endothelial cells, fibroblasts and immune cells and has been reported to be decreased in SSc skin. FLI1 has been identified as one of the factors orchestrating changes seen in SSc myeloid cells. Depletion of FLI1 in myeloid cells has shown to induce CCL2 and CCL7 gene expression [62]. The depletion was also correlated with the upregulation of CXCL10, and CXC11 chemokines and MMP12 and HMOX1, stress inducible protein. Furthermore, macrophages from silenced FLI1 induced collagen production *in vitro*.

Accordingly, macrophage-directed fibroblast activation might be the result of different pathways signaling cascades. A recent study has shown that CXCL4 macrophage stimulation leads to an increase secretion of PDGF-B protein, which has been shown to act on fibroblasts, inducing the expression of pro fibrotic and pro-inflammatory cytokines. Furthermore, fibroblasts treated with macrophage culture supernatants after CXCL4 activation have been shown to have an increased production of collagen and fibronectin. Furthermore, co-culture of SSc macrophages and fibroblast increased macrophage TNF/NFκB signaling and increased the expression of interferon response and αSMA in fibroblasts [54]. Additionally, SSc macrophages-fibroblast cocultures have been shown to induce expression of CCL2, IL-6, MMP1, CCL5, CXCL10, G-CSF, and IL-1Ra [63]. In SSc, this regulation seems to be disrupted, since macrophage secretion of IL-10 seemed to act in a paracrine way, inducing myofibroblast differentiation. Fibroblast activation can feedback and further drive macrophage activation. Exosomes from SSc fibroblast, have been shown to activate macrophages increasing levels of IL-6, IL-10, IL-12p40 and TNF. This further exacerbates fibrosis by activating fibroblasts and inducing collagen and fibronectin deposition. In addition to paracrine stimulation, macrophage and fibroblasts crosstalk might be due to cell-to cell contact. Cadherin, a transmembrane adhesion molecule expressed in SSc skin macrophages, has been shown to create a contact bridge between macrophages and fibroblasts and induce TGFβ signaling between latent TGFβ-producing macrophages and myofibroblasts [64].

As a consequence of the alteration to matrix composition and myofibroblast hyperactivation in SSc, stiffness of ECM increases dramatically at fibrotic niches. The young's modulus of the skin increases from 4 to 14 KPa in healthy controls to 50–80 KPa in SSc patients in the forearm, chest and abdomen [65]. During wound healing, matrix stiffness also increases due to the deposition of the provisional ECM. In rat models of tissue fibrosis, the Young's modulus of skin tissue increases from 1 to 4 KPa up to 20 KPa in granulation tissue. Taken together, these data implicate increased ECM stiffness as a contributory factor in the failure of resolution in the pathogenesis of SSc [66]. Mechanical properties of the ECM have been shown to affect cellular function. Increased expression of MRTF signaling network associated with mechanosensing, has been reported in skin from SSc patients [67]. Macrophages express MRTF-A and are able to sense stiffness and adapt to the mechanical properties [68]. The response to mechanical stimuli has been shown to play a role in cancer. A similar role of macrophages and mechanosensing might feedback in SSc in response to fibrosis [69]. *In vitro* mechanosensing properties of macrophages have been studied using hydrogels, water-swollen fibrillary three-dimensional (3D) networks where collagen type I is the major component. The adhesion of macrophages to soft ECM hydrogels has been shown to inhibit inflammatory activation compared to adhesion to stiff glass or polystyrene culture dishes (~GPa) and is dependent on RhoA kinase signaling [68]. MRTF-A is a transcription factor downstream of RhoA signaling; its inhibition could affect stiffness mediated macrophage pathogenesis in fibrosis and cancer. In fact, in macrophages, MRTF-A, MRTF-B, and SRF regulate cytoskeletal gene expression programs and appear to promote macrophage function, with specificity for proinflammatory macrophages. MRTF-A has also been found to recruit members of the H3K4 methylation complex of inflammatory promoters and activate pro-inflammatory transcription [70].

3. CD206 macrophages as therapeutic targets

CD206 is a mannose scavenger receptor member of the group 6 C-type lectin receptor family. It has eight cysteine-rich domains, which allow it to bind to glycans, monosaccharides and fibronectin type II. It is expressed on the surface of monocytes, macrophages, endothelial and dendritic cells and is encoded by the *MRC1* gene. It functions as a pattern recognition receptor, triggering immunity, although it is not clear which domains or ligands trigger this response. The short cytoplasmic C-terminal domain has a di-aromatic motif that regulates its clathrin-dependent internalization and recycling [71]. Macrophages expressing CD206 have been shown to produce high levels of IL-10, IL-6, TNFα and TGFβ1 and to induce endocytosis. Genetic ablation of CD206 in mice leads to the accumulation of multiple glycoproteins in plasma. In SSc, cells positive for CD86, CD163 and CD206 have been shown to be increased in skin, heart and lung biopsy specimens, and CD206 to be overexpressed in SSc monocytes [54, 72, 73]. A recent study using RP832c, a therapeutic 10 amino acid peptide which targets CD206, has been shown to repolarize macrophages from M2 to M1 signature, suggesting a role of CD206 in the profibrotic macrophage signature [74]. Using the bleomycin mouse model, researchers showed a decrease in fibrosis when injecting RP-832c subcutaneously [74]. Altogether, there is evidence of a potential therapeutic approach targeting macrophages for the treatment of the disease. Further research during clinical trials is needed to evaluate the safety and effectiveness of these approaches in modulating fibrosis in patients (**Figure 1**).

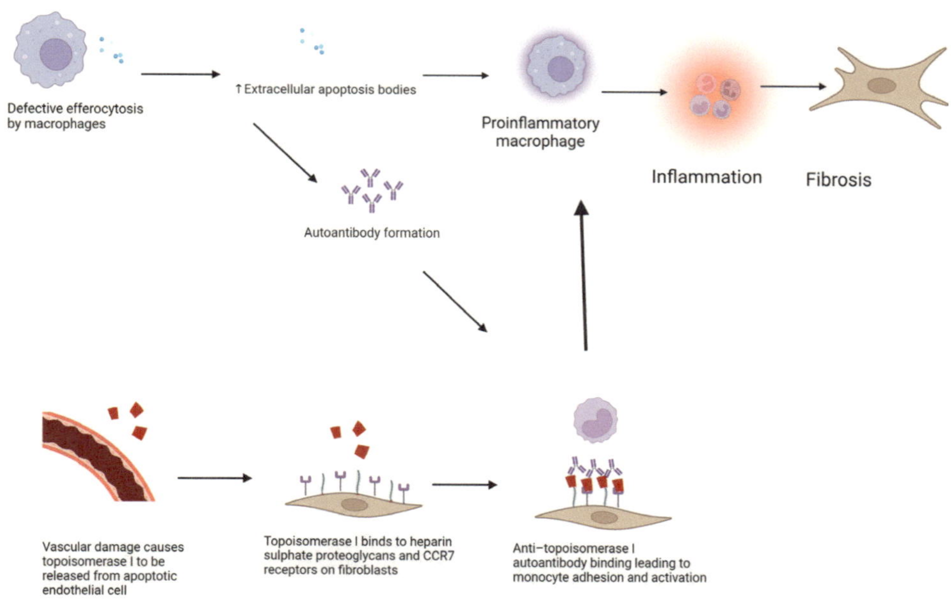

Figure 1.
Schematic summary of proposed role for activated macrophages in promoting inflammatory fibrosis in SSc.

4. Concluding remarks

This chapter has examined the intricate pathophysiology of SSc, a disease marked by severe fibrosis, immune dysregulation, and extensive vascular damage leading to significant clinical heterogeneity and morbidity. We have delineated the clinical subsets of SSc, its global epidemiology, and the current therapeutic approaches, emphasizing the complexity of its management. Particularly noteworthy is the role of macrophages in SSc progression, suggesting that targeting macrophage differentiation and function could offer new therapeutic avenues. The discussion on autoimmunity and vasculopathy in SSc provides further insight into the potential mechanisms driving the disease, presenting opportunities for innovative research aimed at disrupting these processes.

As we look to the future, it is clear that advancing our understanding of the cellular and molecular mechanisms underpinning SSc, especially the roles of macrophages and the specific autoantibodies involved, will be crucial. This could lead to the development of more effective, targeted therapies that not only alleviate symptoms but also potentially alter the disease course. Continued interdisciplinary research and collaboration will be essential in tackling the complexities of SSc, with the ultimate goal of enhancing patient outcomes and providing a framework for more personalized treatment strategies.

Acronyms and abbreviations

ACA	anti-centromere antibody
AECAs	anti-endothelial antibodies
AHSCT	autologous hematopoietic stem cell transplantation
ALK5	activin receptor-like kinase 5
anti-Th/To	anti-RNAse p and mitochondrial RNAse ribonucleoprotein complexes antibodies
anti-U3NP	anti-U3-RNP/fibrillarin antibody
ARA	anti-RNA polymerase III antibody
ATA	anti-topoisomerase antibody
dcSSc	difuse cutaneous systemic sclerosis
ECM	exctracellular matrix
FGF	fibroblast growth factor
IC	immune complex
IGF-1	insulin-like growth factor 1
ILD	interstitial lung disease
lcSSc	localized cutaneous systemic sclerosis
MCP3	monocyte chemotactic protein 3
MERTK	mer tyrosine kinase
MMPs	matrix metalloproteinases
mRSS	modified Rodnan skin score
MRTF-A	myocardin related transcriptor factor a
PAH	pulmonary arterial hypertension
PDGF	platelet derived growth factor
PDGFR	platelet derived growth factor receptor
ROS	reactive oxygen species
RP	Raynaud's phenomenon

SLE	systemic lupus erythematosus
SSc	systemic sclerosis
ssSSc	sine systemic sclerosis
TGF-β	transforming growth factor beta
TIMPs	tissue inhibitor of metalloproteinases
VEGF	vascular endothelial growth factor

Author details

Sandra Lopez Garces[1], Liyang Pan[2] and Richard Stratton[1]*

1 Centre for Rheumatology, UCL Division of Medicine, London, UK

2 Department of Rheumatology, St. Mary's Hospital, London, UK

*Address all correspondence to: r.stratton@ucl.ac.uk

IntechOpen

© 2024 The Author(s). Licensee IntechOpen. This chapter is distributed under the terms of the Creative Commons Attribution License (http://creativecommons.org/licenses/by/3.0), which permits unrestricted use, distribution, and reproduction in any medium, provided the original work is properly cited.

References

[1] Volkmann ER, Andréasson K, Smith V. Systemic sclerosis. The Lancet. 2023;**401**:304-318. DOI: 10.1016/S0140-6736(22)01692-0

[2] Nihtyanova SI, Sari A, Harvey JC, Leslie A, Derrett-Smith EC, Fonseca C, et al. Using autoantibodies and cutaneous subset to develop outcome-based disease classification in systemic sclerosis. Arthritis and Rheumatology. 2020;**72**:465-476. DOI: 10.1002/ART.41153

[3] LeRoy E, Black C, Fleischmajer R, Jablonska S, TR K, Medsger Thomas J, et al. Scleroderma (systemic sclerosis): Classification, subsets and pathogenesis. The Journal of Rheumatology. 1988;**15**:202-205

[4] Poormoghim H, Lucas M, Fertig N, Medsger TA Jr. Systemic sclerosis sine scleroderma: Demographic, clinical, and serologic features and survival in forty-eight patients. Arthritis and Rheumatism. 2000;**43**:444. DOI: 10.1002/1529-0131(200002)43:2<444::AID-ANR27>3.0.CO;2-G

[5] Bairkdar M, Rossides M, Westerlind H, Hesselstrand R, Arkema EV, Holmqvist M. Incidence and prevalence of systemic sclerosis globally: A comprehensive systematic review and meta-analysis. Rheumatology. 2021;**60**:3121-3133. DOI: 10.1093/RHEUMATOLOGY/KEAB190

[6] Royle JG, Lanyon PC, Grainge MJ, Abhishek A, Pearce FA. The incidence, prevalence, and survival of systemic sclerosis in the UK Clinical Practice Research Datalink. Clinical Rheumatology. 2018;**37**:2103-2111. DOI: 10.1007/S10067-018-4182-3

[7] Rubio-Rivas M, Royo C, Simeón CP, Corbella X, Fonollosa V. Mortality and survival in systemic sclerosis: Systematic review and meta-analysis. Seminars in Arthritis and Rheumatism. 2014;**44**:208-219. DOI: 10.1016/J.SEMARTHRIT.2014.05.010

[8] Dupuis J, Hoeper MM. Endothelin receptor antagonists in pulmonary arterial hypertension. European Respiratory Journal. 2008;**31**:407-415. DOI: 10.1183/09031936.00078207

[9] Olschewski H, Simonneau G, Galiè N, Higenbottam T, Naeije R, Rubin LJ, et al. Aerosolized iloprost randomized study group. Inhaled iloprost for severe pulmonary hypertension. The New England Journal of Medicine. 1 Aug 2002;**347**(5):322-329. DOI: 10.1056/NEJMoa020204. PMID: 12151469

[10] Rosenkranz S, Diet F, Karasch T, Weihrauch J, Wassermann K, Erdmann E. Sildenafil improved pulmonary hypertension and peripheral blood flow in a patient with scleroderma-associated lung fibrosis and the Raynaud phenomenon. Annals of Internal Medicine. 2003;**139**:871-873. DOI: 10.7326/0003-4819-139-10-200311180-00030

[11] Tantini B, Manes A, Fiumana E, Pignatti C, Guarnieri C, Zannoli R, et al. Antiproliferative effect of sildenafil on human pulmonary artery smooth muscle cells. Basic Research in Cardiology. 2005;**100**:131-138. DOI: 10.1007/S00395-004-0504-5/METRICS

[12] Shreiner AB, Murray C, Denton C, Khanna D. Gastrointestinal manifestations of systemic sclerosis. Journal of Scleroderma and Related Disorders. 2016;**1**:247-256. DOI: 10.5301/jsrd.5000214

[13] Bose N, Chiesa-Vottero A, Chatterjee S. Scleroderma renal crisis.

Seminars in Arthritis and Rheumatism. 2015;**44**:687-694. DOI: 10.1016/J.SEMARTHRIT.2014.12.001

[14] Denton CP, Khanna D. Systemic sclerosis. The Lancet. 2017;**390**:1685-1699. DOI: 10.1016/S0140-6736(17)30933-9

[15] Khanna D, Denton CP, Jahreis A, van Laar JM, Frech TM, Anderson ME, et al. Safety and efficacy of subcutaneous tocilizumab in adults with systemic sclerosis (faSScinate): A phase 2, randomised, controlled trial. The Lancet. 2016;**387**:2630-2640. DOI: 10.1016/S0140-6736(16)00232-4

[16] Tashkin DP, Elashoff R, Clements PJ, Goldin J, Roth MD, Furst DE, et al. Cyclophosphamide versus placebo in scleroderma lung disease. New England Journal of Medicine. 2006;**354**:2655-2666. DOI: 10.1056/NEJMoa055120

[17] Elhai M, Boubaya M, Distler O, Smith V, Matucci-Cerinic M, Alegre Sancho JJ, et al. Outcomes of patients with systemic sclerosis treated with rituximab in contemporary practice: A prospective cohort study. Annals of the Rheumatic Diseases. 2019;**78**:979-987. DOI: 10.1136/ANNRHEUMDIS-2018-214816

[18] Suleman Y, Clark KEN, Cole AR, Ong VH, Denton CP. Real-world experience of tocilizumab in systemic sclerosis: Potential benefit on lung function for anti-topoisomerase-positive patients. Rheumatology (Oxford). 2021;**60**:3945-3946. DOI: 10.1093/RHEUMATOLOGY/KEAB273

[19] Khanna D, Spino C, Johnson S, Chung L, Whitfield ML, Denton CP, et al. Abatacept in early diffuse cutaneous systemic sclerosis: Results of a phase II investigator-initiated, multicenter, double-blind, randomized, placebo-controlled trial. Arthritis & Rhematology. 2020;**72**:125-136. DOI: 10.1002/ART.41055

[20] Sullivan KM, Goldmuntz EA, Keyes-Elstein L, McSweeney PA, Pinckney A, Welch B, et al. Myeloablative autologous stem-cell transplantation for severe scleroderma. The New England Journal of Medicine. 2018;**378**:35-47. DOI: 10.1056/NEJMOA1703327

[21] Allanore Y, Simms R, Distler O, Trojanowska M, Pope J, Denton CP, et al. Systemic sclerosis. Nature Reviews. Disease Primers. 2015;**1**:1-21. DOI: 10.1038/nrdp.2015.2

[22] Ishikawa O, Ishikawa H. Macrophage infiltration in the skin of patients with systemic sclerosis. The Journal of Rheumatology. 1992;**19**:1202-1206

[23] Higashi-Kuwata N, Makino T, Inoue Y, Takeya M, Ihn H. Alternatively activated macrophages (M2 macrophages) in the skin of patient with localized scleroderma. Experimental Dermatology. 2009;**18**:727-729. DOI: 10.1111/J.1600-0625.2008.00828.X

[24] Higashi-Kuwata N, Jinnin M, Makino T, Fukushima S, Inoue Y, Muchemwa FC, et al. Characterization of monocyte/macrophage subsets in the skin and peripheral blood derived from patients with systemic sclerosis. Arthritis Research & Therapy. 2010;**12**:1-10. DOI: 10.1186/AR3066/FIGURES/4

[25] Lescoat A, Lecureur V, Roussel M, Sunnaram BL, Ballerie A, Coiffier G, et al. CD16-positive circulating monocytes and fibrotic manifestations of systemic sclerosis. Clinical Rheumatology. 2017;**36**:1649-1654. DOI: 10.1007/S10067-017-3597-6/FIGURES/2

[26] Borrell-Pages M, Romero JC, Crespo J, Juan-Babot O, Badimon L. LRP5 associates with specific subsets of macrophages: Molecular and functional effects. Journal of Molecular and Cellular Cardiology. Jan 2016;**90**:146-156. DOI: 10.1016/j.yjmcc.2015.12.002. Epub 2015 Dec 5. PMID: 26666179

[27] González-Domínguez É, Domínguez-Soto Á, Nieto C, Flores-Sevilla JL, Pacheco-Blanco M, Campos-Peña V, et al. Atypical Activin A and IL-10 production impairs human CD16+ monocyte differentiation into anti-inflammatory macrophages. The Journal of Immunology. 2016;**196**:1327-1337. DOI: 10.4049/JIMMUNOL.1501177

[28] Evren E, Ringqvist E, Tripathi KP, Sleiers N, Rives IC, Alisjahbana A, et al. Distinct developmental pathways from blood monocytes generate human lung macrophage diversity. Immunity. 2021;**54**:259-275.e7. DOI: 10.1016/J.IMMUNI.2020.12.003

[29] Cox N, Pokrovskii M, Vicario R, Geissmann F. Origins, biology, and diseases of tissue macrophages. Annual Review of Immunology. 26 Apr 2021;**39**:313-344. DOI: 10.1146/annurev-immunol-093019-111748. PMID: 33902313; PMCID: PMC10786183

[30] Michalska-Jakubus M, Kowal M, Adamczyk M, Krasowska D. Anti-endothelial cell antibodies do not correlate with disease activity in systemic sclerosis. Advances in Dermatology and Allergology/Postępy Dermatologii i Alergologii. 2018;**35**:185. DOI: 10.5114/ADA.2018.75241

[31] Moezinia C, Wong V, Watson J, Nagib L, Lopez Garces S, Zhang S, et al. Autoantibodies which bind to and activate keratinocytes in systemic sclerosis. Cells. 2023;**12**:2490. DOI: 10.3390/CELLS12202490

[32] Kayser C, Fritzler MJ. Autoantibodies in systemic sclerosis: Unanswered questions. Frontiers in Immunology. 2015:6. DOI: 10.3389/FIMMU.2015.00167

[33] Janko C, Schorn C, Grossmayer GE, Frey B, Herrmann M, Gaipl US, et al. Inflammatory clearance of apoptotic remnants in systemic lupus erythematosus (SLE). Autoimmunity Reviews. 2008;**8**:9-12. DOI: 10.1016/J.AUTREV.2008.07.015

[34] Bosurgi L, Cao YG, Cabeza-Cabrerizo M, Tucci A, Hughes LD, Kong Y, et al. Macrophage function in tissue repair and remodeling requires IL-4 or IL-13 with apoptotic cells. Science. 1979;**2017**(356):1072-1076. DOI: 10.1126/SCIENCE.AAI8132

[35] Casciola-Rosen LA, Anhalt GJ, Rosen A. DNA-dependent protein kinase is one of a subset of autoantigens specifically cleaved early during apoptosis. The Journal of Experimental Medicine. 1995;**182**:1625. DOI: 10.1084/JEM.182.6.1625

[36] Ballerie A, Lescoat A, Augagneur Y, Lelong M, Morzadec C, Cazalets C, et al. Efferocytosis capacities of blood monocyte-derived macrophages in systemic sclerosis. Immunology and Cell Biology. 2019;**97**:340-347. DOI: 10.1111/IMCB.12217

[37] Soldano S, Smith V, Montagna P, Gotelli E, Campitiello R, Pizzorni C, et al. Nintedanib downregulates the profibrotic M2 phenotype in cultured monocyte-derived macrophages obtained from systemic sclerosis patients affected by interstitial lung disease. Arthritis Research & Therapy. 2024;**26**:1-13. DOI: 10.1186/S13075-024-03308-7/FIGURES/5

[38] López-Isac E, Acosta-Herrera M, Kerick M, Assassi S, Satpathy AT,

Granja J, et al. GWAS for systemic sclerosis identifies multiple risk loci and highlights fibrotic and vasculopathy pathways. Nature Communications. 2019;**10**:1-14. DOI: 10.1038/s41467-019-12760-y

[39] Tsai S, Santamaria P. MHC class II polymorphisms, autoreactive T-cells, and autoimmunity. Frontiers in Immunology. 2013;**4**:64372. DOI: 10.3389/FIMMU.2013.00321/BIBTEX

[40] Yang ML, Doyle HA, Clarke SG, Herold KC, Mamula MJ. Oxidative modifications in tissue pathology and autoimmune disease. Antioxidants & Redox Signaling. 2018;**29**:1415. DOI: 10.1089/ARS.2017.7382

[41] Hasegawa M, Sato S, Ihn H, Takehara K. Enhanced production of interleukin-6 (IL-6), oncostatin M and soluble IL-6 receptor by cultured peripheral blood mononuclear cells from patients with systemic sclerosis. Rheumatology. 1999;**38**:612-617. DOI: 10.1093/RHEUMATOLOGY/38.7.612

[42] Gourh P, Arnett FC, Assassi S, Tan FK, Huang M, Diekman L, et al. Plasma cytokine profiles in systemic sclerosis: Associations with autoantibody subsets and clinical manifestations. Arthritis Research & Therapy. 2009;**11**:R147. DOI: 10.1186/AR2821

[43] Brkic Z, Van Bon L, Cossu M, Van Helden-Meeuwsen CG, Vonk MC, Knaapen H, et al. The interferon type I signature is present in systemic sclerosis before overt fibrosis and might contribute to its pathogenesis through high BAFF gene expression and high collagen synthesis. Annals of the Rheumatic Diseases. 2016;**75**:1567-1573. DOI: 10.1136/ANNRHEUMDIS-2015-207392

[44] Lescoat A, Bellando-Randone S, Campochiaro C, Del Galdo F, Denton CP, Farrington S, et al. Beyond very early systemic sclerosis: Deciphering pre scleroderma and its trajectories to open new avenues for preventive medicine. Lancet Rheumatology. 2023;**5**:e683-e694. DOI: 10.1016/S2665-9913(23)00212-6

[45] Prescott RJ, Freemont AJ, Jones CJP, Hoyland J, Fielding P. Sequential dermal microvascular and perivascular changes in the development of scleroderma. The Journal of Pathology. 1992;**166**:255-263. DOI: 10.1002/PATH.1711660307

[46] Cossu M, Andracco R, Santaniello A, Marchini M, Severino A, Caronni M, et al. Serum levels of vascular dysfunction markers reflect disease severity and stage in systemic sclerosis patients. Rheumatology. 2016;**55**:1112-1116. DOI: 10.1093/RHEUMATOLOGY/KEW017

[47] Hénault J, Robitaille G, Senécal JL, Raymond Y. DNA topoisomerase I binding to fibroblasts induces monocyte adhesion and activation in the presence of anti–topoisomerase I autoantibodies from systemic sclerosis patients. Arthritis and Rheumatism. 2006;**54**:963-973. DOI: 10.1002/ART.21646

[48] Xue D, Tabib T, Morse C, Yang Y, Domsic R, Khanna D, et al. Expansion of FCGR3A + macrophages, FCN1 + mo-DC, and plasmacytoid dendritic cells associated with severe skin disease in systemic sclerosis. HHS Public Access. Arthritis Rheumatology. 2022;**74**:329-341. DOI: 10.1002/ART.41813

[49] Villanueva-Martin G, Acosta-Herrera M, Carmona EG, Kerick M, Ortego-Centeno N, Callejas-Rubio JL, et al. Non-classical circulating monocytes expressing high levels of microsomal prostaglandin E2 synthase-1 tag an aberrant IFN-response in systemic sclerosis. Journal of Autoimmunity.

2023;**140**:103097. DOI: 10.1016/J.JAUT.2023.103097

[50] Trombetta AC, Soldano S, Contini P, Tomatis V, Ruaro B, Paolino S, et al. A circulating cell population showing both M1 and M2 monocyte/macrophage surface markers characterizes systemic sclerosis patients with lung involvement. Respiratory Research. 2018:19. DOI: 10.1186/S12931-018-0891-Z

[51] Rudnik M, Rolski F, Jordan S, Mertelj T, Stellato M, Distler O, et al. Regulation of monocyte adhesion and type I interferon signaling by CD52 in patients with systemic sclerosis. Arthritis and Rheumatology. Sep 2021;**73**(9):1720-1730. DOI: 10.1002/art.41737. Epub 2021 Jul 31. PMID: 33760395

[52] Manetti M, Guiducci S, Romano E, Ceccarelli C, Bellando-Randone S, Conforti ML, et al. Overexpression of VEGF165b, an inhibitory splice variant of vascular endothelial growth factor, leads to insufficient angiogenesis in patients with systemic sclerosis. Circulation Research. 22 Jul 2011;**109**(3):e14-e26. DOI: 10.1161/CIRCRESAHA.111.242057. Epub 2011 Jun 2. PMID: 21636803

[53] Ganta VC, Choi M, Farber CR, Annex BH. Antiangiogenic VEGF165b regulates macrophage polarization via S100A8/S100A9 in peripheral artery disease. Circulation. 2019;**139**:226-242. DOI: 10.1161/CIRCULATIONAHA.118.034165

[54] Bhandari R, Ball MS, Martyanov V, Popovich D, Schaafsma E, Han S, et al. Pro-fibrotic activation of human macrophages in systemic sclerosis HHS public access. Arthritis & Rhematology. 2020;**72**:1160-1169. DOI: 10.1002/art.41243

[55] Rockey DC, Bell PD, Hill JA. Fibrosis—A common pathway to organ injury and failure. New England Journal of Medicine. 2015;**372**:1138-1149. DOI: 10.1056/nejmra1300575

[56] Broen JCA, Radstake TRDJ, Rossato M. The role of genetics and epigenetics in the pathogenesis of systemic sclerosis. Nature Reviews Rheumatology. 2014;**10**:671-681. DOI: 10.1038/NRRHEUM.2014.128

[57] Cutolo M, Soldano S, Smith V. Pathophysiology of systemic sclerosis: Current understanding and new insights. Expert Review of Clinical Immunology 2019;15:753-764. https://doi.org/10.1080/1744666X.2019.1614915.

[58] Wynn TA, Vannella KM. Macrophages in tissue repair, regeneration, and fibrosis. Immunity. 2016;**44**:450. DOI: 10.1016/J.IMMUNI.2016.02.015

[59] Clark KE, Lopez H, Abdi A, Guerra SG, Shiwen X, Khan K, et al. Multiplex cytokine analysis of dermal interstitial blister fluid defines local disease mechanisms in systemic sclerosis. Arthritis Research & Therapy. 23 Mar 2015;**17**(1):73. DOI: 10.1186/s13075-015-0575-8

[60] Ullm F, Riedl P, de Amorim AM, Patzschke A, Weiß R, Hauschildt S, et al. 3D scaffold-based macrophage fibroblast coculture model reveals IL-10 dependence of wound resolution phase. Advanced Biosystems. 2020;**4**:1900220. DOI: 10.1002/ADBI.201900220

[61] Bhandari R, Ball MS, Martyanov V, Popovich D, Schaafsma E, Han S, et al. Profibrotic activation of human macrophages in systemic sclerosis. Arthritis and Rheumatology. 2020;**72**:1160-1169. DOI: 10.1002/ART.41243

[62] Bujor AM, El Adili F, Parvez A, Marden G, Trojanowska M. Fli1

downregulation in scleroderma myeloid cells has profibrotic and proinflammatory effects. Frontiers in Immunology. 19 May 2020;**11**:800. DOI: 10.3389/fimmu.2020.00800. PMID: 32508810; PMCID: PMC7248379

[63] Bhandari R, Yang H, Kosarek NN, Smith AE, Garlick JA, Hinchcliff M, et al. Human dermal fibroblast-derived exosomes induce macrophage activation in systemic sclerosis. Rheumatology (Oxford). 6 Feb 2023;**62**(SI):SI114-SI124. DOI: 10.1093/rheumatology/keac453. PMID: 35946522; PMCID: PMC9910573

[64] To S, Agarwal SK. Macrophages and cadherins in fibrosis and systemic sclerosis. Current Opinion in Rheumatology. 2019;**31**:582-588. DOI: 10.1097/BOR.0000000000000657

[65] Yang Y, Qiu L, Wang L, Xiang X, Tang Y, Li H, et al. Quantitative assessment of skin stiffness using ultrasound shear wave elastography in systemic sclerosis. Ultrasound in Medicine & Biology. 2019;**45**:902-912. DOI: 10.1016/j.ultrasmedbio.2018.11.015

[66] Tschumperlin DJ, Lagares D. Mechano-therapeutics: Targeting mechanical signaling in fibrosis and tumor stroma. Pharmacology & Therapeutics. 2020;**212**:107575. DOI: 10.1016/J.PHARMTHERA.2020.107575

[67] Shiwen X, Stratton R, Nikitorowicz-Buniak J, Ahmed-Abdi B, Ponticos M, Denton C, et al. A role of myocardin related transcription factor-A (MRTF-A) in scleroderma related fibrosis. PLoS One. 2015;**10**:e0126015. DOI: 10.1371/journal.pone.0126015

[68] Sridharan R, Cavanagh B, Cameron AR, Kelly DJ, O'Brien FJ. Material stiffness influences the polarization state, function and migration mode of macrophages. Acta Biomaterialia 2019;**89**:47-59. https://doi.org/10.1016/J.ACTBIO.2019.02.048.

[69] Reed F, Larsuel ST, Mayday MY, Scanlon V, Krause DS. MRTFA: A critical protein in normal and malignant hematopoiesis and beyond. Journal of Biological Chemistry. 2021;**296**:100543. DOI: 10.1016/J.JBC.2021.100543

[70] Yang Y, Yang G, Yu L, Lin L, Liu L, Fang M, et al. An interplay between MRTF-A and the histone acetyltransferase TIP60 mediates hypoxia-reoxygenation induced iNOS transcription in macrophages. Frontiers in Cell and Development Biology. 18 Jun 2020;**8**:484. DOI: 10.3389/fcell.2020.00484

[71] Cummings RD. The mannose receptor ligands and the macrophage glycome. Current Opinion in Structural Biology. 2022;**75**:102394. DOI: 10.1016/J.SBI.2022.102394

[72] Rudnik M, Hukara A, Kocherova I, Jordan S, Schniering J, Milleret V, et al. Elevated fibronectin levels in profibrotic CD14+ monocytes and CD14+ macrophages in systemic sclerosis. Frontiers in Immunology. 2021;**12**:642891. DOI: 10.3389/FIMMU.2021.642891/BIBTEX

[73] Schneider L, Marcondes NA, Hax V, da Silva Moreira IF, Ueda CY, Piovesan RR, et al. Flow cytometry evaluation of CD14/CD16 monocyte subpopulations in systemic sclerosis patients: A cross sectional controlled study. Advances in Rheumatology. 2021;**61**:1-11. DOI: 10.1186/S42358-021-00182-8/FIGURES/4

[74] Ghebremedhin A, Salam AB, Adu-Addai B, Noonan S, Stratton R, Ahmed MSU, et al. A novel CD206 targeting peptide inhibits

bleomycin-induced pulmonary fibrosis in mice. BioRxiv [Preprint]. 29 Jul 2020:2020.07.27.218115. DOI: 10.1101/2020.07.27.218115. Update in: Cells. 26 Apr 2023;**12**(9): PMID: 32766584; PMCID: PMC7402041